A MEDICAL HISTORY OF SKIN:
SCRATCHING THE SURFACE

STUDIES FOR THE SOCIETY FOR THE SOCIAL HISTORY OF MEDICINE

Series Editors: *David Cantor*
                  Keir Waddington

TITLES IN THIS SERIES

A MEDICAL HISTORY OF SKIN: SCRATCHING THE SURFACE

Edited by

Jonathan Reinarz and Kevin Siena

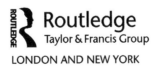

Routledge
Taylor & Francis Group

LONDON AND NEW YORK

First published 2013 by Pickering & Chatto (Publishers) Limited

Published 2016 by Routledge
2 Park Square, Milton Park, Abingdon, Oxfordshire OX14 4RN
711 Third Avenue, New York, NY 10017, USA

First issued in paperback 2015

Routledge is an imprint of the Taylor & Francis Group, an informa business

© Taylor & Francis 2013
© Jonathan Reinarz and Kevin Siena 2013

BRITISH LIBRARY CATALOGUING IN PUBLICATION DATA

Reinarz, Jonathan.
A medical history of skin: scratching the surface. – (Studies for the Society for
the Social History of Medicine)
1. Skin – Diseases – History – 18th century – Case studies. 2. Skin – Diseases
– History – 19th century – Case studies. 3. Skin – Diseases – History – 20th
century – Case studies. 4. Skin – Diseases – Treatment – History – 18th century
– Case studies. 5. Skin – Diseases – Treatment – History – 19th century – Case
studies. 6. Skin – Diseases – Treatment – History – 20th century – Case studies.
I. Title II. Series III. Siena, Kevin Patrick.
616.5'009-dc23

ISBN-13: 978-1-138-66226-1 (pbk)
ISBN-13: 978-1-8489-3413-9 (hbk)

Typeset by Pickering & Chatto (Publishers) Limited

CONTENTS

LIST OF CONTRIBUTORS

Gemma Angel is an interdisciplinary doctoral researcher in History of Art at University College London, UK. She is currently working in collaboration with the Science Museum, London, on a historic collection of 300 preserved tattooed human skins. Her publications include 'The Tattoo Collectors: Inscribing Criminality in Late Nineteenth Century France' in a special issue of the German journal of science and technology studies, *Bildwelten des Wissens*, 9:1 (Spring 2012), addressing 'prepared specimens'.

Mechthild Fend is Reader in History of Art at University College London, UK. She specializes in French eighteenth- and nineteenth-century visual culture and art theory, and has a particular interest in images of the body, including medical imagery and specimens. Fend's publications in this area include 'Bodily and Pictorial Surfaces: Skin in French Art and Medicine, 1790–1860', in *Art History*, 28 (2005); and 'Emblems of Durability: Tattoos, Preserves and Photographs', in *Performance Research*, 14:4 (2009). A book entitled *Fleshing Out Surfaces: Skin in French Art and Medicine 1650–1850* is forthcoming with Manchester University Press.

David Gentilcore is Professor of Early Modern History at the University of Leicester, UK. His current interest in maize and pellagra emerged out of a Leverhulme Trust-funded research project on the reception and assimilation of New World food plants in early- and late-modern Italy. His most recent books are *Pomodoro! A History of the Tomato in Italy* (New York: Columbia University Press, 2010) and *Italy and the Potato: A History, 1550–2000* (London: Continuum, 2012).

Anne Kveim Lie is Associate Professor in Medical History and Medical Anthropology at the University of Oslo, Norway. Her recent publications include (with Hilde Bondevik) *Rødt og Hvitt* (*Red and White*) (Oslo: Akademika, 2012); *Tegn på sykdom* (*Signs of Illness*) (Oslo: Unipub, 2009); and *Radesygens tilblivelse* (*The Coming-into-being of the Norwegian Radesyge*) (Oslo: Unipub, 2008).

Richard A. McKay is a Wellcome Trust Research Fellow at the University of Cambridge's Department of History and Philosophy of Science. His current research explores the process by which 'the homosexual' became the focus of venereal disease prevention efforts in the mid-twentieth century. Following graduate studies at the University of Oxford, he was an ESRC Postdoctoral Fellow at King's College, London, where he organized the lecture series 'AIDS@30: Three Decades of Responding to HIV/AIDS' (2011). He is currently working on a manuscript exploring the emergence of the 'patient zero' concept for University of Chicago Press.

Adrien Minard is currently completing a doctoral thesis on the struggle against syphilis in France, 1860–1970, at Sciences Po, Paris. He has published (with Michael Prazan) *Roger Garaudy: Itinéraire d'une négation* (Paris: Calmann-Lévy, 2007), and co-edited a recent special issue of the journal *Tracés*, 21 (2011), on 'Contagions'.

James Moran is Associate Professor in the History Department at the University of Prince Edward Island, Canada. Recent publications include (with Leslie Topp and Jonathan Andrews) *Madness, Architecture and the Built Environment: Psychiatric Spaces in Historical Context* (London: Routledge, 2007) and (with David Wright) *Mental Health in Canadian Society: Historical Perspectives* (Montreal: McGill-Queen's University Press, 2006). He is currently finishing a book manuscript comparing the history of lunacy investigation law in England and the United States.

Matthew L. Newsom Kerr is Assistant Professor of History at Santa Clara University, California, USA. He researches primarily in the social and cultural history of medicine and public health, and is currently completing a book on infectious disease hospitalization in late Victorian London. An article on fears surrounding contagious transport appeared in the *Journal of British Studies*. A chapter on the experiences of smallpox isolation is forthcoming in *Residential Institutions in Britain, 1725–1950: Inmates and Environments* (London: Pickering & Chatto).

Lynda Payne is the Sirridge Missouri Endowed Professor of Medical Humanities and Bioethics and a Professor of History at the University of Missouri, Kansas City, USA. Her publications include *With Words and Knives: Learning Medical Dispassion in Early Modern England* (Aldershot: Ashgate, 2007) and 'What Would William Hunter Think of Bodies Revealed?', in J. Lantos (ed.), *Controversial Bodies: Thoughts on the Public Display of Plastinated Corpses* (Baltimore, MD: Johns Hopkins University Press, 2011). Her current research projects include completing a monograph on the life and legacy of the eighteenth-century surgeon Percivall Pott, and preparing an annotated edition of the illustrated travel journals of the anatomist Sir Charles Bell, 1774–1842.

Jonathan Reinarz is Reader and Director at the History of Medicine Unit, University of Birmingham, UK. His recent publications include (with Graham Mooney) *Permeable Walls: Institutional Visiting in Historical Perspective* (Amsterdam: Rodopi, 2009) and *Healthcare in Birmingham: The Birmingham Teaching Hospitals, 1779–1939* (Woodbridge: Boydell Press, 2009), which contains a chapter on the Birmingham Skin Hospital. Forthcoming publications include a special issue of the *Journal for Eighteenth-Century Studies* on 'the Enlightenment and the Senses', a history of smell, and an edited collection on medicine and the workhouse.

Kevin Siena is Associate Professor at Trent University, Canada. He is author of *Venereal Disease, Hospitals and the Urban Poor: London's 'Foul Wards' 1600–1800* (Rochester, NY: University of Rochester Press, 2005) and editor of *Sins of the Flesh: Responding to Sexual Disease in Early Modern Europe* (Toronto: Centre for Reformation and Renaissance Studies, 2005). His articles explore the eighteenth-century histories of gay transmission of syphilis, hospital visitation, suicide, workhouse medicine, searchers of the dead and the plebeian body. He is currently writing a book on class and contagion in eighteenth-century London.

James F. Stark is a Research Fellow at the University of Leeds, working as part of the university's major Arts Engaged project. His recent publications have focussed on the global history of anthrax, particularly in Britain, France and Australia, and the regulation of disease in Victorian factories. His current research explores the importance of patenting and ownership in the history of medical technologies, the provision of clean drinking water to nineteenth-century Leeds, and the changing practices associated with chemical disinfection in British households.

Kathleen Vongsathorn is a Postdoctoral Research Fellow at the Max Planck Institute for the History of Science in Berlin. She recently completed her doctoral thesis at the University of Oxford, entitled '"Things that Matter": Missionaries, Government, and Patients in the Shaping of Uganda's Leprosy Settlements, 1927–1951'. Her recent and forthcoming publications include an article in the *Journal of Eastern African Studies* on mission and government priorities for the treatment of leprosy in Uganda, and an article in the *Journal of Imperial and Commonwealth History* on the rhetoric of leprosy as a humanitarian cause in the British Empire. Currently, she is undertaking research on the role of women in the spread of biomedical knowledge in colonial Uganda.

Philip K. Wilson serves as Professor of Humanities and Director of the Doctors Kienle Center for Humanistic Medicine at Pennsylvania State University's College of Medicine in Hershey, Pennsylvania, USA. His earlier work on skin disease appeared as *Surgery, Skin and Syphilis: Daniel Turner's London (1667–1741)* (Amsterdam: Ropodi, 1999). More recent scholarship includes his co-edited (with Elizabeth A. Dolan and Malcolm Dick) *Anna Seward's Life of*

Dr Erasmus Darwin (Studley: Brewin Books, 2010), his co-authored (with W. Jeffrey Hurst) *Chocolate as Medicine: A Quest over the Centuries* (Cambridge: Royal Society of Chemistry, 2012), and his forthcoming *Glaciers, God and Geography: Neuchatel's Arnold Guyot (1808–1884) at Princeton* (Swiss American Historical Society).

Tania Woloshyn was recently Postdoctoral Research Fellow in the Department of Art History and Communication Studies, McGill University, Canada, funded by SSHRC, Canada. Her contribution to this volume emerged from research undertaken during this Fellowship (2010–12). She is currently a Postdoctoral Research Fellow in the Centre for the History of Medicine, University of Warwick, funded by the Wellcome Trust (2012–15). Her recent publications include '*Le Pays du soleil*: The Art of Heliotherapy on the Côte d'Azur', *Social History of Medicine* (2012), and 'Aesthetic and Therapeutic Imprints: Artists and Invalids on the Côte d'Azur, c. 1890–1910', *Nineteenth-Century Art Worldwide*, 11:1 (2012).

LIST OF FIGURES AND TABLES

SCRATCHING THE SURFACE: AN INTRODUCTION

Kevin Siena and Jonathan Reinarz

On 5 December 1739 in London, Elizabeth Bradshaw stood trial for killing her tenant, greengrocer Richard Challenger, who was behind with the rent. Witnesses testified that on the night of 10 November, Bradshaw refused to let him enter. In spite of his plea – 'I can't give it you To-night, but if you'll stay till Morning, when I have sold my Greens, by G-d you shall have it' – she shoved him down the stairs. He tumbled into the street, hit his head and died the next day. Despite numerous witnesses and claims to Challenger's previous good health, Bradshaw walked free.

Something spoke more forcefully in the courtroom that day: Challenger's skin. A witness seeing his body washed for burial exclaimed with revulsion: 'how they can touch him, he's all over Scabs and Sores'. John Row, the surgeon who examined the body for the coroner, drew further attention to his skin. He believed Challenger's head wound was insignificant because his skin was only abraded. 'There was no Contusion through the Flesh – only through the Skin, or in the Way of rubbing, as by a Brick.' Instead of head trauma, Challenger's skin suggested a different cause of death. Row's final words close the trial record: 'there were Blotches all over his Body, through the Instigation of the Venereal Disease. Acquitted'.[1] Challenger's blemished skin provided the most critical evidence of the day.

This admittedly dramatic example points towards the historical importance of reading the skin. While not all instances of interpreting skin lesions had life and death hanging in the balance, the following studies suggest that medical interpretations of the skin have never been disinvested of enormous and complex meaning. They are premised on the notion that the skin speaks, and that throughout modern history people have listened intently. This is not a history of dermatology per se. Rather this volume aspires to provide case studies with the wider ambit of exploring the cultural history of skin through the prism of its diseases. Dermatology has some thorough, if dated, historical surveys.[2] However, a spate of recent studies has the potential to coalesce into a new field, which is as yet unnamed but could easily be termed 'skin studies'. Typified by the work of Claudia Benthien and Steven Connor, this scholarship applies insights from such diverse fields as psychology, anthropology, biology, art history and cultural studies to issues like tattooing, scarification, piercing, cosmetics, disease, tanning, ageing and nudity, to place the skin at the centre of investigations into the self.[3] We hope that medical historians can offer another layer to this conversation. Medical historians have not ignored the skin; to the contrary, blemishing diseases like leprosy, syphilis and smallpox have rich histories. However, those studies tend not to situate the skin as a primary focus of investigation, leaving contributions on the skin frequently pigeonholed within various sub-fields.

We explore the eighteenth century onwards, in part because the dawn of modernity may witness a shift in the meaning of skin. Both Connor and Benthien see the skin as central to the self, and historians of the self have pointed to the Enlightenment as a transformative moment. Applying the ideas of philosopher Charles Taylor, Dror Wahrman suggests that the eighteenth century brought a closed, fixed sense of personal identity, characterized by an inward-looking sense of self, unlike earlier constructions of identity that were externally constituted, based on relations with others, and much more mutable.[4] Connor and Benthien rely more heavily on theories of psychoanalysis, especially Didier Anzieu's notion of the 'skin ego',[5] but they arrive at the same place – the eighteenth century, from which point a self-contained, healthy self required closed (read: unpenetrated), healthy skin. This narrative draws on and fits well with work by historians of the body, perhaps most importantly Mikhail Bahktin, who presented a grotesque, porous early modern body yielding to the modern, individuated, closed body by the nineteenth century.[6] Barbara Duden demonstrated that eighteenth-century German patients still understood their bodies as porous and connected to the world around them by fluid exchanges that moved in both directions.[7] Mieneke te Hennepe suggests that early nineteenth-century microscopy studies of the skin's many strata enhanced the emerging sense that the skin provided a thick boundary demarcating an individuated body.[8] From a feminist perspective, Elizabeth Grosz concurs that the ideal modern body, the 'body in control', is hermetically sealed and male,[9] and Dorinda Outram's dating of the emergence of that body in the French Revolution places this development in roughly the same period.[10] This modern body and its skin may already be an historical artefact, as studies of the postmodern body point to the extreme plasticity of its skin,[11] something histories of cosmetic surgery bear out.[12] Nevertheless, histories of the modern body gel well with the work of skin-scholars like Benthien, who offers the rise of dermatology as a new specialist field and shifts in cosmetics – away from baroque styles of masking and towards more natural-looking make-up – as indications that attitudes to skin altered with the Enlightenment.[13] The new importance placed on transparency, which changing make-up fashions seem to signify, is bound up in the abrupt decline in baroque masquerade that Wahrman independently suggests further demonstrates a shifting identity regime.[14]

If these related premises hold – that skin is key to identity, and identity changed in the late Enlightenment – we can speculate that damage to skin took on greater psychic and cultural weight as the nineteenth century dawned. Thus the stigma associated with the conditions explored in this book may have intensified with modernity, as closed skin became more important than ever. That said, the subtitle of this book makes apparent that it aspires only to begin a conversation. In that spirit, the first suggestion for future work must entail a companion volume on the medieval and early modern periods – eras central to the histories of such blemishing (and stigmatized) conditions as leprosy, plague and syphilis – to test whether the late Enlightenment brought such a dramatic shift, or if longer continuities prevailed.[15] Until then, we hope readers will benefit from Philip Wilson's Afterword, which gives some taste of medical thinking on skin over a longer period.

Regardless, Connor, Benthien and other skin-scholars have established beyond a doubt the utility of exploring the skin as something to be read. Although Connor's title *The Book of Skin* utilizes the metaphor of text, he also employs the allegory of the cinema screen, a surface on which messages are broadcast, often whether we like it or not.[16] Nina Jablonski thinks along similar lines, employing Philippe Di Folco's suggestion that skin functions as an 'advertising billboard'.[17] Such an approach highlights the utility of applying the tools of linguistic and visual analysis to skin and helps explain why the dermis has received such attention in cultural studies. So too does skin's role as a border.[18] As Benthien notes, skin marks where we end and the world begins. Skin fascinates because, like other borders, it is routinely crossed. Pathogens make their way in; sweat and effluvia exit. We assure ourselves with fantasies of safely closed skin and revile at wounds and lesions opening our skin and rendering us vulnerable. Thinking of the skin as a border holds potential for analysing elements of liminality and processes of transgression that have proven fruitful in studies of other frontiers.[19] The very concept of the skin as a border brings to the fore the influence of geographic thinking – for, if skin has been read as a kind of text, then surprisingly often that text has been a map.

In a theme explored more fully in Wilson's Afterword, physicians borrowed tactics from geographers. Spatial thinking and geographers' techniques for visual representation played vital roles in the development of a science of skin, as early dermatologists tried to make sense of corporeal landscapes, or what one scholar has termed the 'skinscape'.[20] Wilson suggests that geo-historical thinking helps explain why physicians appropriated a geographer's tool – the dermatological *atlas* – to render skin diseases visible and meaningful. Skin lent itself well to this technique. Despite the greatest efforts, 'skin surface will always fail to be smooth'.[21] Pimples, pustules, spots and scales transformed complexions into variegated landscapes. Skin, like the earth's surface, is also 'temporal in the sense that it is affected by the passage of time', expanding, contracting, eroding and gradually acquiring wrinkles and creases with age.[22]

Indeed, the study of skin was one of the most visual of all medical specialties. Images have always influenced medicine. Vesalius's anatomical drawings offer only the most famous example that one need not await modernity for images of bodies to transform medicine.[23] Yet one can still argue, as Katherine Ott has, that visual material played a greater role at an earlier point in dermatology than in almost any other medical field, anatomy excepted.[24] Text was clearly secondary to imagery in dermatological atlases, a genre Barbara Stafford suggests demonstrates an epistemic shift whereby visual evidence gained considerable ground in the nineteenth century.[25] That the skin is the most evident organ, one whose illnesses do not hide but announce themselves, sometimes shockingly, meant that early dermatology lent itself especially well to visual analysis. The coincident rise of pathological anatomy augmented this development by concentrating medical attention on lesions.[26] Skin specialists may have been ahead of the curve, having focused for more than a century (and potentially longer) on the fine distinctions between different types of sores.[27] The size, shape, colour and texture of *internal* lesions mattered little before medicine's capacity to explore the subcutaneous body without significantly damaging it, and when doctors usually only saw such lesions at autopsy. Skin lesions were another matter entirely. Doctors trained to evaluate the subtle differences in skin lesions' characteristics recognized that 'a strange alphabet ha[d] to be learned' before atlases could be utilized optimally.[28] According to te Hennepe, this visual language 'took shape in Great Britain and France between 1790 and 1840',[29] initially comprising four 'Orders' in the 1808 volume *On Cutaneous Diseases*, published by the British physician Robert Willan (doubling to eight 'Orders' six years later when Thomas Bateman completed Willan's work), which defined diseases according to morphological appearance.[30] Under the French physician Jean-Louis Alibert, who in addition to signs and symptoms took into consideration cause, course and duration of skin diseases, these were arranged into two classes and twelve separate families.[31] Though these classifications varied and changed over time, their appearance improved communication between doctors discussing skin. Above all, the era of the dermatological atlas ushered visual material to centre stage in medical presentations of skin

Smallpox provides a powerful example both of skin's capacity as a text and of the centrality of visuality to the contested readings levelled on it. Matthew Newsom Kerr maintains that smallpox may hold a unique place amongst diseases, because the affliction and its associated procedures, inoculation and vaccination etched into the skin potent, often permanent, symbols that signified little less than life and death. The shift he detects in the visual culture of smallpox in the early nineteenth century further supports seeing the period as a key moment in skin's history. Before vaccination, Newsom Kerr describes an 'ocular tolerance' for smallpox, characterized by a culture of display whereby the disease was ever-present in survivors' scarred skin. Inoculation conveyed the actual disease and thus could mark patients dramatically. In the eighteenth century, however, the pustules of the inoculated and the scars of survivors conveyed comfort rather than horror, normalizing the disease and suggesting safety.

Vaccination changed this, largely through contesting images of the skin. Vaccinators contrasted the arbitrary spread of inoculation's pustules with their orderly sores that confined the disease to a single discrete mark on the skin. Natural smallpox was like a wild animal, erratic and dangerous. Vaccination tamed that beast, bringing it under scientific control and offering unblemished skin as proof of its promise for the British nation. Ironically, as smallpox became more hidden it became more terrifying. Emerging fears of disfigurement suggest that vaccination's advantage lay partially in the realm of aesthetics.

Mechtild Fend's chapter demonstrates the importance of aesthetic considerations differently. She considers Scottish pathologist Robert Carswell, who published an authoritative dermatological atlas in 1838 and sketched or painted more than a thousand works on skin pathology. Simultaneously artist and physician, Carswell advocated the importance of painting to dermatology. If interpreting the size, shape and colour of lesions mattered, then his watercolours were superior teaching tools to the pickled specimens in museum jars that might fade or shrivel.

Fend concurs that the rise of pathological anatomy's emphasis on lesions influenced dermatology deeply. Yet some of Carswell's aesthetic choices complicate one of the most important claims about the rise of pathological anatomy. Medicine's newfound fascination with lesions is said to have realigned the doctor-patient relationship, as sufferers were objectified and silenced before a medical gaze that no longer saw patients, only diseases.[32] Certainly, close-up images of dermatological wounds isolated from discernible bodies covey that sense.[33] However, Carswell did not occlude patients but rather drew intimate attention to them through the conventions of portraiture. Dermatological images differed from other kinds of morbid anatomy because they were sketched *pre-* rather than *post*-mortem: they portrayed living patients. As Schnalke has argued for moulage,[34] Carswell's depictions told the second story of an individual, including details like clothing or hairstyles that initially seem medically irrelevant. One senses not a detached physician objectifying his patient, but rather a relationship in which the physician is emotionally involved to a greater degree than scholars like Foucault allowed. The presentation of heavily blemished faces through portraiture was nonetheless confounding. The face was meant to be legible, but blemishing diseases terrified because they disfigured. Some dermatologists crafting atlases sought to elicit emotional reactions like fear, as when they drew images in purposefully 'terrifying colours', not unusually obscuring the facial features of young women and children. But Fend suggests that Carswell's addition of tiny details may have softened the shock of his images – calling close attention to widespread facial lesions while simultaneously trying to mitigate their power to dehumanize.

The skin could be marked in other ways that fascinated scientists. The nineteenth century saw rising interest in new dermatological markings, especially tattooing, among the destitute and so-called deviants.[35] As Gemma Angel's chapter shows, dermatologists and criminologists came to focus on tattoos roughly simultaneously, making these stigmata objects of study for both the biological and social sciences. The fields cross-fertilized in their attempts to pathologize tattooing as 'an innate degenerative tendency'.[36] At first glance the tattoo and the lesion seem unrelated: the one voluntary and aesthetic, the other involuntary and pathological. However, like the ulcers of so many skin diseases, tattoos were considered signs of deeper pathology, in this case social pathology. Moreover, tattooing, which penetrated the skin and introduced foreign substances, shared qualities with biomedical processes like contagion or inoculation. Indeed, worries that diseases were transmitted via the tattoo-needle invited physicians to join criminologists in exploring tattooing's social dangers. Perhaps unsurprisingly, given the low status of most tattoo-bearers in the period, syphilis figured importantly in these discussions. At times tattoos became lesions, because the site of infection and inscription were one and the same. However, the triumph of vaccination that Newsom Kerr charts may have made itself felt beyond smallpox, as dermatologists began using tattooing practices, reminiscent of acupuncture techniques, for therapeutic and cosmetic purposes, a development fuelled perhaps by popular myths about the tattoo's healing power. These folk traditions appear to originate in non-Western cultures, including Egypt and Morocco, offering further evidence that the transmission of medical knowledge is not unidirectional when it comes to skin.[37] As in other medical fields, the potential of a traditional technique, namely manual tattooing, was augmented through the symbolic power of improved technologies,[38] like electric needles and an emerging faith in the curative powers of chemical and biological substances such as carbolic acid and vaccines. Angel further demonstrates that many of the representative strategies that Fend explores framed clinical images of tattoos.

Images of many kinds were thus central to the science of skin. Carswell was neither the first nor the last doctor who created images of skin. Both Tania Woloshyn and Jamie Stark describe early twentieth-century physicians who similarly straddled the line between artist and healer. In Stark's case, University of Leeds physician Frederick William Eurich studied anthrax among woolworkers. The success of pathological anatomy in linking diseases to lesions was such that anthrax came to be identified almost exclusively by a particular 'characteristic' black lesion. However, Eurich knew the disease was tricky, sending a bevy of variegated signs to the body's surface that did not always correspond to typical lesions in textbooks.

If the skin was a text, then one had to decipher its visual grammar, full of inflection and subtle intonation. Eurich's tool for promoting skin-literacy was a poster so that workers could recognize the signs quickly. Timing was crucial, because anthrax advanced rapidly and lesions changed by the hour. Eurich's depictions of anthrax lesions – like vaccinators' presentations of smallpox pustules – showed them evolving over time, bearing out some of the temporal dimensions of Wilson's attention to geo-historicity. Unlike Carswell, Eurich had a camera available to him, yet he still chose the paintbrush because colour photography was too expensive. Though photography had its advantages,[39] older techniques like painting and moulage retained value because they captured the colour and texture of skin disease's complex visual language.[40]

Woloshyn explores forms of light therapy – the controlled exposure of patients to natural and artificial light – in the same period, a practice that again depicts the physician-as-artist, in this case the photographer. Research by Niels Finsen on ultraviolet light for treating tuberculosis, especially lupus, provided such therapy with a scientific basis. Doctors thus promoted sun-tanning on medical grounds long before it became popular for its aesthetic qualities. Yet physicians kept tanning's aesthetics closely in mind; proponents of light therapeutics made crucial aesthetic choices, crafting images that implied that tanning bestowed health. One might echo media theorist Laura Marks in noting that these images operated through 'a distinctive visual register of touch', encouraging viewers to 'discern texture' rather than just form.[41] As argued by Connor, in this way a 'fantasy' was constructed in the minds of sun worshipers of the tan's ability to construct a 'protective second skin' that shielded the body.[42] It may seem ironic that doctors advocated intense sunbathing, given current warnings about melanoma.[43] However, doctors were convinced that a tan was a visual indicator of healing; light therapy generated an 'inner luminance', to use Connor's expression,[44] leading physicians to claim that those who tanned best healed best. As in almost every incident examined in this book, the skin's signs were assumed to reflect what occurred much deeper in the body. Health was rarely ever only skin deep. Photographs of the tanned, unblemished skin of visually fit people advocated powerfully for light therapeutics, especially when set against 'before' pictures of blemished sufferers that emphasized paleness by such photo-rhetorical techniques as using dark backgrounds. Finally, Woloshyn offers a fuller account of a patient's perspective. Nobel Prize winner André Gide's accounts of his own treatments similarly portrayed his skin in illness as weak and penetrable, and revelled in the sensual, quasi-sexual quality of sunbathing. In a telling passage, he expressed shame at his skin, not because it was blemished but merely because it was pale, resolving only to sunbathe 'where I knew no one can see me'.

Gide's embarrassment raises a central issue in the history of skin and its diseases: stigma. Erving Goffman's foundational study on stigma long ago identified disfigurement as one of its fundamental forms, pointing repeatedly to the scarred, blemished or facially marked.[45] Stigmatization – whether physical branding, in Goffman's example of Greek slaves, or a disfiguring disease – begins on the skin, with material marks indicating a 'spoiled identity'. The visibly stigmatized 'must suffer the special indignity of knowing that they wear their situation on their sleeve' (or we might say their skin), 'that almost anyone will be able to see into the heart of their predicament'.[46] Again, one must look back centuries for a full account of this tradition, starting at least as early as the treatment of medieval lepers and likely earlier.[47] As Sander Gilman and others have attested, graphic artists have used skin lesions as symbols of immorality for centuries,[48] a practice kept alive into our period by William Hogarth, who time and again used spots – understood to be syphilis sores – to demarcate disreputable characters.[49] Moreover, as moral tales like the *Rakes Progress* or the *Harlot's Progress* advanced, Hogarth drew those spots growing from tiny points to large black marks, suggesting that the graphic sequencing of lesions over time predates the dermatological atlas and served as a powerful didactic tool to make ethical claims about the blemished.

Hogarth's visual trick worked because Connor's insight was already accurate in the eighteenth century. The skin was a screen that broadcasted messages about the person wearing it, allowing for 'the "epidermalization" of inferiority'.[50] It certainly was for Richard Challenger, whose death we recounted at the outset and whose blotches suggested syphilis and all its related assumptions. Indeed, syphilis, along with leprosy, cast an enormous shadow over thinking on the skin in the eighteenth century. Kevin Siena studies a ubiquitous skin disease that Enlightenment Britons called 'the itch'. It was likely scabies, and some early microscopists identified a parasite as its cause.[51] However, majority opinion held that it was a disease of the blood assumed to be related to syphilis or leprosy. Itch sufferers tried to conceal their condition, because they understood all too well the degrading assumptions they might face. The itch was a lowly disease, and like leprosy and the pox it was assumed to strike lowly people.

It is thus worth reflecting on issues of public and private when thinking about the history of skin disease. The walls of the bourgeois home have provided perhaps the most common boundary for thinking about the public and private spheres. However, the skin may provide an even more intimate boundary between what is personal and what is publicly consumed. Indeed, anxieties about hiring domestic servants whose skin suggested infection – a development discussed here in three separate chapters – suggests how these different formulations of the frontier between public and private could conflict. It is important to note that skin diseases were frequently assumed, sometimes wrongly, to be contagious, amplifying their terror and driving forms of policing and exclusion. The isolation of lepers and quarantining of pox sufferers offer the most notorious examples.[52] Participation in the urban public sphere became all the more important as the Enlightenment took form, yet it was precisely publicity that frequently anguished the blemished. We will never know the feelings of the impoverished hospital patients who sat while Carswell painted their portraits – literally with warts and all – but it is difficult not to speculate that for some such intimate attention to their facial lesions may have been unwelcome, if not downright agonizing. Considering that these images were made public in the most dramatic way then possible – by being literally 'published' – it is hard not to see the process as a kind of public stripping. Speculating on why that might be, Connor points out the blatancy of skin diseases:

> Skin markings, especially when they are associated with disease, have the flagrancy of the blatant; they blur out what the tongue might prefer to keep secretly veiled. They are shameful and disgusting, not only because they inspire fear, but also because they are shameless.[53]

Connor reflects on the roots of the term 'blatant', from the Latin term that also gives us a verb for loose speech, 'to blatter', and which we might add, not coincidentally, also supplies the root for the German term for syphilis's pustules (*'Blattern'*) and early hospitals (*'Blatternhaus'*).[54] Unable to hold a secret, the skin makes public what one hopes to keep private. It speaks with a very loose tongue.

In the case of AIDS, the lesions associated with Kaposi's sarcoma quickly became signs that advertised the afflicted. Originally described in 1872 by the Hungarian-born professor of dermatology at the University of Vienna, classic Kaposi's sarcoma was a rare skin cancer affecting older men of Mediterranean and Eastern European ancestry. From its first description in 1981, however, AIDS-related Kaposi's sarcoma steadily increased with the incidence of a new epidemic, manifesting itself in 15 per cent of AIDS' American victims.[55] As a result, Kaposi's sarcoma rapidly became a key diagnostic marker of this deadly sexually transmitted infection. As Richard McKay's chapter suggests, the public wanted a stigmata of AIDS, and they found it in Kaposi's sarcoma.

McKay illustrates how this once rare form of skin cancer was inscribed with new meaning as it marked the bodies of young gay men. In particular, he explores the implications of this blatant stigma for one well-known AIDS victim, French-Canadian flight attendant Gaétan Dugas, the oft-maligned 'patient 0'. Dugas's early symptoms led him to commence his illness thinking of himself as a cancer patient, initially consulting dermatologists. In his history of the American AIDS epidemic, *And the Band Played On* (1987), journalist Randy Shilts portrayed the flight attendant as a sociopath, 'an AIDS Aggressor',[56] allegedly revealing his lesions after sex and telling partners that they too might acquire 'gay cancer'.[57] In contrast to Shilt's 'bourgeois novelistic form', McKay challenges the chronological assumptions made by those accusing Dugas of irresponsible sexuality, denial and ultimately murder.[58] McKay's more nuanced reading of Dugas includes his meticulous efforts to conceal his cancerous lesions in order to continue leading a normal life at a time when ideas about AIDS transmission were yet to be definitively determined.

KS lesions thus served as visual markers with profound implications for identity, and McKay demonstrates that physicians played no small role in this development. In this way, KS had many historical antecedents. We can reflect again on the itch, for example, which Siena suggests was also framed by doctors with repercussions for identity. Physicians advanced what he calls a 'moral biology', suggesting that certain bodies were disposed to pathogenesis. The unhygienic lifestyle of the poor, along with their diet, drinking or sexual immorality, allegedly rendered their blood putrid and capable of generating the itch. Such putrid blood could even be passed hereditarily, allowing for a deeper inscription of class on the body. The Scots fared no better, as English doctors similarly blamed northern diets, climates and hygiene for making the itch endemic there. Physicians voiced popular prejudices that had seized the rhetorical power of the itch to smear Englishmen's new compatriots. The geo-historical locating of the itch to Scotland went a step further in suggesting that Scotland had a skin disease all its own, a related ailment called 'sibbens'.

Sibbens was linked to numerous diseases, including the disease explored by James Moran that ravaged eighteenth-century Quebec, one that also carried powerful implications for identity. British colonial authorities saw 'St Paul's Bay Disease' as a major threat and mounted the largest public health campaign theretofore witnessed in colonial Canada, working through the church and pressing local priests into public health service. This medical missionary strategy bore resemblances to the clerical visitations still occurring in parts of Europe during the long Reformation. As in the Old World, priests withheld sacraments and used other punishments to force peasants to abide by British colonial health mandates. This again raised public/private tensions. Peasants clearly saw the heavily blemishing disease as dishonourable, yet the state required that the names of the infected be made public. Only by identifying who had the disease could authorities monitor it, launching a campaign to map it numerically and geographically. Their campaign was geopolitical as much as geo-historical, for the epidemic raged at a precarious moment. The fortunes of one of Britain's last North American colonies seemingly hung in the balance, creating anxiety about the disease's implications for empire and speculation on the racial degeneration of the French colonists that made them prone to such a gruesome malady.

Kathleen Vongsathorn's chapter also charts skin disease in a colonial context, but it issues a reminder that, Goffman notwithstanding, stigma is not a universal reaction to blemished skin, even for that most stigmatized disease, leprosy. She finds that attitudes towards the disease varied between Ugandan indigenous groups. If the Bakiga people of south-western Uganda, for example, stigmatized leprosy, it was because it disabled, not because it disfigured. Nevertheless, when British missionaries conducted medical safaris to search for lepers – ventures not unlike the visitations of Moran's Quebec priests, and which might be thought of as a kind of skin-surveillance mission – they brought with them long-held Western assumptions, especially that skin diseases arose from lack of hygiene, morals or other markers of 'civilization'. Vongsathorn finds that indigenous attitudes towards leprosy began to harden, though she speculates that the fear and loathing of the disease might have been driven more by the associations that accompanied quarantine and segregation. In this respect, and to complement the discussions of other contributions to this volume, Vongsathorn's unravels the process through which the skin *becomes* rather than simply *is* meaningful. Revealingly, missionaries did not only judge their colonial subjects' skin. They also judged their *attitudes* to skin, arranging Ugandan peoples hierarchically based on their attitudes towards lepers: more intense stigmas suggested cultural advancement. Civilization was thus marked not just by healthy skin, but by a healthy *hatred* of leprous skin.

Skin was thus a marker of identity. This claim is hardly novel given the importance of pigmentation to racial thinking, as outlined by Franz Fanon, for example, in his classic study *Black Skin, White Masks* (1967).[59] However, skin has other qualities than colour, and its predilection for disease deserves more attention within the histories of scientific attempts to categorize people. The chapters that follow show that classes, nations and races have at various times been denoted by their tendency towards blemishing ailments. The tradition of linking race to skin disease is of course quite old, as evidenced by Benjamin Rush's infamous suggestion that Africans were dark due to congenital leprosy.[60] Adrien Minard demonstrates the further possibilities of exploring race through dermatology in his exploration of what French doctors in North Africa termed 'Arab syphilis', a heavily disfiguring disease that was likely one of the four treponematoses (yaws, syphilis, bejel and pinta). It ravaged the face in ways unfamiliar to European doctors trained to spot venereal syphilis. The doctors concluded that they were looking not just across the sea, but backwards in time, assuming that the disease reflected the true, ancient syphilis of Renaissance legend. Framing colonial subjects as vestiges of an ancient past had been common since the Enlightenment, when Rousseau speculated on noble savages living out a bygone era that Europeans could visit through imperial adventures.[61] French physicians commenting on the uniqueness of Arab syphilis thus robustly embody a geohistorical perspective, mapping the disease in a multidimensional schema that situated it in both space and time.

Minard's research bears out leprosy scholar Rod Edmond's insight that colonial practices naturalized hierarchies by advancing binaries between healthy whites and unhealthy natives.[62] In ways that recall claims about poor Londoners, Quebec peasants or native Ugandans, French colonial doctors presented the disease as evidence of degeneracy. And while they could have ascribed the disease's uniqueness to North Africa's climate, they insisted it reflected poor hygiene and cultural retardation. Minard's chapter also marks where the themes of stigma, identity and visuality conjoin, for photography powerfully framed the disease. The decision to concentrate heavily on the face was no accident. Facial deformities conveyed a shocking sense of racial degeneration to consumers in the metropole, where the photographs fuelled anti-immigrant diatribes. Such photographs figured the colonial subject as monstrous, incapable of governing and desperately in need of the historical progress that required forces like Western biomedicine. The skin's health – not just its colour – was a vital barometer of civilization.

French doctors had considerable trouble interpreting lesions on differently coloured skin, as did doctors in colonial settings trying to diagnose anthrax on darkly pigmented patients by using posters showing lesions on white skin, as Stark discusses. Their difficulties raise a final theme that several chapters convey, namely the diagnostic confusion that pervaded within dermatology for a very long time. It seems counterintuitive that diseases sitting on the body's surface and visible to the naked eye could be so perplexing. Influencing this may have been the tendency to interpret the unknown by way of the known, an understandable drive that may have led to more confusion than clarity. Doctors made sense of new and confusing diseases by linking them to well-known ones, and David Gentilcore's study of such a disease, pellagra, reveals confused attempts to make sense of a baffling disease that eroded the skin. Pellagra is today considered a vitamin deficiency. However, its nature was debated well into the twentieth century,[63] and its names derived from its symptoms: *pellarina* for 'peeling skin', or more commonly, *pellagra* for 'rough skin'. On the one hand, it seemed like a new disease. But, as in instances described in other chapters, physicians tried to render it manageable by suggesting it might be a new form of an old disease, in this case leprosy or scurvy. These debates expressed the professional aspirations of Italian doctors seeking fame by mastering a 'new' disease, and Gentilcore reminds us that dermatology, like all branches of medicine, was framed by the socio-economic and political forces governing doctors and patients. However, whether it was a form of leprosy or scurvy mattered, because Italian doctors thought the former was primarily a skin disease and the latter more deeply rooted. The diagnostic confusion Gentilcore tracks was thus partially a debate about whether the disease sat on the body's surface or rose from deeper within.

The timing of that debate is potentially important, because – occurring as it does across the turn of the nineteenth century – it lies right when skin-scholars suggest formulations of the skin shifted with important ramifications for its diseases. Whereas skin lesions on the porous early modern body were usually interpreted as surface-level manifestations of deeper systemic ailments, nineteenth-century skin diseases were increasingly seen as eroding the body's outer layer, now understood as a thicker boundary.[64] Debates on pellagra, therefore, occurred during a period of epistemic flux. Gentilcore shows that into the early nineteenth century, the older model held; pellagra remained a systemic disease. Doctors focused on the poverty of patients, employing the same theories that explained the itch and arguing that poor diet and inactivity rendered the blood putrid. By focusing on diet, doctors actually laid the groundwork for eventual success against the disease. But by suggesting that the inactive became sick by not sweating out impurities, they said a great deal – they propelled the idea that blemished skin was a marker of poverty. Furthermore, they perpetuated the early modern understanding of skin as a porous portal controlling an economy of fluids that connected bodies to their environment, with massive ramifications for health.

These themes echo loudly in Anne Kveim Lie's exploration of a disease with links to those explored by Siena and Moran, and one that, like Gentilcore's 'Italic scurvy', was framed geographically in terms of nation. Before Norway was even its own country, it laid claim to a nasty, disfiguring sickness called radesyge. Diagnostic confusion abounded here, too. Eighteenth- and early nineteenth-century Norwegian physicians, like their Italian and British counterparts, rummaged through the same old chest of diseases – syphilis, leprosy and scurvy – trying to find one that fit. Eventually radesyge was recast as tertiary syphilis, and Norway's unique disease disappeared. However, the debates leading up to that re-classification dated roughly from 1770 to 1850, offering another look at the shift from early modern to modern notions of skin and confirming the development detected by Benthien and Connor. Initially, and like the itch or pellagra, radesyge represented inner putridity and was accordingly linked to the poor, whose wretched ulcers and rank odour were read to bespeak bodily corruption. However, by the mid-nineteenth century radesyge had transformed, just as the skin itself had done. It now became a disease *of* the skin, rooted in the body's thick, closed, exterior layer. Lie also charts representations of radesyge in dermatological atlases, and explores how early doctors tried to assist the body in its efforts to expunge its inner foulness through the porous skin.

Managing that all-important membrane was a major component of early doctors' work. Philip Wilson's work on skin specialist Daniel Turner demonstrated how skin formed a different kind of boundary in the eighteenth century – a professional one. For centuries physicians and surgeons struggled in a jurisdictional turf war that came down to the skin. Surgeons could handle the body's exterior, but the mysteries beneath the skin were the physician's domain.[65] Lynda Payne's exploration of eighteenth-century surgery demonstrates how central skin was to surgeons' work, much of which focused on supervising the passage of material through its surface. Often they created artificial wounds. Payne details surgeons' efforts to perforate the skin by creating blisters and issues, draining boils, letting blood and a bevy of other strategies that opened the skin. The early modern body was porous, but Georgian surgeons clearly believed that sometimes it was not porous enough. Surgeons took charge of the skin, mastering how to open it, close it and shepherd corrupt matter through it. Though at times brutal, such skin work allowed surgeons to hone their skills, monitoring the root causes of conditions manifested on the skin and minimizing the procedures in their repertoire, including suturing and scarring. Commanding the processes of drainage and flow that many believed governed health, surgeons positioned themselves as Enlightenment managers of Nature. With its eruptions, eminences, papillae and suppurations, surgeons described the body's surface in the manner of a landscape that became so familiar to practitioners in the eighteenth century it often rendered the skin medicine's 'invisible backdrop'. Too familiar to attract the attention of practitioners, whose focus was on the deeper causes of disease, it was often cast off, like the flayed *pellis* draped over the arms of the early figures populating the first anatomical atlases.[66]

It would be foolish for any edited collection to make claims for comprehensive coverage, especially when the topic touches as many related issues as skin clearly does. We have mentioned a few of the areas deserving of more study, such as the pre-modern period and the patient's perspective. Related to the latter, we regret that despite concentrating little on the institutions where medical practitioners first confronted these conditions, including hospitals, workhouses and prisons, our book focuses mainly on physicians' and surgeons' thoughts about the skin. However, non-professional interpretations of skin may have been just as important. For example, in London up until 1837, elderly women termed 'searchers of the dead' examined corpses to report causes of death; they would present just one opportunity to explore non-professional actors reading the flesh.[67] Of course one should resist dichotomies between professional and popular, because topics like cosmetics or the skin-care industry complicate such divides nicely. Joan Jacobs Brumberg's chapter 'Perfect Skin', charting the gendered history of acne in America, suggests the potential for such endeavours.[68] The same can be said for histories of hygiene that have spotlighted the skin.[69] In addition, our chapters do not address the skin's ability to feel, but medical historians taking up the skin could potentially offer a great deal to the emerging historiography on the senses.[70]

We have arranged the chapters in three sections: on the period when skin work was emerging as a field, on skin diseases' stigmas and their implications for identity, and on the relationship between dermatology and visual culture. The chapters are then followed by an Afterword that weaves some of this material together through a lively exploration of the geo-historical framing of the skin over many centuries. However, we consciously resisted organizing this introduction according to these sections or discussing the chapters in the order that they appear. Many chapters speak across the synthetic sections that we created for them, and themes similarly stretch across the three centuries we chart. Thus despite the fact that the early nineteenth century may provide an epochal moment in the history of skin, it made little sense to sequester the chapters on opposite sides of that divide. When Gaétan Dugas concealed his KS sores with make-up to avoid the labelling and scorn that they were likely to generate, his actions and motivations bear striking similarities to those of eighteenth-century syphilitics and itch sufferers who acted similarly, notwithstanding the massive contextual gulf separating them. There are thus many ways that these histories could have been sutured collectively. We nevertheless hope that however readers choose to stitch them together, these case studies will, like a healthy dermis, appear sufficiently layered and convince them of the need to make skin a central focus in medical histories to come.

1 DRAIN, BLISTER, BLEED: SURGEONS OPEN AND CLOSE THE SKIN IN GEORGIAN LONDON

Lynda Payne

> ... are your olfactory nerves so delicate, that you cannot avoid turning sick when dressing an old neglected ulcer? or, when, in removing dressings, your nose is assailed with the effluvia from a carious bone? If you cannot bear these things, put surgery out of your head, and go and be apprentice to a man milliner, or perfumer.[1]

From Mr Peters, a surgeon:[2]

> [On] Dec. 28. 1737. *James Channon*, aged about 14, was accidentally shot in his Back by another Lad at the Distance of Two Yards from him; so that the whole Load of [Gun]Shot, not having Space to scatter, enter'd like a Ball, by the Edge of the Left Scapula, which it splinter'd ... [it then] pass'd between the two superior Ribs, and fractur'd the Clavicle – with a Touch of the Incision-Knife ... I took out about a dozen shot.[3]

Mr Peters then bled James and bandaged the wound on his back. A week later, he expressed satisfaction at the development of 'healthy suppuration'. But then the suppurating pus became so copious that 'When the dressings were removed, I frequently made him force a Cough, and try if he could not throw out any Pus by his Mouth; but, instead of passing that Way, it flew out thro' the Wound like Water from a Pump ... and the "Air which was forc'd thro" the Wound by Coughing, would blow out a Candle, which I often experienced – I thought he would die'.[4]

This went on for eight weeks, during which time James coughed up twenty-five gunshots; he became emaciated; his skin was hot and dry. A cannula, or gum elastic catheter, was inserted to drain the wound, but the shivering from the boy's high fever kept causing it to fall out. James waxed and waned over the next few months, occasionally coughing up yet more gunshot and often running high fevers.

In November 1738, nearly a year after the shooting, a frustrated Mr Peters used a caustic – a hot iron – to burn a hole through the scar of the gunshot wound, and then 'kept it open with a large Bean, to try if a Discharge ... might divert the Matter from coming by the Mouth ... [The boy] weather'd out the Winter tolerable well'.[5] This method of keeping a wound artificially open by inserting a foreign object, such as a pea, bean or bead, created what was known as an issue.

In March 1739 James complained of a pain in his side and Peters applied a 'warm Plaister [or poultice] and drew off ten Ounces of Blood ... A few Days afterwards an Abscess formed between the Ribs ... which I opened, and discharged about four Ounces of ... fetid matter, and 18 Shot'.[6] Excited by the possibilities this new wound offered to drain yet more pus, the surgeon removed the bean from the original gunshot wound and allowed it to heal; he then kept the new wound open with a cannula. But after ten days the matter had stopped flowing, the patient had a high fever, and Peters reported: 'I threw aside the Cannula, and healed the Wound between the Ribs, it answering no End to keep it open longer'.[7]

The patient lingered on, through 1740, 1741 and 1742 – James generally got sick every spring and autumn and coughed up pus and even more gunshot. But the surgeon cheerfully added that 'Between these grand fits of Coughing ... the boy would gain Strength, grow fat, and work at his Trade of Glove-Making'. In 1743 James became very ill and coughed up a two-inch bone fragment that was presumed to be part of his shoulder bone. Old pieces of dead bone were known as sequestra and were regarded as indicative of a major infection. Peters admitted James to the local hospital. There he was bled repeatedly, put on a milk diet and confined to bed – and after fifteen months was proclaimed to be 'healthy, strong, and fat'.[8] Finally in 1745, eight years after being shot in the back by another adolescent boy, James Channon, now aged twenty-two, was discharged from Peters's practice as successfully cured.

The case of James Channon demonstrates several of the tools and techniques used by Georgian surgeons in attempts to heal their patients' wounds – knives, cannula, caustics, issues, poultices and dressings. It validates research that has shown that a lot of surgeons' work in the eighteenth century was the surgery of trauma, especially related to wounds and broken bones. They set simple fractures and amputated for compound or open fractures, with probable mortality rates of 5 per cent and 50 per cent respectively.[9] Surgeons trephined or drilled into the skull for open and closed head injuries. Most of their surgery went septic, and as in Channon's case, wounds suppurated, resulting in copious amounts of pus.[10] But what the case of James Channon does not demonstrate is the theories behind the choices Mr Peters made in treating the boy's wound.

With this narrative in mind, I would like to consider the advice given in hospital surgical training to young apprentices and pupils about – to quote a leading Georgian surgeon – 'the most common business of surgery',[11] which was the care of wounded skin. How did a wound heal? What kind of wounds should a surgeon treat, and what should he leave alone as necessarily fatal? What was an abscess? What treatments were available for skin wounds, and what were the challenges and controversies surrounding them? Did early modern surgeons discuss pain control, or is this, as some historians have claimed, a modern concern? And what can all of this tell us about the history of skin? In short, does evidence from clinical encounters support contentions put forward by scholars on the nature of pre-modern skin – that it was 'a sort of porous tissue that could potentially have an opening anywhere',[12] and/or a 'cushion touched from beneath by a delicate webbing of "sensitive" and "irritable" nerve fibers'?[13]

Many of the surgical cases in mid- to late eighteenth-century London came to St Bartholomew's Hospital, one of the English capital's seven teaching hospitals. Patients there often came under the care of Percivall Pott (1714–1788), considered by his peers to be the best practical surgeon of his day. Born in London in 1714, he was apprenticed at the age of fifteen for £200 to Edward Nourse, a surgeon and lecturer at St Bartholomew's Hospital.[14] Despite the nauseating nature of the work, Pott credited his early training in cutting up rancid human body parts to make Nourse's teaching specimens with giving him the dexterity – and the strong stomach – that a surgeon needed.

Pott was a prolific author, and in 1756 he used the recovery time following a riding accident to write his first book, *A Treatise on Ruptures*, or hernias. It covered one of the most common ailments a surgeon treated, and began a stream of publications that give a glimpse of the workaday existence of a Georgian practitioner of surgery: a second book on ruptures and treatises on head wounds, cataracts, spine curvature and testicular cancer all followed. As a senior surgeon at St Bartholomew's Hospital from 1749, Pott trained hundreds of future surgeons, including the three on whom I focus in this chapter: John Abernethy (1764–1831), Peter Clare (1738–86) and John Heaviside (1748–1828). They in turn became successful surgeons and authors of medical texts and, in the case of Heaviside, anatomy museum owners. At St Bartholomew's Hospital, pupils followed Pott on his ward rounds, wrote up cases, attended lectures on surgery and anatomy, and admitted patients. Michael Crumplin estimates that between 1728 and 1820, 60–90 per cent of all hospital students were surgical trainees.[15] Dressers such as Abernethy, Clare and Heaviside paid extra to obtain ward experience with Pott.[16] In addition to other skills, Pott taught them to open and close the skin. They learnt how to let blood by lancet, fleam or leech, to apply wet and dry bandages, to mix up poultices, to apply heated cups and to make an issue with a pea or a bean to create a persistent sore. Along with the pupils, they observed but also often assisted at operations that generally took place on Saturdays between 11 a.m. and 1 p.m., when the light was presumably at its best.[17]

Lectures and publications by Pott and his former dressers, Abernethy, Clare and Heaviside, reveal the theories, practices and fierce arguments behind treating even the simplest of skin wounds. The initial question was how a wound to the skin naturally heals; according to eighteenth-century surgeons, there were three stages involved. The first was called digestion, and to quote Clare from his 1779 treatise on skin ailments, 'digestion involved the formation of a quantity of good pus on the surface';[18] he addressed good and bad pus later in the chapter. The second stage of natural healing was known as incarnation, and here the wound fills up with 'granulations of tender flesh and becomes florid'.[19] Clare referred to this granulation as a fungus, which had to be protected at all costs – perhaps with oil, 'as it is an artificial pus that protects and comforts the tender wound'.[20] Cicatrization was the third and last stage, and 'compleats the cure'.[21] This was the formation of a hard dry scab on the wound.

Anatomical and physiological descriptions of the skin were limited in lecture and in print. In 1789 James Moore discussed some aspects of the skin in a prize-winning treatise on wounds. The cutis or outer layer of the skin was described as growing hair and being full of 'eminences', named papillae, which ran in waving rows, triangles or whorls (fingerprints, in modern parlance). Under the cutis lay the rete-mucosum, which appeared furrowed on dissection from the papillae above it. The rete-mucosum could be white, yellowish, brown or black, and so gave colour to the skin. Moore explained that scars were whiter in white men because they were less vascular than the original cutis had been, but 'in negroes the reverse takes place, their scars being generally blacker than other parts, owing to a darker rete-mucosum forming'.[22] Scars were unable to grow hair or create papillae because these were only 'formed in the first organization of the body, and are never afterwards produced'. Moore added that anatomists and surgeons were joined in the opinion that papillae were the source of feeling in the skin, and therefore the lack of them was why scars had no feeling.[23]

With this analysis in place, what skin wounds could be treated? Surgeons attempted to provide guidelines on when it was worth trying to save a patient's life and when it might be futile. Pott instructed his students that wounds to the brain, the heart and major thoracic vessels 'may be fairly reckoned' as fatal, while chest and abdomen wounds were 'not necessary fatal but always attended with some hazard' to treat, and wounds to the extremities were usually not fatal.[24] However, as Abernethy lectured in 1810, 'People will die under trivial Operations – even in opening a common Abscess they will lie down & die – (and) we should (always, therefore) give a doubtful prognosis'.[25]

This brings us to one of the most common and problematic skin issues treated by Georgian surgeons, namely the 'common' abscess. Clare described an abscess as 'a collection of matter betwixt the muscles and the skin and their formation was usually attended with great pain and fever'.[26] The matter he referred to resulted from the process of inflammation. When inflammation first occurred in any injury to the skin, it was called the adhesive type. A buff-coloured membrane, generally believed to be made up of lymph, filled up a wound. Blood vessels then grew through the cavity made by the wound, resulting in what was known as 'healing by first intention'. Many surgeons theorized that if the wound was exposed to air, this somehow deprived the blood of the power to unite the parts by first intention;[27] therefore they covered an exposed wound with plasters and/or stuffed it with lint in order to absorb any blood and enable the wound to form a hard dry skin on top of the cavity. But this practice was a matter of debate:

> Mr. Potts would not advise as a great many of our Practitioners do, to cram the wound with Lint, as it hinders the parts from coming together ... A Farrier will stick his knife into an abscess of a Horse let out the matter dressing it superficially & the Horse gets well.[28]

If the wound did not heal by first intention within two to three days, the second and final stage of inflammation developed, known as the suppurative.[29] This was known to be hard on the body, but beneficially could expel foreign bodies from wounds. Pott gave the following directions in lectures on how to treat gunshots:

> The method I make use of, after, having enquir'd what kind of fire arms the wound had been inflict'd with and in what position he was in & likewise what the piece was load'd with, you are then carefully to extract all extraneous bodys ...

He continued that the wound may have to be enlarged to grasp the shot with forceps, and if it had entered the body 'violently', a counter opening could be necessary. Pott recommended using a very soft dressing:

> free from any irritable quality, the digestive bals.m of Barth,w Hosp.l, cover'd with a soft cooling Cataplasm will prove the most serviceable and must be continu'd for some time.[30]

Pott firmly warned his audience of eager young men not to rush to get the ball out unless it was visible to the eye and not entangled in bones or near a large vessel. They should wait until suppuration is established – 'when one of two things undoubtedly will happen it (the shot) will unite with Callus or come away with suppuration'.[31] This method was all too clearly used in the case of James Channon.

Essentially, suppuration was the process of forming thick pus to fill a cavity; if it developed in a cavity with no external opening, a cyst or abscess developed. Surgeons recognized suppurative inflammation through several cardinal signs – hot flushed skin, pain, rigours and cold fits:

> The discharge from a wound during this period is principally, the putrid serum and crassamentum; this is soon mixed with a thin serous secretion formed on the wounded surfaces. This discharge by degrees, acquires a whiter colour and thicker consistence; and about the fourth or fifth day, pure pus is discharged, and the inflammation abates.[32]

If the wound was not healing, a patient would have a violent prolonged fever and the granulations of new flesh would be white like a cauliflower, rather than a good red. Most ominous of all, the pus would not be of the good suppurative type, which was yellowish white and of a thick ropey consistence, but of the bad type, which was serous, bloody, thin, of an offensive smell, curdled and cheesy.[33]

Heaviside noted Pott's instructions in a lecture on wounds to the head on differentiating between good and bad inflammations of the scalp. How did the scalp take the impression of a finger, how puffy was it, what colour was it, how much delirium and pain did the patient have, were they shivering and/or sweating?[34] In 1768 Pott published a large treatise on head injuries and related cases where he cut through the scalp, removed skull pieces, drained blood, and attempted to stitch up the scalp after swelling to the brain was relieved:

> Case 18: A Girl about sixteen was knocked down by her mother with an iron poker of considerable weight; the latter immediately ran away and the former was brought senseless to the hospital. She had a large wound on top of her head, with a considerable fracture of the sagittal structure. The broken pieces were so large, and so loose, as to be easily removable without any perforation.[35]

After Pott removed the shattered pieces of her skull, the girl was left with a two-inch hole and was 'perfectly and absolutely senseless'. Five days later, Pott became increasingly concerned that the girl was not waking up and decided to drain the blood collected around the wound. A nurse held a dressing in place while he visited his other patients. Pott returned to discover the girl coming round. By the next day she was asking for a drink, but despite these positive signs the outcome was not good – seventeen days after being brought to the hospital, she convulsed and died. Pott opened her skull and was not surprised to discover a massive abscess full of 'bad' pus.[36]

Abscesses were complex to treat. Eighteenth-century London surgeons agreed that they should not be removed until they reached their full inflammatory and suppurative maturity, because an abscess could potentially be the crisis of an internal disease. It was good to allow pus to accumulate. As a result, abscesses were left to ripen and could become enormous. Abernethy jovially lectured that 'To give an idea of one – I let out 4 "Alehouse quarts" of pus from an abscess on the back of a patient'.[37]

> The old Surgeons were terribly afraid of opening large abscesses – Hence Mr. Pott used to say – The Man who escaped with a lumbar abscess was as fortunate as the Man who drew a £20,000 prize.[38]

To demonstrate he was unafraid of operating on large infected abscesses, Abernethy described the case of a woman with a two-foot circumference swelling on the inside of the knee. Over four years it had grown from the size of an egg into an enormous and debilitating soft tumour. Bedridden for two years, the woman was hospitalized at her family's plea when the swelling:

> ulcerated, sloughed, and left a cavity of the size of a pint-bason. From the sides of this cavity poured forth a most copious and foetid discharge: she had frequently lost blood from the vessels laid open by ulceration or sloughing.[39]

Ultimately Abernethy amputated the leg, injected and inspected it, and was surprised to discover that the abscess had not arisen from an infected bone.

Poultices or formentations were formulated and reformulated in eighteenth-century hospitals to encourage abscesses to come quickly to fruition. The recipes for these were elaborate, and surgeons took pride in making soft pulpy bread poultices as opposed to lumpy doughy ones. Abernethy, somewhat defensively, lectured that 'it is attention to these little things that qualifies a Man to become a good Surgeon'.[40]

> Scald out a bason (to make it hot) pour in some boiling water – then throw in as much coarsely crumbled bread as you want for a poultice – let it stand for a time, and then pour off the superabundant water & you will have left a soft pulpy poultice which you may beat up together & spread on double linen about ⅛th of an inch thick.[41]

Abscesses that burst but then refused to heal were classified as indolent or lazy sores, and, according to Abernethy, required 'nothing but whipping & spurring' with further stimulants, such as carrot juice, yeast, oatmeal, fumigation with carbonic acid gas, and metallic salts as a tonic mixed with fresh burnt charcoal. Arsenic could be tried, but only as a last resort as 'it produces a strong slough'.[42] According to Clare, all these substances worked because their subtle vapours penetrate the pores of the skin, which 'being very minute, refuse the admission of the grosser fluids, oil, or water'.[43]

While they may have agreed on what an abscess was and the substances used to heal a lazy one, Abernethy and Clare vehemently disagreed in letters and print on how to open and drain the skin. Abernethy advocated the use of a lancet and:

> hav[ing] an assistant apply firm pressure so no bubble of air gets in the abscess as it drains as this can result in horrible putrefaction and this being penned up in the abscess, some has been absorbed & the patient has died of the most violent putrid fever imaginable ...[44]

Clare disagreed. He supported caustics rather than the knife for opening abscesses. Caustics were burning chemicals, like silver nitrate or copper sulphate, applied to the skin for several hours in a dressing oiled with lard or beeswax in order to cause a deep blister. Clare advanced several reasons for this preference – it was 'less terrifying' to the patient than the knife, and could be administered with opium. 'Those surgeons who have joined opium with their caustics affirm, that their patients have fallen asleep during the operation.'[45]

Using knives or caustics, however, was as much the choice of the patient as the surgeon. The knife was so strongly and negatively identified with surgeons that Pott began his first lecture on surgery by stating, 'we ought never to have recourse to the knife when a gentler Method will succeed'.[46] Getting patients to submit to the knife was difficult and often impossible. Even in cases of cancer, where cutting out a tumour offered a much better prognosis than burning it with caustics,

> patients would sooner suffer the Caustic [applied by some quack] than submit to the knife, and all arguments us'd to persuade them of the great difference of pain and time of the operatn., are often fruitless so great is their dread of the knife.[47]

Moreover, Pott continued that knives enable a surgeon to save skin and minimize scarring, 'which with the Caustic you cannot do, as it totally destroys the skin'.[48] He did, however, encourage the use of caustics *if* the patient refused the knife. In his notes from Pott's lecture on 'Cancer of the Breast' (1767), Heaviside reports Pott claiming:

> I cannot see a reason why the Surgeons should be afraid to do it by Caustic as well as the Quacks. The Caustic is tedious in its Operation, inefficacious, & horridly painful ... From this Quackery Destruction has happened to thousands, & probably will to many more.[49]

To complicate matters, Pott was a pioneer in using caustics on children with paralysis of the limbs, most likely from tuberculosis spondylitis of the skeleton, which caused massive deformities and contractures. He believed that the scarring caused by caustics would over several weeks pull the backbone into alignment. Heaviside wrote up 'Case 7th Paralysis' from Pott's lectures in January 1786 about a 14-year-old boy paralyzed in his lower extremities. Pott advised a caustic to be applied to each side of the spinous processes of the backbone, and then an 'issue was made so large as to admit 12 pease [peas], after it had discharged for 3 weeks the boy began to find a numbness with a gentle perspiration attack'.[50] Seven weeks later the boy was walking with a stick. 'Case 8th', a 16-year-old boy named Thomas Barker with a history of spasms in his legs, whooping cough, falling down repeatedly, a hacking bloody cough and anorexia, did not fare so well: 'when the issues stopped draining ... all his complaints returned redoubled' and 'he fell – a victim to his last enemy [death]'.[51]

Pott's experimental use of caustics on the skin of at least ten patients with lower limb paralysis and deformed spines was widely publicized. Dr Johann Hunczovsky (1752–98), the personal surgeon to the Emperor of Austria and director of the prestigious military surgical teaching institute, the Josephinum in Vienna, observed and questioned Pott during his tour of the major hospitals in Europe. In a letter of 11 June 1779 to Alexander von Brambilla, the chief surgeon of the Austrian Army, Hunvzovsky reported on Pott's treatment of several patients with paralysis of the lower limbs:

> Two of these patients are being treated at the moment, one aged 37, the other 14; the former fell on his spine three years ago and became paralysed in the lower limbs; the tumour which is now formed by the vertebrae developed imperceptibly. The latter

suffered the same accident in infancy ... both patients are improving and particularly the boy is starting to walk unaided.[52]

Several themes emerge in surgeons' debates between knives or caustics. First, caustics are at times associated with quacks, especially cancer quacks, whether because they could not wield a knife skilfully nor apply caustics properly. Second, patients were difficult creatures and frequently refused to submit to the knife, even if they died from the consequences of this decision. For example, in 1780 Pott treated several women who were accidentally shot during the Gordon Riots.[53] One of them was Alice Kent, who, according to an anonymous physician on Bart's Watt Ward, 'seems to have lived rather an irregular life':

> 12, June, Alice Kent 48 Years of age a married Woman was admitted on Wednesday night into the Hospital for a Compound fracture of the leg about an inch and a half above the ankle Joint ... She was shot by a musket ball about an hour before her admission on the inside of the leg which shattered both Tibia and Fibula passed obliquely through the Joint, out of the Heel, both bones were broke in many places and directions and the Joint seemed to have been very particularly concerned – She was advised to suffer amputation which she positively refused – and her leg was laid up ... with splints ... Saturday the 10 – ... a black beginning mortific.n took place – a Poultice was put on and she took freely of opium and Bark ...
> Dead
> The woman died from mortification.[54]

The debate of caustic versus knife also raises the issue of pain and its mitigation in the treatment of skin wounds. Knives might be much quicker, but caustics could be mixed with opium, as Clare indicated and as Pott administered to patients with paralysed legs. Essentially, little evidence appears to survive in eighteenth-century records of how pain was measured qualitatively or quantitatively by patient or surgeon. Pott does refer occasionally to pain in relation to the cutting of skin in his lectures:

> If it is a large breast, it is necessary to make six or seven Motions with the Knife, each being equall [*sic*] in Pain, because equal in Duration – sh.d remember that the Patient do not measure pain by the Incision but of the operation.[55]

Pott then proceeded to describe how to remove a presumed cancerous breast with the knife, remarking that:

> The only pain of any Consequence in this Operation is in the Division of the Skin, & here Celerity [or quickness] is perhaps most required, & of whatever size the Breast may be, it is always best to divide the skin by two semicircular Incisions, which should be deep enough; Young surgeons are sometimes embarrass'd from the great depth they appear to cut this, but it is nothing but skin, teat & cellular membrane.[56]

In contrast to mastectomies, he waxed lyrical in a lecture concerning gunshot wounds on the miracle of opium:

> These Wounds soon become extremely painful, the Pain is 1ˢᵗ to be appeased by means of Opium – Opium (that heavenly medicine – I think I may without Vanity say, that the Gentlemen of this Hospital are entitled to the Honor of ... giving it in much larger doses than had before been tried ...[57]

Patients, at least in the minds of their surgeons, thus viewed pain in terms of the kind and length of their operation rather than by the number of cuts, blisterings and insertion of irritants into wounds. It seems surgeons believed pain increased in proportion to the age of a wound, whether made by themselves or a foreign object. The process of opening the skin was not supposed to be as painful as that of encouraging it to close. This attitude can be contrasted with the well-known case of Fanny Burney (1752–1840), who provided a rare account of mastectomy from the patient's view in 1811. In a letter to her sister Esther, Fanny described her lengthy scream as the knife cut through the skin and the excruciating pain of the air rushing into the wound as the knife was withdrawn. She graphically recalled her sense of the surgeon changing hands as he tired from having to saw 'against the grain', as it felt to her, of the flesh.[58]

Opium was being used more at St Bartholomew's Hospital. We can add to this the knowledge that alcohol or cordial (comprising largely alcohol) was given after surgery as a stimulant, rather than before surgery to sedate the patient. In fact, alcohol is a poor analgesic at best and causes prolonged bleeding.[59] It was not seen as a sedative but a stimulating tonic, and was often prescribed for breakfast on the wards. The side effects of opium were well known – vomiting, constipation, depressed respiration – and Pott makes reference to the need to keep increasing the dose as the patient developed tolerance.

Pott also lectured repeatedly on the age-old problem of surgeons causing pain unnecessarily just to be seen to be doing something, for example in the cases of children who were unable to pass faeces due to an imperforate anus. This was a congenital problem that Pott frequently encountered; he instructed students to resist making any kind of opening in the skin:

> I know of nothing surgery can do for it – I mention this to you on your Guard, & to enable you to resist a Proposition often made in this State of things; the People belonging to the Child will say, the Child is certainly dying, give it the Chance of Life by pushing in your Knife or Trocar ... I never would do what must give pain ... even if you should happen to thrust the Instrument within it, it can only afford a temporary Relief, the child has no Rectum ... & therefore it could answer no end, & I have seen a trocar pushed up as high as possible to please the Parents, from which a Gush of Urine has flowed & no feces & the infant has soon died, I wont say from [what] but with a wounded bladder ...[60]

We have no evidence that Mr Peters ever gave James Channon any opium, and he never mentions the use of an anodyne, the early modern medical term for a moderate painkiller. Nor do we have evidence that Mr Peters was troubled by how James's skin would look after his eight years of treatment concluded. Yet Heaviside does record rare moments in Pott's lectures when some passing mention was made of what a patient would look like following surgery. This included the case of head wounds:

> Lecture 8: On injuries of the scalp: The removal of the scalp in Women, ought to be prevented as much as possible, as Hair will never grow on that Part again ...[61]

Another was in the case of operating for harelip, where gold pins with points that could be screwed off were to be inserted, rather than straight steel pins, as the latter attracted a crust when pulled out and so left behind larger scars. The pins were placed around the edges of the wound before waxed linen thread was woven around them in a figure of eight.[62] It is interesting that both examples involved women and children.

Skin suturing was actually rare in Georgian surgery, as it was believed to intensify inflammation and perhaps cause haemorrhaging.[63] This theory led to stitches being applied reluctantly, as Abernethy recorded in his work on tumours. Case three in the book involved an Oxfordshire man who presented himself at the hospital with three diseased lymphatic glands of the neck, each the size of a large plum. Sir Charles Blicke, a surgeon, removed the diseased gland and 'the external maxillary artery was unavoidably divided'. The patient's wound was sutured (with one suture) and closed with sticking plasters. Fortunately, Abernethy noted, the suture broke and the plasters fell off once the patient was taken back to the ward, as the man was close to choking due to their abnormally tight application.[64]

In fact suturing more often involved dead bodies than live ones. For example, James Wilson included the following information in the inaugural lecture at the Great Windmill Street Anatomy School in London in 1798:

> In sewing up the body again you turn down the sternum and fasten some of the cartilages in their situ.n to keep all the parts natural either by stitches of a bit of wood across under the sternum. Then sew the angle together at the navel & then sew till you get to the breast of 2 Ilii. A flat sided needle preferable to a Glovers and use as large a thread as the needle will carry easily, to prev. blood etc from oozing out afterwards & making the shroud be bloody. Put the needle in the inside of the skin always\ /\/\/\ and be careful that no flesh or cellular membrane be let to appear.[65]

On a patient's discharge from hospital, sutures do appear to have been occasionally used as a restraint measure to keep a wound together when nothing else worked, the patient 'due to the restlessness and intemperance or obstinacy' having failed to keep dressings on.[66]

Gangrenous wounds presented a particularly pressing problem and source of debate for surgeons working with skin. Thomas Kirkland addressed the question of when to amputate when gangrene developed. He was trying to establish a middle ground in a heated debate that had been raging for six years, involving two major surgeons, M. Bilguer, the Surgeon General to the Armies of Prussia, and Pott, London's best known surgeon.[67] Kirkland had been Pott's pupil, but like most good students did not agree with everything his teacher proposed. Bilguer opposed amputation in nearly every injury, while Pott recommended amputation when gangrene first appeared or was likely.

As part of Kirkland's argument that amputation was only necessary when mortification arose from a gangrenous disposition of the juices versus from a local and external injury, he gave a detailed explanation of how the skin reacts to wounding. First, lymph stagnates about the wound and immediately inflames. This corrodes the vessels, which contain the lymph, and air 'bubbles' into the membrane adipose and other membranes. They instantly form more bubbles, which increases the inflammation. These then spread and extend over the injured limb. Fever is often precipitated with the onset of delirium, and patients experience a great dejection of spirits, often accompanied by a wild demeanour. Finally the 'scene is frequently closed with a rapidity that will not admit of assistance'.[68]

How did surgeons acquire this detailed knowledge of the stages of skin breakdown and responses to injury? Kirkland stated that such information came from making incisions in the wound over several days. Incising the skin when bubbles first form produces a discharge of blood; however, if incision is made when the skin inflates, one gets a large discharge of wind and frothy matter. Later, if one pierces the skin, the blood will be black and the muscles putrid. Finally, the skin becomes livid and putrid. The rotting of wounds thus progressed from the inside to the outside of the skin.

Kirkland argued that hospitals hastened and aggravated this series of events for three reasons. First, the air that was breathed in by patients was 'destitute of its vivifying spirit, so necessary for the preservation of life, [and] it really becomes putrid from being confined, and repeatedly inspired, and from being loaded with the putrid exhalations arising from mortifications, different kinds of sores, diseased bodies, &c.'. Second, the hospital diet was problematic because many of the 'unfortunate' patients have been used to 'drink plentifully of drams, beer and the like, [and] will sink even under the full diet of the Hospital, and die for want of some indulgence in these bad habits, which are now, from custom, become necessary assistants in supporting the strength of the body'. By contrast, patients from the country often had different diets and, importantly, they breathed purer air. Kirkland stressed that hospital physicians often ignored their patients' usual regimens at their peril: 'I have repeatedly seen the most salutary effects follow a due allowance of ale, wine or brandy'.[69] Finally, hospitals were unsuited to wound treatment because hospital surgeons were too inclined to operate rather than let nature take its course, or even to treat the wound with milder actions. Operating was easy and required little talent; coaxing an abscess to fruition, healing a chronic ulcer and setting an open fracture was more challenging. Similar claims by rural surgeons such as Kirkland became increasingly common in the eighteenth century as urban surgeons made their reputations and fortunes by inventing new operating techniques or instruments. The mundane work of setting bones and lancing boils offered little opportunity to gain fame or fortune from patrons or pupils:

> I know, indeed, Operations often make a great noise, and prejudice people in favour of the abilities of the Operator; and some, with very little knowledge in Surgery, have raised themselves great reputation by this mechanical part of the profession, which requires no great genius, as it depends only upon a knowledge of anatomy, and a practical dexterity of the hand ... Nevertheless, notwithstanding this part of practice is so readily acquired, it has of late years been more attended to by the student, and cultivated with more assiduity, than the treatment of Fractures, Luxations, Wounds, Abscesses, Ulcers, etc ...[70]

Kirkland was particularly concerned that surgeons appeared to believe, and largely to publish, that there was nothing more to be learnt about or to improve upon in the treatment of 'the most common business of surgery', skin wounds. Kirkland called this 'that part which cures without the assistance of the knife, except the opening of abscesses, sinus's [*sic*], and the like'.[71] This was the difficult process to manage, not operations where surgeons could surmount any problem 'if you can *preserve a calmness and a presence of mind*'.[72]

To conclude, what does the treatment of wounds by Georgian surgeons in London tell us about the history of the skin? First, it demonstrates that skin was a tissue made up of minute pores that many substances such as water and oil could not penetrate; and second, that manifestations on the skin were seen as signs of internal disturbances. One could draw these out in numerous ways through injuring or stimulating the skin. Apply a hot iron, a burning chemical, create an issue, attach a leech – Georgian surgeons employed many methods to work the skin. But there was not widespread agreement on what to try and when. Arguments were put forward in lectures and print on the most successful and efficient methods to release substances from under the skin. This made sense given that wounds healed from below, the last stage being a formation of a cicatrix or hard scar on the skin. Most agreed it was best to keep wounds open to allow material to rise to the surface and be discarded, but air was seen as a potential poison that could cause blood to corrupt and mortify. Alternative and competitive exit routes on the skin were carefully dug with fingers and knives, and peas, beans and cannula inserted in order to allow pus to flow from the primary and covered wound. Pain from cutting and burning the skin was of concern to surgeons, and some particular attention was paid to how women and children would appear after surgery, especially their heads and faces.[73] Skin was a complex and challenging theoretical and practical substance, one that surgeons wrestled with daily. In lectures, on rounds in the wards, and in print, they argued about its meaning both to them as healers who drained, blistered and bled, and to their patients who suffered the opening and closing of their skin in Georgian London.

2 ABOMINABLE ULCERS, OPEN PORES AND A NEW TISSUE: TRANSFORMING THE SKIN IN THE NORWEGIAN COUNTRYSIDE, 1750–1850

Anne Kveim Lie

> Even the plague, at present so humiliating and devastating to the Turks, seems to intro-duce a kind of mildness compared to the hideous radesyge. The first cuts the process short, and immediately delivers death one prey after another. The latter torments slowly, kills tardily, destroys unborn generations, and disfigures well formed bodies.[1]

In June 1781 the physician Nicolaus Arbo, practising in the district of Strømsø in eastern Norway, received a letter from a chamber councillor in the neighbouring county of Telemark.[2] The councillor requested that Arbo take compassion on two poor, single male peasants, whom he had met in a 'most miserable and lam-entable state'. Both of them had been discharged from the hospital as incurable, and they now dwelled in a tiny peasants' hut, entirely ostracized by the commu-nity, which feared infection. The councillor[3] pitied these two unfortunates, and their 'utterly deplorable fate' had triggered his request to the physician. One of them, named Hans, was thirty-six years old. His health had begun deteriorating five years earlier, and the infirmity reappeared a few years later, with ulcers in the throat and under the nose. Eventually the whole lower part of the nasal cartilage and most of the upper lip were completely destroyed by the disease. He looked 'extraordinarily repulsive', but his health was otherwise good. The other, John, was thirty years old. His suffering had commenced three years earlier with ulcers in the throat and loss of the uvula. He had also contracted a disease of the chest, and his speech was severely impaired due to shortness of breath and increasing hoarseness. The colour of his face was pale and yellowish. The chamber council-lor requested a physician's judgment and promised to cover the medical expenses personally. Arbo, the physician, examined the 'wretched' patients and proclaimed that although their recovery was uncertain, he nevertheless wished to commence treatment. Hans was prescribed several medicines, including pills and drops, to cleanse the blood. John received Ethiopian pills, a decoction of sarsaparilla root and sassafras, juniper and china bark. The treatment had a striking effect. Two months later both patients were declared 'happily cured'. They resumed their usual work and were 'thereby once more included in the community'.

The case of Hans and John is from the early history of radesyge in Norway, which emerged as a public threat from the late 1760s. The disease was particularly prevalent in the south-western part of the country, but was increasingly found in other areas. In 1772 the Copenhagen-based Collegium Medicum, the highest medical council in the absolutist state of Denmark–Norway, informed the chancellery that Norwegian radesyge was a dangerous disease, both common and damaging to the people.[4] As the case above reveals, the main symptom of radesyge was skin ulceration. This chapter will focus on the changing perceptions of radesyge. In the eighteenth and early nineteenth century, these surface manifestations were perceived as the result of the body's efforts to rid itself of peccant matter, whereas by the middle of the nineteenth century, these cutaneous lesions constituted the defining features of the disease. Initially radesyge was understood as a disease located within the body, a body open to its environments, and the surface symptoms were indicative of the skin's porous opening that enabled poisonous matter to exit. During this period the skin was regarded as nothing but the exemplary projected surface, a flat screen on which the trained clinician could read the hidden malaise of the body. A century later, radesyge became a disease that lay in the skin, the new organ that came into being in the beginning of the nineteenth century and that fundamentally changed the perception of radesyge.

The Norwegian Radesyge

Towards the end of the eighteenth century, Norway was not yet an independent nation and did not possess a proper university. What the Norwegians did have, however, was their own disease, the radesyge. Indeed, in the eighteenth century it was called 'the Norwegian radesyge'; radesyge had become a national disease in the midst of a growing patriotism. The story above touches many of the themes central to its history. One issue involves the diseased patients, who generally belonged to the lowest strata of society; another relates to the authorities, who were concerned and introduced curative and preventive measures. Their concern was not unambiguously defined by pity, however. Radesyge was not only a disease detrimental to the patients' health and function. Like the St Paul's Bay disease described in Moran's chapter, it was also increasingly regarded as a threat to the nation.[5] As the physical health of the population was considered a relevant factor for economic management in the absolutist state of the twin realms Denmark–Norway, measures were taken at a public level. It is thus not coincidental that the patients' restoration of working capacity led the narrator in the story above to rejoice. The engagement with radesyge as a threat to the nation is also evident in one of the first written statements concerning this new disease – a 1769 letter to the Danish king from the district commander (stiftsamtmann) in Christiansand diocese,[6] Hans Hagerup:

> In recent years, a 'saltzfluss'-like, contagious disease, ruining the country, has begun to infect the commons in this district. People in this area have given the disease the name of Radesyge, and many people succumb in the prime of their life ... – it is steadily increasing, and if remedies are not taken immediately ... more than half of the population will be demolished.[7]

Hagerup had been present at an examination of men liable for military service, and witnessed how the 'most beautiful and healthiest young men' had to be demobilized and 'reduced to hospital patients.'[8] The concern was thus not primarily about people's suffering, but also about the state's need for able bodies, as many were transformed from sturdy contributors to feeble dependents.

It was when physicians like Nicolaus Arbo concentrated on radesyge that they first assumed a central role in hospital management, making this disease an important one for the history of the medicalization of Norwegian hospitals. When radesyge first made its appearance, Norway had only five officially appointed physicians and no hospitals dedicated to short stay and treatment.[9] However, in this period sixteen so-called 'radesyge hospitals' were constructed – the first hospitals in Norway with a therapeutic role.[10] The largest of these was the hospital in Bratsberg, where Hans and John had been treated. Most would be rebranded a century later as municipal hospitals, and thus literally constituted the foundation of the modern health care system in Norway. In the same period the number of officially appointed civilian medical officers (physicians and surgeons) increased from about ten to forty-seven, and most of the new officers were appointed specifically to handle the radesyge epidemic.[11]

Hans's and John's stories reflect another important aspect of the history of radesyge in Norway: their cases are narrated in one of the books constituting the so-called radesyge literature,[12] Norway's first medical literature in the vernacular. Radesyge later became the topic of several doctoral dissertations, including the first dissertation to be defended at the newly founded (1811) university in Norway in 1817.[13]

Etymologically, the name radesyge derives from two words: *rada* and *syge*. Rada was a word used among the peasants at the west coast of Norway to mean bad, wicked or evil:[14] a rada man would suggest an evil man, a rada thing a bad, harmful thing. Radesyge thus literally signified a wicked, bad or evil disease (syge). While many colloquial expressions have been used to denote diseases in local communities, radesyge is unusual in that it did not remain confined to these localities; it travelled from the Norwegian countryside via medical literature into Latin dissertations.[15] By the mid-nineteenth century, it had even settled in the Latin vocabulary and became an accepted entry in Latin-German dictionaries.[16]

The story of John and Hans touches on another, material aspect: the large, abominable ulcers, which gave the disease its name. In the medical literature these ulcers were described as having their own agency; they were 'devastating' and 'consuming', they would 'seize' bodies, in particular the face, 'dig' into bones, and leave behind eroded noses and decayed bodies. Patients with an advanced stage of the disease were, according to contemporaries, a spectacular and miserable sight. The metaphors used to describe the disease often evoked images of death. In his recommendations to the king on how to manage radesyge, the physician Rasmus Frankenau claimed that the disease created 'living corpses' who resembled 'bugbears to their fellow human beings'.[17] The priest Andreas Faye described the diseased as 'excessively spectacular and miserable' and 'true prisoners of death'.[18] Such imagery recalled metaphors of leprosy in the Middle Ages. Roy Porter emphasized how ecclesiastical leaders in Europe portrayed leprosy as a living death.[19] As we shall see – and much like the diseases explored by Gentilcore and Siena – physicians debated whether radesyge was a kind of leprosy, as the latter disease, in contrast to the rest of Europe, had not disappeared from Norway.

A Porous, Open Body

The medical literature on radesyge shows a profound ambiguity. On the one hand, authors struggled with how to define it. Radesyge was a new disease, nowhere to be found in contemporary nosological texts. Was it a new disease, or a known disease in disguise? In disease classifications, skin colour played a prominent part, as it did in the nosologies of Cullen and de Sauvages.[20] Most authors held it to be related to scurvy in one way or another, either by being a kind of land scurvy or by being frequently associated with and aggravated by scurvy. But radesyge was also regularly associated with leprosy, either by being classified as a species within the more general class of leprosy, or as a stage in a process leading up to leprosy. Some also held it to be a kind of venereal disease, complicated by land scurvy. Tellingly, English physicians made all of these assumptions about the itch, as Siena's chapter indicates.

Most authors were less concerned with how to define the disease, and more with providing guidance on how to treat it in the remote areas of south-western Norway where it was most prevalent. Clearly, determining how to deal with the problem in practice was a priority. In these discussions it becomes obvious that skin colours, so crucial for nosology, were only superficial, outward manifestations of the disease. The real theatre of disease took place inside the body. Although radesyge showed itself on the outside of the body, its devastating ulcers and effect on skin colours bore witness to disease-processes taking place deep inside the body, inaccessible to the observer. The descriptions of the causes and treatment of radesyge evoke images of the body reminiscent of those portrayed by Barbara Duden.[21] Using the journals of a women's doctor in eighteenth-century Eisenach, Duden is able to show that the early modern body was invested with a meaning very different from that which it has today. Body fluids were constantly in motion, and the skin was understood as a porous layer with a multitude of possible openings. As part of this body, the skin was a place of permeability and mysterious metamorphoses.

One aspect of this open bodily surface that Duden does not mention, but which is crucial to the literature on radesyge, is the concept of insensible perspiration, where innumerable skin pores play a prominent role. Hans Møller's treatise on radesyge, for example, referred to the seventeenth-century Padua physician Sanctorius and his *Medicina Statistica*. More than one thousand years earlier, Galen had claimed that in addition to the discernible sweat, an insensible perspiration was continuously emitted from the body. Sanctorius tried to measure the insensible perspiration by weighing himself, his intake of food and drink, and his waste products over the course of thirty years. He concluded that more than half his normal weight loss arose from insensible perspiration through the pores of the skin. To Hans Møller, this perspiration was 'the greatest foundation of health and the most fertile of all mothers of disease'.[22] Such theories were vital to early medical thinking on skin diseases, as evidenced by their roles in early formulations of the itch and pellagra analysed elsewhere in this volume. When perspiration became hindered, the body's renovation system failed. This perspiration consisted of water, but also of 'impure, briny and sharply parts'.[23] And when these were held within the body, they destroyed both the solids and the fluids. In addition to referring to the scholarly literature, Møller was appealing to the common experiences of the bad smell and salty taste of sweat, and to the facts that long-worn clothes became dirty and long periods without cleaning the body caused itching. This proved, argued Møller, that insensible perspiration contained bodily waste products. Sweat was excrement. Frederik Holst, who wrote the first dissertation to be defended at the new university of Christiania (present-day Oslo) in 1817, remarked that 'a cause is only sufficient in so far as it manages to damage the distinct function of the skin, that is the insensible perspiration'.[24] To Holst, the other predisposing causes of radesyge involved the obstruction of insensible perspiration: the Norwegian fishermen's laborious work, bad hygiene and cramped quarters all instigated occlusion of the pores and obstructed perspiration.

The pores not only caused radesyge when they were blocked; Holst argued that they also drew the disease into the body when they were open, especially in stinking air: 'Smoke and other impurities pollute the common people, locked up in their small cottages ... The moist stench is absorbed by the breathing pores in the skin, and due to the uncleanliness it is inflicting damaging matter to the body'.[25] Alain Corbin has argued how a sudden increase in sensitivity and collective concern about smell took place in the latter part of the eighteenth century, which ultimately produced modernity's 'deodorized environment'. Between 1750 and 1850 '[o]dours simply began to be more keenly smelled. It was as if the thresholds of tolerance had been abruptly lowered'.[26] To Norbert Elias, the growing intolerance towards smell, stench, dirt and waste was an essential component in the civilizing process.[27] In the discourse on radesyge, smell became a central medical issue. Møller claimed that 'the stench which is to be found in most people's houses, shows that the air is filled with rotten vapours, often of a numerous family and servants, of rotten old cheese, meat, fish and other impurities'.[28] Alternatively, Christoph Elovius Mangor described how patients developed such a 'reeking breath, that they can fill the whole house with an almost intolerable stench, wherein their stinking sweat plays an important part. Their saliva is sticky and has a foul smell'.[29]

Although the medical literature on radesyge reflects the proliferation of medical theories in the eighteenth century, the authors agreed that a successful cure depended on bringing balance to the body. In the different medical texts, this imbalance was characterized either in iatromechanical terms by sharpness of the fluids, or in iatrochemical terms by too much salt or bile, but all of them considered radesyge primarily as an internal ailment characterized by imbalance. This disparity had to be treated. In this context the notion of the healing powers of nature, or *vis medicatrix naturae*, was fundamental. [30] It was an image of nature as an inner power, a force; nature as a norm.[31] The nature of the human body was to maintain internal balance and prevent its disturbance. The nature of disease, however, was to destroy this balance. If the balance was disturbed, the body tried to re-establish an original state of equilibrium. If the disease was too strong and the body unable to restore its balance alone, then the physician had to assist its natural healing process. A guiding principle was to observe how the nature of the body fought the nature of disease and the spontaneous disease-processes occurring on the skin, which often indicated how to proceed therapeutically.[32] For instance, spontaneous bleeding could indicate a general surplus of fluids, whereas ulcers were a sign that the body was attempting to expunge harmful matter it could not eliminate through ordinary channels. This healing excretion was crucial to medical practice, as Payne's chapter explores in detail. Exclusively concentrating the healing processes on the manifestations on the skin – for example, only treating the ulcers themselves – could result in an accumulation of peccant matter in the body. Therapeutic intervention thus consisted primarily in clearing a path to the surface for internal impurities in order to achieve purification. If the body did not open on its own, an exit was created through bleeding or a blistering dressing. Wounds and bloody discharges from the skin were thus seen as the body's own healing processes, something to be assisted rather than prevented.

Thus in late eighteenth- and early nineteenth-century discourse, radesyge was a disease interacting with the surrounding world. It was inseparable from the rural districts of south-western Norway, from rotten fish, stationary air and impure clothing. The skin was the open barrier mediating between the inside and the outside. In a bidirectional process – through its open pores – poisonous matter penetrated to the body's inner reaches, causing radesyge. The same invisible pores, however, also brought stench, foulness and sweat out of the body, passing radesyge back into the environment, affecting other bodies, other ambiences. The body suffering from radesyge was open to its surroundings, somewhat reminiscent of Starobinski's descriptions of the body in Montaigne's time.[33]

Towards the mid-nineteenth century, views regarding bodily suffering from radesyge fundamentally changed. The disease moved into the skin, which in turn had become established as a separate organ, containing diverse layers and different components. This new radesyge was not a disease communicating with the outside world; it was a disease situated within this new organ of the skin.

Radesyge Becomes a Skin Disease

After an initial rise in the numbers of radesyge cases during the first two decades of the nineteenth century, the disease was reported to be in decline from the 1820s onwards.[34] Its diagnosis and etiology were no longer perceived as a *fait accompli*, but increasingly problematized and eventually discarded as old-fashioned, vague and unspecific. In 1840 an important article on the condition was published in the first issue of the Norwegian medical journal *Norsk Magazin for Lægevidenskaben* by Johan Hjort, an assistant physician in a hospital in Christiania. Hjort argued that radesyge had been incorrectly confused with scurvy, leprosy and venereal disease. In order to avoid these confusions, he contended that it needed a new name, and his suggestion was *theria*, the Greek word for malignant ulcers. To Hjort, radesyge, or theria, was an inflammation localized in a particular tissue: 'the essential symptoms of radesyge are constituted by a chronic inflammation or infiltration of the outer as well as of the inner skin (through all its layers), as well as of the neighbouring cellular tissue'.[35] Crucially, everything, including the symptoms, formerly connected to the patient's experience, had moved into the skin.

The difference between this and earlier texts is evident; pathological anatomy and the new discipline of dermatology provided a new way of perceiving radesyge. Between this and the older texts, a fundamental change had taken place. The era of the all-encompassing classification endeavour in medicine was gone, and the focus now was on the localization of disease in individual bodies. The findings at autopsy now became fundamental to descriptions of disease.[36] Also, in the nineteenth century dermatology was emerging as a new discipline within medicine, a discipline closely connected to pathological anatomy. The skin was no longer a porous surface, bearing witness to processes within. Now it had become a proper organ, with a defined structure and depth, where pathological processes could be observed. In the first decade of the nineteenth century, the English physician Robert Willan had already formulated a new classificatory system based on the morphology of skin eruptions.[37] Instead of describing diseases, Willan based his system on providing an alphabet of skin diseases by describing eight primary lesions: papules, squama, exanthemata, bullae, pustules, vesicles, tubercles and macules. In the same way that letters in the alphabet constitute a restricted number of combinable basic elements, these eight primary lesions could be variously combined in different diseases. The method he proposed to identify skin diseases, describing the basic elements and classifying the disease according to the commingling of these elements, was adopted by the majority of the nineteenth-century dermatological community.[38] However, Willan also introduced a new form of graphic presentation, the dermatological atlas, discussed in Fend's chapter and Wilson's afterword. Willan's edition contained a set of hand-coloured engravings, with descriptions of the elementary lesions presenting in the most important skin diseases. Thus elementary lesions essentially constituted a visual alphabet that could be used in the classification of disease. For the first time skin diseases appeared as a distinct medical subject, with a characteristic set of lesions. In Hjort's description of theria, several of Willan's elementary lesions – pustula, tubercles and ulcers – are present. These constituted the basis for the classification, in addition to the question of how far the lesions extended into the skin's tissue. Theria was then divided into subgroups depending on the form of its lesions and how deeply they infiltrated the skin.

To Hjort, the skin had become complex and layered; it comprised the outer and inner skin, and contained diverse elements, such as glandular tissue, hair follicles and blood vessels. This is why radesyge, although revealing different symptoms, was nevertheless one and the same disease.[39] The attacked tissues were related, for they shared a similar anatomopathological structure.

To modern readers it may appear as if medicine had finally begun to recognize what is obvious to our eyes. Hjort pretended simply to write down his sensory impressions. However, this way of seeing is historically conditioned, relying on a complex way of seeing. Pathological-anatomical changes in the skin are not immediately given to the observer. They demand an interpreter who reads the outer manifestations of the skin with a gaze that knows the structure within and has learned a particular way to interpret that which is visible. Hjort, unlike the eighteenth-century authors on radesyge, was not concerned with the ever-changing surface of the human body.

Earlier, radesyge was a disease characterized by changes in the fluids deep inside the body, which became visible only when putrid matter was discharged through openings in the body's surface. Now the disease was actually located in a new organ, the skin. In eighteenth-century radesyge texts, the skin was a sheet surrounding the body. Now it had become layered and thickened significantly. As a consequence this new disease also lost any association with fluids inside the body, the poor living conditions of the Norwegian peasantry, the hard work at sea and the eating habits of the common people. Now the disease was firmly located within the skin, and what differentiated varying types of radesyge was the extent to which they penetrated the skin. The radesyge in Hjort's text had been cut with sharp knives, literally and metaphorically speaking.

Between the earlier texts and this one, another fundamental change had taken place – the coming into being of the clinic. The hospital played a major role in these transformations. Hjort emphasized his opportunities to study numerous cases of the disease on the patients in hospital wards, both at home and abroad. Whereas eighteenth-century authors like Mangor or Møller did not gain their credibility by referring to extensive clinical experience, Hjort repeatedly referred to his experience of observing and detailing skin changes on patients in the hospital ward. Not only did he observe these patients, he also counted, arranged and made calculations based on their lesions. The clinic gave him the opportunity to make use of another of the peculiarities of the new medicine: the technology of numbers. Hjort informed the reader of the number of radesyge patients he had seen (400), and several times used statistics to substantiate his claims on the location of ulcers, the extent of lesions and even their colours. The individual patient had become a case, to be observed, compared with others, and counted.

The End of Radesyge

With the advance of the studies of diseases of the skin and the syphilitic disease, the names of Radesyge and Theria will disappear.[40]

In 1860 Norway's first professor of dermatology, Carl Wilhelm Boeck, published a book called *Traite de la radesyge*, with the subtitle *syphilis tertiare*. The subtitle was placed within parentheses on the title page, but what really happened in this text was that radesyge was bracketed. Boeck himself proclaimed that he had become convinced that 'radesyge is nothing other than an offspring of syphilis'.[41] In this text, radesyge exfoliates; it is not recognized as a proper disease, but is defined as advanced syphilis. Boeck was appointed professor of medicine at the university in Christiania in 1851, with responsibility for teaching surgery, dermatology and syphilis. It was the new discipline of dermatology, and in particular the sub-discipline of syphilology, that was Boeck's main field of interest. From 1850 he ran his own specialist clinic, where he began to experiment with syphilization, a mode of treatment centred on repeated inoculations, on multiple locations on the skin, of syphilitic matter taken from primary sores.[42] Auzias-Turenne, the French dermatologist who established the method, was never allowed to implement the practice in French hospitals. However, in Norway syphilization was the most common treatment for venereal disease between 1852 and 1875.

Boeck largely accepted Hjort's descriptions of the tissue changes in radesyge. The problem with earlier studies on radesyge, according to Boeck, was that they lacked exact descriptions of the disease, but this knowledge gap had been filled by Hjort. Nonetheless, Boeck argued, these very same descriptions convinced him that radesyge could not be a disease of its own.[43] To Boeck, radesyge was a development of tumours in the subcutaneous tissue, analogous to the gummous tumours described by French venereologists.

Boeck was referring to an international literature that had changed since Hjort published his text. Whereas Hjort cited dermatological texts, Boeck primarily engaged with venereology, a sub-discipline of dermatology that had been maturing since the time Hjort was active. In particular, Boeck drew heavily on Philippe Ricord, who is best remembered for having established gonorrhoea and syphilis as separate diseases. In this context, however, it is more relevant that he introduced the division of syphilis into three stages – primary, secondary and tertiary. The first stage was a local affliction, comprising the primary ulcer on the genitals. In the second stage the disease had disseminated in the blood, causing a general affection with exanthema of different forms all over the body. The third stage consisted of manifestations of the skin, bone and muscles, so-called *gummata*, which were soft, large tumours that could erode the skeleton and lead to deformations. Boeck compared Hjort's descriptions of radesyge with Ricords's depictions of syphilis, and concluded that the slight differences could not warrant categorizing radesyge as a proper disease. The symptoms in the third stage of syphilis, argued Boeck, were to a large extent concurrent with 'our own Radesyge'.

In his work, Boeck devoted considerable space to case studies, which had become an important element of medical discourse during the period.[44] Yet most of the patients whose stories he presented were not his own, but rather derived from Hjort's old hospital records. Hjort, however, had consciously chosen not to present any of his own patient histories, because he did not have sufficient knowledge of dermatology at the time he produced the records; he had not yet 'attended the school of a certain Rust and Biett'. Therefore his own case histories were insufficiently detailed and contained too little observation to be worthy of inclusion in the text. Boeck thought otherwise, and included them along with his own. In total, his section consists of sixteen cases. Although the original author of the cases had rendered diagnoses of leprosy, radesyge, theria or syphilis, Boeck argued that all of them were one and the same disease, namely syphilis.[45] The rhetorical effect of this arrangement was that the radesyge cases that Boeck observed in his own practice, as well as all the previous diseases known under that name, were reinterpreted as syphilitic cases.

Because venereal disease was regarded as a disease arising from sexual contact, in one sense Boeck re-established the old connection between disease and environment. In the nineteenth century radesyge alias syphilis had become a disease arising from impure sexual relations, firmly rooted in the urban problems of prostitution and its moral discourse. However, as we have seen, Boeck largely accepted Hjort's descriptions of the cutaneous lesions, and radesyge, having entered the body, was still a disease characterized by skin changes. When Boeck published his atlas of skin diseases, radesyge figured prominently.[46] This atlas also includes an important element in nineteenth-century dermatology and venereology that Hjort's text lacks: illustrations, all of different skin lesions, made by the painter Johan Ludvig Losting. In the hundred years that had passed since radesyge first made its appearance, medicine had become visual, a development explored in greater detail by the chapters in the third section of this volume. Whereas none of the eighteenth-century radesyge treatises contained any graphic elements, the watercolours in Boeck's volume constitute an essential part of the argument and define the scope and size of the atlas. Earlier, the inner, invisible body played the main role in the theatre of the disease; now the skin had moved centre stage.

Conclusion

Boeck's text marks the end of the radesyge era. After the 1850s radesyge ceased to be a phenomenon of the real world. In the first part of the nineteenth century, it had also ceased to be a Norwegian disease. Through its redefinition as a particular affliction of the skin, radesyge lost its former close connections to the living conditions of the poor peasants in the Norwegian countryside. The body suffering from radesyge was no longer a body defined by individual conditions. The coming-into-being of the universal body, a body essentially uniform in all human beings, enabled comparisons of Norwegian radesyge with other diseases in other places. The epithet 'Norwegian' was used until 1814, when Norway, as a result of the Napoleonic Wars, separated from Denmark and entered a Swedish–Norwegian union under the Swedish crown. In the first dissertation defended at Norway's new university, radesyge also became a Swedish disease. But then, radesyge gradually became associated with other previously unrelated diseases, like the Dietmarsch disease in southern Germany, the Jutland syphiloid, Skerljevo in Slovenia and the sibbens in Scotland,[47] the latter explored in Siena's chapter. All of them had been diseases with skin manifestations, firmly rooted in their local environments. Now, however, their description in the new vocabulary of dermatology caused them to disappear as separate entities.

That, however, does not mean that the old descriptions of radesyge lack value. That they evoke images of a body foreign to us does not mean that they can be discarded as products of insufficient knowledge, or of speculation gone astray. 'One has first to learn to look in order to be able to see that which forms the basis of a given discipline', as Ludwik Fleck argued in 1935.[48] To Fleck, the complexity of human disease makes necessary the coexistence of incommensurable thought styles dealing with pathological phenomena. As a case in point, he emphasized that specialists in bacteriology, like himself, could not differentiate and recognize dermatological changes: 'at first he listens to the descriptions of the dermatologist as if they were fairy tales, as much as he has the described object lying in front of him'.[49] Fleck's point is that the apparatus of sense – touch, vision and perception in general within medical practice – is historically conditioned, and that separate training in the perception of specific forms is absolutely crucial. During the process of specialization in medicine, the capacity to recognize some phenomena was necessarily accompanied by the loss of the ability to perceive others. Hjort, Boeck and their contemporaries in the nineteenth century were clearly trained to see in a new way. Their bodies learned to be affected by hitherto imperceptible differences through the mediation of an artificially constructed context: hospitals where the patients could be observed side by side and their diseases classified, and autopsy tables where skin lesions could be identified, extracted and inspected. But this process also implied that other, older ways of seeing and knowing became obsolete. It is indeed a very long way from the sufferings of John and Hans and the medical theories surrounding them to Boeck's practices of syphilization and the descriptions of the ulcers traversing the layers of the skin in Hjort's and Boeck's medical texts. But that does not make the world of Hans and John any less real. The main difference is that the skin had been transformed. Previously a place of encounter between self and the other – a world fraught with tentativeness, intimacy and potential repulsion, through the open pores and the body openings – the skin in the nineteenth century became a sealed membrane that confronted the world.[50] In this sealed and layered membrane, there was no longer a place for radesyge as it was previously understood. Radesyge was made irrelevant as an object of medical knowledge, but that transformation did not make it disappear from history.

3 PROTECTING THE SKIN OF THE BRITISH EMPIRE: ST PAUL'S BAY DISEASE IN QUEBEC[1]

James Moran

St Paul's Bay disease was a greatly feared infectious illness in late eighteenth-century Quebec. From 1775 to 1790 it was a health problem of major proportions in dozens of parishes in Quebec – one that appeared to be both endemic and epidemic in nature. Considered by contemporaries (and by more recent medical historians) as a form of non-venereal syphilis, or perhaps another of the treponematoses (pinta/yaws), St Paul's Bay disease was prominent throughout the colony, affecting thousands of colonists directly and indirectly.[2] By 1785 it had created enough concern to elicit an ambitious response that brought to bear the combined energies of the British colonial government, the Catholic clergy and the medical profession upon the physically unwell peasantry of Quebec. Leading the medical charge was the physician James Bowman, who was instructed by Governor Henry Hamilton to create an effective plan for the eradication of the disease.[3]

The widespread nature of the disease (its epidemiological scope), its prominent skin-deep manifestations and its geo-imperial context explain much about how it was identified, approached and negotiated by various social groupings in late eighteenth-century Quebec. British colonial authorities understood the vulnerability of French colonists to this disease in much the same way as they understood the precarious position of their newly acquired French colony, situated as it was beside a North American population to the south that was increasingly hostile to British interests. The geopolitical context of North American imperialism, marked by the British conquest of Quebec in 1760 and the American Revolutionary War twenty years later (1775–83), directly influenced the meaning of St Paul's Bay disease. Colonial officials combined geo-military considerations with the metaphor of racial decline to come to terms with the presence and timing of St Paul's Bay disease. The concerns of British authorities that Quebec was threatened by invasion from belligerent American colonists to the south (as happened, for example, in the 1775 invasion of Quebec) paralleled their concerns about the spread of St Paul's Bay disease. Their medical response was conditioned by reports about the severity of its symptoms on the skin, and about the extent to which the disease invaded and debilitated the bodies of their francophone colonial subjects. In the case of this disease, the progression of skin-deep symptoms was read as a kind of cutaneous barometer of the fortunes of the British colony. The threat of St Paul's Bay disease gained traction among British officials and among French religious authorities as its symptoms were seen to be wreaking havoc on the skin of its sufferers, as the number of its victims seemed to be increasing across the Quebec colonial map, and as the weakening francophone population was perceived as a further threat to the geographical integrity of British North America.

This understanding of the medical geography of St Paul's Bay disease led to a medical response in eighteenth-century North America hitherto unprecedented in scope. The nature of this response – various forms of mercury treatment – left its own impact on the skin. Furthermore, the response helped to reshape social relationships in Quebec by making local priests responsible for the administration of treatment and for evaluating its rate of success. Bishops and local priests expressed concerns about St Paul's Bay disease that were separate from yet closely tied to the imperial concerns of their new colonial masters. Their struggle to maintain social cohesion at the height of this disease's spread highlights other preoccupations related to balance between British imperial rule and French parish life.

This crossroads of empire, disease, skin and locale resonates analytically with authors like Steven Connor, who suggests that during the eighteenth century the Western medical world began to see skin as more than just a protective envelope for the body, but rather more metaphorically as a 'membrane' that governed 'interchanges of substance between the body and its environment'.[4] This, argues Connor, helped eighteenth-century medical observers to understand diseases like syphilis, and, I would argue, St Paul's Bay disease, 'as arising from deeper and more systemic disorderings of the body, despite the fact that their manifestations were primarily on the skin'.[5] Moreover, as Connor suggests, these interchanges between the body and environment could be read externally as well as internally, linking anxieties about the spread of St Paul's Bay disease to the broader geographies of British imperial concern. Just as some eighteenth-century physicians were busy mapping the parameters of the body's skin,[6] so too did the consideration of the skin's condition extend outward from colonists' bodies to the condition of the colony itself. For a historical moment in Quebec, the 'geo-pathology' of colonist and colony were mapped onto the same surface. Further helping to place disease, medicine and colonial rule on the same plane of understanding for a time in Quebec was, as Kevin Siena has termed elsewhere, a kind of 'moral biology'[7] that in this case was articulated by medical and administrative officials to help explain and justify their response to Quebec's 'vulnerable francophone race' in the face of St Paul's Bay disease.

The first official reports of St Paul's Bay disease appeared in the spring of 1775,[8] although the problem likely existed earlier, as the term St Paul's Bay disease had clearly become familiar usage by 1775. In fact this was only the most commonly used term for the disease, which was also variably called *la maladie des Eboulements*, Sibbens, *la maladie de Chicot, vilain mal, mauvais mal, gros mal, la maladie Allemande, mal Anglois* and Molbay disease.[9] Most, but not all, medical authorities considered it to be a form of syphilis, and there was disagreement about its mode of transmission. Dr James Bowman's description of the disease makes clear the striking effects that it had on the skin. The first symptoms appeared as small ulcers on the lips and tongue, and in the mouth and 'secret' parts. 'The ulcers', he continued:

> are small pustules full of white coloured pus, a poison so subtle that only a small amount can communicate the infection to another. Drinking from a glass, or smoking from a pipe infected by this poisonous matter is enough to result in a small blister on the lips filled with the same white pus that drains, dilates the sore, and corrodes the surrounding flesh creating a larger ulcer ... For some the initial ulcers disappear but they come back quickly, and the illness is thus at its second stage. Hereafter, larger ulcers appear in the mouth, throat, private parts, and at the foundations. The glands of the throat, armpits and groin become inflamed, occasionally discharging pus. Often these become hard and insensitive and change position when touched. Before long pain takes hold in the head, shoulders, arms, hands, thighs, legs and feet. During this phase the sick person thinks that it is his bones that are affected. These pains sometimes get worse with exercise, in humid conditions and in bed when it is hot, and they diminish in the morning ... The third degree of the illness can be recognised by itchy scabs on the skin that appear and disappear in turn. Thereafter, the bones in the nose begin to rot, as do the palate, teeth and gums; then lumps appear on the head, the clavicles, on the leg bones, on the arms and on the fingers. Then, ulcers form all over the body which subsequently disappear, then reappear. Finally, chest pains, difficulty in breathing, cough, loss of appetite, hair loss, blindness, loss of hearing and of smell are the symptomatic precursors to death.[10]

From this description, it is clear that each stage of St Paul's Bay disease could be measured according to its effects on the skin of its victims. According to most observers, the disease was chronic and debilitating, but did not result in an especially high mortality rate. This further accentuated the visual implications of the disease, as its sufferers exhibited symptoms over a long period of time.

Because most medical practitioners agreed that St Paul's Bay disease was a form of syphilis, their recommendations for its eradication were likewise unanimous at a general level. The best form of treatment, they concurred, was mercury-based medicine. Mercury was one of the oldest treatments used in regular medicine, and it was considered effective against syphilis as early as the 1500s. Yet as Jay Cassel points out, it is not clear that mercury had a curative effect, because the 'sores and eruptions' of the skin caused by syphilis and related treponematoses 'cleared up' whether mercury was administered or not. Further-more, if it was in fact syphilis, mercury would have had an indeterminate effect on the disease-causing organism. Mercury was a punishing form of therapy. As Cassel notes, depending on how it was administered, mercury led to various 'skin disorders ... disorders of the digestive system – inflammation of the stomach and the intestines accompanied by nausea and vomiting, diarrhoea, abdominal cramps, and heavy salivation'.[11] Mercury treatment itself thus likely added to the litany of skin (and other) problems suffered by patients. These negative consequences of mercury therapy led to 'a bewildering diversity of preparations' in efforts to enhance its performance and mask its effects, and this diversity was reflected in the debates about which mercury compound was the best for this particular disease.[12]

There were two overlapping phases to the state's response to St Paul's Bay disease.[13] The first involved the use of military surgeons and assistant surgeons to treat the disease. This was the logical extension of extensive military activity in the colony; it was the likeliest source of orthodox practitioners in Quebec between 1775 and 1783, and it reflected the centralizing governing tenden-cies of colonial governors Guy Carleton and Frederick Haldimand. Beginning with John Stephen Dan in 1775, and after his death with William Menzie and Philippe-Louis-Francois Badelart, Governor Guy Carleton ordered these surgeons to treat St Paul's Bay disease in the area of St Paul's Bay and in other Quebec parishes. Other military surgeons and doctors involved during this period included Dr Hugh Alexander Kennedy and surgeons Francois Suzor, Charles Blake and Robert Jones.

By 1783 there was growing concern among Montreal's medical elite that the disease was becoming an epidemic that the medico-military measures of Carle-ton and Haldimand were unable to control. Haldimand responded by issuing a call through the bishop of Quebec, Jean-Olivier Briand, to local parish priests to make a list of the numbers of infected persons in each parish, so that they might be treated. However, by the spring of 1784 Haldimand considered that the number of patients sick with St Paul's Bay disease was less than had been previously thought.

When Governor Henry Hamilton replaced Haldimand in 1784, a second phase in the official response to St Paul's Bay disease began to unfold. Hamilton issued an order to Dr James Bowman to create a strategy for curing the epi-demic in the most economical way possible. Bowman decided that this should involve a heavy reliance on local parish priests. This was, by 1785, not a new idea, but Bowman's plan was of a scale not previously considered. Beginning in 1785, Bowman took two tours of Quebec. His first was several months long and consisted of a considerable entourage of carriages, buggies, hired help and some medical assistance. He travelled from parish to parish, identifying victims of St Paul's Bay disease and organizing their treatment by local priests. Bowman typically sent individuals ahead of his entourage to the next parish to alert local authorities to identify and prepare patients for treatment. He brought with him a written programme of advice, and treatment guidelines for local priests. He examined patients and tried to determine the scope of the disease in each parish. The priests were instructed to administer the drugs that Bowman made available to them to their afflicted parishioners. Bowman, with the backing of the bishop of Quebec, also ordered priests to make a record of all those infected, their symptoms, whether they were cured as a result of treatment, and other potentially useful observations. During these two tours, Bowman also solicited the help of surgeons to monitor and treat patients in various parishes. The government also ordered all militia captains to assist Bowman on his tour and to identify potential patients.[14] This second initiative, then, consisted of giving extraordinary powers to Dr Bowman to organize the combined energies of military officials, military surgeons, medical doctors and local priests in a concerted response to St Paul's Bay disease.

This convergence of medicine and religious authority made sense for several reasons, in Quebec and elsewhere. First, priests and nuns had longstanding traditions of charitable work with a variety of groups, including the poor, the neglected and the unhealthy.[15] Second, they were by and large a literate group who could become conversant with the rudiments of orthodox medical practice, interact successfully with patients and medical authorities and, when necessary, record the progress of patients. Third, local religious figures were in principle invested with cultural and social authority, thereby increasing the chance of success of the orthodox treatment regimens issued by the state and by organized medicine.

British colonial officials exhorted the bishop of Quebec to make his priests aware of the government's wishes concerning their expected role in the treatment and understanding of the illness. But the importance of the parish priest and of the networks of religious and familial customs of which he formed an essential part long predated the arrival of the British. When the strategy of using the priests as the front line of defence against St Paul's Bay disease was invoked, the colonial state was inserting itself into a set of relationships over which it exerted only partial control. Control over the diagnosis, treatment and understanding of disease was contested and mediated by the negotiations of everyday parish life, just as the power of the local priest was contested at the crossroads of state, religious and customary powers. Evidence that St Paul's Bay disease was causing a serious disturbance can be found in the bishop's circulars, which were sent to instruct local priests about their role in its cure. In his circular, written in 1783, Bishop J. Oliver Briand noted that a:

deadly illness by the name of St Paul's Bay Disease that has devastated this region for many years, continues to do so. It makes greater and greater deplorable progress: there are almost no parishes in this diocese where it has not spread. It is beginning to harm business and social gatherings; it restrains visitors to be inconveniently vigilant; I even know that it has already been harmful to the functions of the Holy Ministry: the administration of the Sacrament of the Eucharist, and even Confession, can become dangerous to the priest.[16]

Two years later Briand's successor, Louis Philippe Mariaucheau d'Esglis, reiterated the point, noting that the disease was 'so dangerous in certain functions of the ministry'.[17] These bishops were acknowledging the major social disruptions that the disease was having at the local level. Ollivier Hubert notes that social regulation in Quebec parishes during this period was dependant on the 'ritual of Sunday Mass' – an event that reinforced the connections between the patriarchal family and the family of God, and also the socio-economic hierarchy of families within the parish itself. Through a process of spatial inclusions and exclusions within the church and in the public sphere, behaviour was 'normalized'. Central to this process was the priest's punishment of sin through the process of confession, and 'a fairly lengthy process of reintegration, with an obligatory period spent standing at the rear of the church'.[18] The withholding of communion performed a similar regulatory function by publicizing the extent of a parishioner's sins. In a social environment held together in great measure by the 'ritual performance' surrounding religious practices at the micro-level, a serious and long-term disruption to key markers of social regulation – mass, communion, confession and the like – such as that effected by a major chronic epidemic like St Paul's Bay disease was indeed great cause for concern.

Further compromising established patterns of sociability was the nature of the disease itself. According to Bishop Briand, 'those attacked by this deadly illness regard it, mistakenly, as dishonourable, and do not dare to declare it, or they don't want to submit to the regime that is prescribed for its cure. His Excellency, aware of this obstacle, believes that there is no better way to defeat this disease then by praying us to enjoin you to enter into their views of charity and humanity. Here is what we prescribe ...'[19] Briand's message merged the concerns of the state and those of the church. Hubert contends that 'the church recognized that honour was fundamental to the standing of families', but that honour was subject to the vagaries of scandal and gossip.[20] Because of its perceived links to illicit intercourse, its disfiguring and debilitating symptoms and its contagious nature, St Paul's Bay disease would have greatly compromised the honour of families unlucky enough to contract it. It also likely had an impact on the numbers of sufferers who elected to identify themselves for treatment.[21] Yet according to the orthodox community of doctors and surgeons in Quebec, effective treatment with mercury and the collection of statistical knowledge required that those living with the disease be put on public notice in the parish. Sufferers would also be required to submit to a prolonged period of treatment supervised by the local priest.[22]

An examination of the surviving correspondence between Bowman and parish priests highlights the preoccupations and concerns they had about their role as gatekeepers and mediators in the response to St Paul's Bay disease. In some cases, priests informed Bowman that the medication he had sent to them had been consumed and that more was needed to complete the course of treatment. At other times, priests identified new cases that were not apparent during Bowman's visit.[23] The correspondence indicates that Bowman responded to these requests by sending more medication.[24] These examples, along with the massive inventory made by Bowman of the medications he sent to various priests, suggest that clergymen were actively involved in patient treatment, that they were concerned about identifying new cases, and that they were prepared to identify which patients were still in need of medication.

A final theme in the correspondence that deserves attention is the extent of gratefulness expressed by several priests for Bowman's good services and the benevolence of the colonial state. At a superficial level, the number of letters that express an exaggerated thankfulness is striking. This can be seen, for example, in the letter of Father Morin from St Anne, who noted that 'the patients of my parish not less sensible to your attentions, than to the generosity of the respectable government ... received great comfort in following your [treatment] regimen'.[25] Perhaps the most effusive vote of approval belonged to Father Lorimier of St Cuthbert, who summarized Bowman's visit as follows:

> I could never express with what sentiments of gratefulness I had the honour of your [last letter]. To be esteemed by a person commendable for such manners was something that will make me overjoyed to deserve until the end of my days.

As complimentary as letters might be, they were likely intended to serve many purposes. First, it is entirely possible that many priests were in fact overjoyed by the attention that Bowman gave to what was in some parishes an intractable medical problem. Moreover, in a colony with about 2,000 British people representing merely 1.6 per cent of the population,[26] Bowman would have appeared interesting and perhaps even exotic to some priests – a representative of British rule worthy of ritualized forms of praise given to any authoritative figure of his ilk. Second, because priests might soon ask Bowman for more medications or advice about treatment, employing the language of deference and gratefulness could never hurt.

But in some letters a more sophisticated form of 'gratefulness' is clearly at play – one that links the specific strategies of fighting St Paul's Bay disease with the subtle relationships linking pastoral, state and episcopal power in the eighteenth-century colony. These links are made by Father St Germain, who, after praising Bowman for his good work, exclaimed:

> but your hand which brings upon us these favours, does not conceal from our view the source from which they derive; these traits of humanity are the production and the natural inclinations of the friendly domination, under which we have the good fortune to live ... and under a government free and generous, we now carry only the chains of public love and of the gratitude to second in the future your beneficent visions ...[27]

Clearly this was no ordinary parish priest. In this expression of appreciation of Bowman's medical interventions, St Germain draws on the complex connections between medical intervention and the powers of English colonial governance. Father St Germain and other priests – who were operating from within the contexts of individual parishes and the Catholic hierarchy – were balancing their wish for the continuation of medical aid for an illness that threatened the stability of local religious and social life, with the need to ingratiate themselves to new colonial masters.

The colonial government's desire to gather statistics to track the disease, and to maintain the efficacy of Bowman's therapy, reflected both the increasing concern about the consequences of this disease and an inclination to respond to it as a problem of colonial governance. In his orders to Bowman, Governor-General Hamilton stressed the importance of quantifying the course and treatment of this disease. He made Bowman responsible for keeping:

> an exact diary of your journey and a correct list of the parishes you shall have visited, with a faithful return of those persons who shall undergo your inspection, distinguishing their age, sex, and condition; stating the progress of each, and procuring (if practicable) a certificate from the respective Curates of the number whose cure shall have been undertaken by you.[28]

To this end, priests were given medical forms to indicate the patient's name and sex, the date at which Bowman's recommended treatment began, the date at which the patient was cured and any additional observations peculiar to the case.

This strategy reflected a period of transition in the medical response to epidemic disease. As Ulrich Tröhler explains, by the end of the eighteenth century, there existed in British medicine an older therapeutics of rational deduction and a newer one of empiricism. The much older tradition of rational deduction – by which 'the rationalist physician explains [the patient's symptomatology] within a framework of pathogenic and pathophysiological theory, whence he deduces, by good argument, his therapy which does not need testing' since it is theoretically based – is evident in the use of mercury as the main course of treatment.[29] The newer method of empirical induction, relying less upon medical theory and more upon 'feedback, based on the assessment of one's own observations',[30] was reflected in the desire to quantify the results of the mercury-based treatment, to see if it actually worked regardless of its theoretical basis. This statistical strategy could also be an early example of an increasingly modern approach to governance – the imposition of order and the expression of power through the acquisition of empirical knowledge.[31] Moreover, collecting data by parish enabled the authorities to sense the geographic spread of the epidemic, allowing them to frame the disease numerically as well as spatially. The plan for curing St Paul's Bay disease thus straddled epistemologies of treatment and social regulation. Gaining control over the visible symptoms of individual patients might entail using an age-old remedy (mercury), but the delivery of this treatment, and its efficacy, would be measured scientifically – the retreat of symptoms from the skin and the speed of recovery could be documented on the medical forms, and the rates of recovery in the population as a whole could be measured by counting them. This was an attempt at a rational approach to safeguard Quebec from the threat of invasion at multiple levels.

The surviving records from this grand initiative allow for a partial epidemiology of St Paul's Bay disease. The numbers affected by this disease can be counted by examining the returns of the parish priests and Bowman's own return of patients. What is immediately evident from the returns is the high incidence among members of the same household. Sometimes priests indicated that entire households were infected. But it was also Bowman's policy to treat all members of a household in which more than one person was infected, as he was certain that the contagious nature of the disease, along with the eating and living customs of rural Quebecers, would lead to the spread of the disease to all household members. This of course makes it very difficult to assess the returns. At the very least it gives some idea of those infected and a better idea of those undergoing treatment. It is also reasonable, given the awful side effects of treatment, to argue that most of those receiving treatment would not have done so unless they were themselves feeling symptoms of the disease, or convinced about its contagious nature.

Just before Bowman and the parish priests made their returns, the census of 1784 was taken of parishes in Quebec. Table 3.1 indicates the percentages of the population affected by St Paul's Bay disease in parishes listed by Bowman, and by parish priests, that could be cross-referenced with the 1784 census. This table suggests that the percentage of parish populations affected could range from an unusually high 39.6 per cent in Berthier, to a negligible 0.73 per cent in Point Claire. Yamaska, St Paul's Bay, Berthier and St Charles sur la Rivière Richilieu all had percentages that were 20 per cent or higher, and there were significant numbers of parishes (eight parishes on this table) with between 10 and 20 per cent of their inhabitants identified as having St Paul's Bay disease. Table 3.1 suggests that this illness would have generated more alarm in some parishes than others, although a thorough spread of St Paul's Bay disease seems to have occurred throughout the population of Quebec.

This epidemiological fragment of St Paul's Bay disease suggests that it was a legitimate cause for concern among medical, military and government officials, as well as local priests and the 'ordinary' inhabitants of the colony. Although there were certainly other worrisome diseases in late eighteenth-century Quebec, most notably smallpox epidemics and various 'fever' outbreaks, the lingering chronic and endemic nature of St Paul's Bay disease, its slowly developing and often grotesquely disfiguring symptoms, and its infectious nature spurred Quebec observers to dwell on its potential consequences at the local and colonial levels. The intrusive and painful treatment strategies of surgeons and doctors no doubt added to the fear surrounding St Paul's Bay disease.

Table 3.1: Percentage of people treated for St Paul's Bay disease in selected parishes.

Parish	Priest/Bowman Return	Parish Population	% Treated
Beloil	214	1188	18.0
Berthier	248	625	39.6
Boucherville	112	1315	8.0
Cap Santé	28	803	3.4
Chambly	161	1881	8.0
Chateau Richie	2	545	0.36
Dechambault	70	698	10.0
Ile Perrault, Les Cedres	26	478	5.4
Isle aux Coudres	9	486	1.8
La Chine	14	678	2.06
La Prairie	55	4659	1.1
Les Eboulements	67	395	16.9
La Petite Rivière	33	185	17.8
Masquinongé	40	457	8.75
Nicolet, La Baie du Fevre	61	760	8.1
Pointe Olivier	89	1150	7.7
Pointe aux Trembles	39	718	5.43
Pointe Claire	7	955	0.073
Pointe du Lac	7	350	2.0
Repentigny	140	854	16.39
Rivière du Loup	133	1364	9.75
Sorel	50	1158	4.3
St Anne	28	329	8.5
St Assomption	83	1340	6.1
St Charles sure la Riv. Richilieu	194	862	22.5
St Charles and St Gervais	217	2301	9.4
St Croix and Lobbiniere	58	961	6.0
St Cuthbert	127	1136	11.1
St Denis	53	981	5.4
St-Ferréol-les-Neiges	7	240	2.9
St Hyacinthe	55	765	7.1
St Joseph and St Francois	90	1021	8.8
St Laurent	17	879	1.9
St Michel	15	284	5.2
St Nicholas	29	553	5.2
St Ours	163	1158	14.0
St Paul's Bay	295	966	30.5
St Philippe and St Constant	234	4659	5.0
St Sulplice	65	628	10.3
St Thomas	193	1373	14.0
St Valier	45	1340	3.3
St Vincent	54	1201	4.4
Terrebonne	55	1066	5.1
Varennes	64	1684	3.8
Vercheres	83	1535	5.4
Yamachiche	64	1449	4.4
Yamaska	228	1011	22.5

This climate of concern coincided with a growing preoccupation among Quebec officials about the future of the colony at a macro level. In fact, in late eighteenth-century Quebec there was a real historical 'conjuncture' that combined concern about the spread of this disease with a fear among colonial authorities about the future of Quebec in an unstable geopolitical context. This interplay of the politics of disease with the politics of colonial rule is logical at a general level when one considers that the first official reports of St Paul's Bay illness appeared just over a decade after the conquest of Quebec by Britain, and that the perceived peak of its spread coincided with Britain's permanent loss of the colonies south of Quebec with the American Revolutionary War. As Britain focused its energies on retaining what remained of its British North American colonial holdings, the peculiarly French nature of Quebec shaped an imperial view of St Paul's Bay disease. Although medical experts largely agreed that this disease was a variant of venereal disease (one possibly brought to Quebec from Britain), by the mid-1780s many began to view it as unique in its characteristics, as growing at an alarming rate and as a real threat to the francophone population of the colony. Apocalyptic language was used in accounts of English doctors and colonial authorities in predicting the consequences of St Paul's Bay disease. For example, in 1782 a grand jury presentment in Montreal noted that this disease threatened 'the ruin and destruction of the rising generation within the province'. In a similar vein in the same year, four Montreal surgeons had this to say about the impact of the disease: 'we are now beholding the last race of Canadians remarkable for bodily make and strength'.[32] Here we can see a proto-social Darwinism that is familiar to those who have studied predictions of racial decline and extinction among African-American slaves[33] and North American First Nations peoples.[34] In these cases, as in Quebec, groupings of people observed to be especially susceptible to disease were regarded by those in authority to be on the verge of extinction, and thus by definition weaker and not entitled to govern.

This mode of reasoning reinforced ideas of racial superiority and further legitimated the power of, in this case, the British ruling authority. Yet as with African slaves and the First Nations, the end of the race was not necessarily in the best interests of imperialism. As the smallpox vaccinations of Plains Indians in nineteenth-century Canada and the efforts of slave owners in the southern colonies in combating malaria show, ruling elites did not view the wholesale loss of imperial subjects as necessarily conducive to their hold on economic and political power.[35] Likewise, in the late eighteenth century, a major threat to the existence of the francophone majority in the colony of Quebec was perceived as a real threat to the maintenance of British authority and control. It is in this context that we see the fashioning of a major state initiative under the auspices of James Bowman in medical statistics gathering, treatment and eradication of the disease.

In Quebec, this racialization of disease, and its links to the politics of colonial rule, can be seen in the writings of prominent medical authorities in the response to St Paul's Bay disease. Bowman wrote about the challenges to his treatment created by the 'prejudice, the persuasion of self interested persons, reluctance to be treated until the last extremity, and the manner of life of the canadians, joined with their ignorance, [which] have thrown in the way many obstacles interrupting complete success'.[36] This 'manner of life', including 'all the family eating, drinking, sleeping, and the male part smoking together', quickly led the disease to afflict 'the whole family'.[37] For Bowman and others, it was the primitive way of life of the French peasants in Quebec, their 'communal living spaces, their sharing of the glass, the pipe', etc., that led to the virulent spread of this disease and to the decline of the French-Canadian race. Their reluctance to embrace the treatments of orthodox medicine (and therefore to acknowledge its authority over their own knowledge and treatment of illness), along with more civilized modes of living, were signs of their inferiority, an inferiority that broadcast itself in horribly disfigured skin.

Such rhetoric could of course be considered more a reflection of prejudices stemming from differences of rank and race, rather than a reflection of the social relations of colonial rule. But in the full articulation of Bowman's sense of his role in the eradication of St Paul's Bay disease, the connections between the response to disease and imperialism become clear. In an appeal to government in 1785, Bowman warned that if he was not properly financially compensated for his work, 'I shall not be able to fulfil my Engagements, I shall lose the public confidence and the further promises of Government through the Channel of circular letters of Bishops will be but little respected among the Priests or the People who being twice disappointed will not be disposed ... to engage in serving so immediately their duty and this country may sink into a wretched state'.[38] With less evident self-interest, surgeon Robert Jones made essentially the same point in suggesting that local priests and seigneurs could be used as conduits for a state response to St Paul's Bay disease. 'By this means', he argued:

> Government will be greatly assisted in their endeavour to extirpate the Disease ... by their mutual endeavours without any great expence, or any extensive professional assistance the Country may yet be recovered from a calamity more destructive than war or famine; the sword even when most fatal, destroys life without the horrors of lingering in pain and poverty, and bounteous nature generally repays a year of famine, with a succeeding one of plenty. But disease renders the poor inhabitant unable to guard against the one or take advantage of the other; by stopping its ruinous career, this province under his auspices who formerly long governed it with honor will again be the most flourishing in the world; and the citizens who perceive, and the peasantry who feel the advantage will bestow additional blessings on the name of [Governor] Carleton.[39]

Both Bowman and Jones make clear links between the successful treatment of St Paul's Bay disease and the maintenance of stability and good order during a period of uncertainty in colonial Quebec. Although Quebec's peasant population was, by some accounts, racially implicated in its own plight by dint of its primitive social mores, this view only made the eradication of an infection that threatened the stability of the colony more of a priority. The threat represented by St Paul's Bay disease led colonial officials and the medical elite to launch an extensive medical response (by the standards of the day) out of concern for the decline of the French-Canadian race, and its consequences –the loss of yet another colony. The emphasis placed on statistics gathering of patients' responses to mercury-based therapy also formed a part of a rational approach to colonial rule – a scientific study of a medical problem plaguing the colony's welfare.

British officials' worries about the effects of the disease on England's hold on power in Quebec were matched by the episcopate's worries about the impact of St Paul's Bay disease on religious control of its parishioners. For Quebec priests, the social regulation of parishioners in the face of many disruptions, including the disruptions of epidemic disease, was more important than how St Paul's Bay disease might affect imperial struggles on the North American continent. Yet, the peculiarities of this disease, and the response of British colonial officials who eventually perceived it as a threat, clearly determined how priests and the Catholic hierarchy negotiated the complex social relationships of colonial Quebec. Although the precise nature of the stigmatizing effects of this illness are hard to tease from existing records, it is clear that a combination of physical debility from St Paul's Bay disease and its unpleasant and obvious effects on the skin were keeping parishioners away from the daily ministrations of the church. This in itself was a crisis worthy of attention from the Catholic hierarchy, which after the conquest of Quebec was the predominant form of French-speaking authority left from the '*ancien regime*'. Yet their efforts to maintain the integrity of traditional parish life (as they saw it) were in turn shaped by the peculiarities of Governor Hamilton's ambitious medical response through the auspices of James Bowman. Its main course of treatment – mercury dosing – further complicated the effects of this disease on patients' skins, while its principle method of delivery and assessment put priests in the unusual position of protecting the skin of the British Empire in Quebec.

4 'ITALIC SCURVY', 'PELLARINA', 'PELLAGRA': MEDICAL REACTIONS TO A NEW DISEASE IN ITALY, 1770–1815

David Gentilcore

Introduction: Padua's San Francesco Grande Hospital, 1789

In 1789, a twenty-five-year-old student doctor at Padua's hospital of San Francesco Grande reported on his first encounter with a new disease:

> I came across it quite by chance in the hospital, having resumed my customary practice of going there, as the real and only source of medical observations. It so happened that one day I was present when a young sick woman was admitted. The attending physician was asking her different questions as usual, to which she replied haltingly, evidently in a daze. I happened to gaze at her hands, and saw that they were of a blackish colour, as was also part of her arms. I proceeded to examine her more carefully, and I noticed that the cuticle there was dried and rough, and that here and there it was starting to peel off, whilst the skin underneath remained white and shiny. In addition, the [woman's] mother related how an extreme weakness, particularly in her legs, had reduced the poor young woman to a state where she was incapable of performing her country labours, and how these complaints had afflicted her the past two years, at the start of the spring season. Pausing to think about the three observed phenomena, that is her dizziness, extreme weakness and especially the morbid alteration of the cuticle, I was immediately reminded of *pellagra*, a disease pervasive in the territory of Milan [Lombardy], and I believed there was a very great similarity to it. The attending physician, seeing me particularly attentive in the examination of this sick woman, told me that for the last few years, but especially this year, similar patients had been coming to the hospital, about whom only general ideas had been reached hitherto.[1]

At the time of his writing, our young doctor Francesco Fanzago (1764–1836) had just returned from two years' training at the hospital in Pavia, at what was Lombardy's university. There he had studied under Johann Peter Frank, the noted German scholar of hygiene and legal medicine and proponent of public health reforms. Fanzago returned to his native Veneto, to Padua where he had taken his degree, full of curiosity and crusading zeal, which he applied to his study of pellagra. His committed and methodical examination of hospital cases and his undogmatic presentation of his findings were also consistent with the approach outlined by the Scottish physician John Gregory, whose work on medical ethics Fanzago had just translated into Italian.[2] From the start Fanzago's concerns were as much social as nosological, and he would spend the next twenty-five years of his life studying and writing about the disease.[3] More than anyone else in the Veneto, he was the physician who put his name to pellagra; not that there weren't other claimants to the title, as we shall see.

Most of Fanzago's 1789 *Memoria* on the subject consists of a description of sixteen pellagra case histories observed in Padua's San Francesco Grande hospital. The hospital setting allowed Fanzago to follow the course of the disease and observe the effects of treatments more systematically and in greater detail than previously, in addition to carrying out autopsies on patients who died there. His observations meant that he was the first to be able to identify *pellarina* ('peeling-off') in the Veneto and *pellagra* ('rough skin') in Lombardy as one and the same disease. As Fanzago puts it, both names were 'derived from the affliction observed in the epidermis' that constitutes one of pellagra's 'most evident signs'. Sunburn triggered something: 'Burns to the epidermis on the parts exposed to the sun', which represented the first stage of the disease, and which 'more than any other symptom serves to remind the physician of the nature of the disease'.[4] As Fanzago points out, in all of his hospital patients the skin eruptions appeared on areas of the body normally uncovered: the back of the hands, the neck and the feet, '[they] having worked in the fields barefoot'.[5] Fanzago never fails to relate the condition of the patients' teeth and gums, as he was convinced of pellagra's close links with scurvy. The second and third stage of the disease were numerous and varied, according to the patient's 'morbid dispositions'.[6]

In this chapter I would like to focus on the exploration of pellagra as a new disease and the character of the medical debates that ensued. If pellagra in Italy can be characterized as a disease of the 'long' nineteenth century, this study will examine its first phase, from 1770 to 1815. There is no specifically medical history of pellagra in Italy.[7] At least as regards the early phase, this chapter will attempt to fill this gap. I propose to explore what we can consider the three phases characterizing the reaction to the 'new' in late eighteenth-century medicine, which will take us from clinical history, through to the nosological 'problem', and end with aetiological polemics. The focus will be on debates over the cutaneous nature of pellagra as a key to investigation and understanding its causation and nosology. The extent to which the different authors considered the disease's skin manifestations to be important will provide the focus. This is far from a history of linear progression, there being as much diversity of opinion in 1815 as there had been forty years earlier. Even when medical investigators had reduced the skin lesions to but a 'stage' of pellagra, by the mid-nineteenth century they continued to haunt the social construction of the disease, to the extent that the somewhat bizarre and confusing medical label 'pellagra *sine* pellagra' had to be coined to refer to those cases where dermatitis was not manifest.

Belluno, 1776

When it came to understanding the 'new' in medicine, Fanzago's 1789 investigations into pellagra typify the clinical history phase, with its emphasis on direct experience over doctrine, observation of hospital patients and detailed description of case histories. Fanzago republished his 1789 investigations into pellagra in 1815, together with all the work he had published on the subject in the intervening years.[8] But the collection began with the first known work on the disease, published in 1776 in the Veneto by Jacopo Odoardi. Fanzago staked a claim for the study of pellagra in the Veneto, beginning with an implicit presentation of himself as the direct heir to Odoardi, offered as a pioneer of the clinical history phase.

The earliest notions of the new disease, even the names given to it, relate to its nature as an affliction of the skin. This is what particularly struck those who first came across it – the peasants of the Veneto, who called it *pellarina*. According to Odoardi, 'first physician' in the town of Belluno, the disease appears first as a roundish mark (*macchia*) on the back of the hands in March or April, accompanied by mild itching. Sufferers say they have been sunburnt. The next year it is worse, itchier, and the skin does not return to its previous colour, but peels off. In addition, in women their already scarce menses stop altogether. During the third and fourth years, the feet and shins suffer like the hands, the skin there peeling off as well; in consecutive years, the scabs on the hands and feet become so large as to resemble the scabs of lepers. The disease can also affect the mouth, Odoardi wrote, causing gums to swell, teeth to blacken and pieces to fall out. Ulcers may appear on the lips and tongue, and the breath becomes smelly.[9] For Odoardi, the new disease was a 'particular kind of scurvy', although it differed in some important details, as we shall see.

Odoardi's accurate and detailed clinical description of the disease, evidently based on direct observation in and around his native Belluno, became the standard, and his work was always referred to by successive investigators. His concerns about the origins, nature (nosology) and cure of the disease would become standard approaches. Debates centred on how to classify it, as reflected in decisions over what to call it. Much depended on whether it was a form of scurvy or leprosy. Odoardi noted that the name first assigned to the disease in the Veneto, 'Alpine scurvy' (*scorbuto alpino*), coined by Giuseppe Antonio Pujati, is something of a misnomer. Odoardi did not object to the adjective 'Alpine', because he was convinced that the disease was a regional one, affecting 'this our wide valley [Belluno] and our Alps'. Odoardi was not entirely happy with the label 'scurvy', however, since scurvy does not affect the brain, unlike pellagra. He nevertheless chose to retain the label because the other symptoms, as well as the cure, were so similar.[10]

For Odoardi, the surface of the body reflected what was happening inside it. Late eighteenth-century medicine had not completely jettisoned its Galenic underpinnings; indeed with physicians like Pujati, and his disciple Odoardi, they were positively re-embraced. If scurvy was then seen (at least by Odoardi) as a kind of food poisoning affecting the blood, caused by a subsistence on floury foods, a peasant diet based largely on unsalted maize polenta, combined with the forced inactivity of the winter months and close living conditions, led to the formation of a 'scorbutic sluggishness' (*lentore scorbutico*) in the blood.[11] Utilizing Pujati's peculiar mixture of humoralism and iatromechanics, Odoardi argued that these factors interfered with the process of 'insensible transpiration'. The resulting blockage in the blood then manifested itself the following spring, with marks on the backs of the hands 'that announce the start of the disease'.[12] Through hard labour in the fields, sweating and a diet rich in seasonal fruits, 'the perverted humours are spent' during the summer months and the marks disappear. However, scabs and eruptions form on the skin in successive years, like those of lepers. This happened due to 'the gradually increasing acrimony of the scorbutic sluggishness' stagnating and corroding in the blood, which 'eventually breaks down the links with the epidermis, more or less causing the skin to become detached and lift it off, like lepers' scabs'.[13] Later, because of the different specific gravity of the mouth related to the hands and feet, it settles in the vessels of the mouth and affects the gums.

Padua, 1792

In addition to republishing his 1789 *Memoria* and Odoardi's pioneering 1776 study, Fanzago also included a more extensive essay, the *Paralleli* (1792). Here, he compared pellagra to other known diseases.[14] The self-congratulatory element came in the form of letters of encouragement from two doctors, Fanzago's mentor, Johann Peter Frank, and a physician investigating pellagra, Giovanni Videmar. Because both were active in Milan, not the Veneto, they posed no threat to Fanzago, and indeed seemed to sound an objective note of praise.[15] With this publication, Fanzago took the social construction of pellagra in the Veneto into a new phase, the nosological, where the concerns of classification shaped investigation and debate.[16]

Fanzago took the opportunity to elaborate on his assertion that pellagra was a new disease, since the few previous authors on the subject, such as the Milanese doctors Francesco Frapolli and Gaetano Strambio, had not gone so far.[17] Its novelty seemed evident, because only in recent years had it made itself felt and caused significant harm. We lack sufficient information to make a judgement on its existence earlier; but if it did, it is strange that no one refers to it.[18] If it is new, how to approach and investigate novelty? It is a nosological question: Fanzago defers to (the ancient Roman doctor) Celsus that when an unknown disease is first encountered it should be reduced to a disease already known and described. This presents the medical author with a paradox, Fanzago writes: if a new disease neatly fits in with one that is known, then it is hardly worth writing about, but if it exhibits specific characteristics, then it will be hard to match it to a pre-existing illness.[19] And to which pre-existing illness should pellagra be compared? There are different opinions, from scurvy to leprosy, from hypochondria to a 'distinct illness'.

The question is a serious one, Fanzago argues, for our answer will determine the kind of cure most appropriate. If pellagra is a form of scurvy, then 'it will be necessary to choose those antiscorbutic medicines which can be best adapted to the specific degeneration of the humours'; if pellagra is leprosy, then we must treat it as a disease of the skin, 'as the most obstinate and essential symptom'; if hypochondria, then we have to treat 'the system of the nerves'; and if we consider it to be 'a disease of a distinct type, then the measures we take must be likewise distinctive'.[20] The problem is that every investigator sees something different when looking at the description of a disease.[21] This is particularly true of pellagra, with its diversity of symptoms. Fanzago's solution is to explore each of the parallels in turn, comparing how closely the analogy fits, so that each reader 'will be able to discover the truth for himself and reach a candid and impartial judgement'.[22] The fact that Fanzago stresses the discontinuities between the three different parallels over the similarities leaves us in little doubt as to where his sympathies lie – that is, with the distinctiveness of pellagra.

The first and longest discussion is the 'parallel' between pellagra and scurvy. As Fanzago notes, for some investigators the two seemed one and the same, to the extent that they considered it a mistake to see a difference. For Odoardi there was a resemblance but not a complete one, which is why he added the adjective 'Alpino' to the noun 'scorbuto'. However, 'Alpine scurvy' is a misnomer for Fanzago, since the disease strikes both upland and lowland inhabitants. And even Odoardi was struck by the differences between scurvy and this new form, such as the unique series of 'metamorphoses or successions'.[23] The attraction of scurvy as a possibility lay in its open-endedness: despite the many recent English studies into the disease, there were many different 'kinds' of scurvy and resulting confusion and contradictions about its causes.

More specifically, pellagra seems to have many symptoms in common with scurvy, first of all its effects on the skin; but although similar, those of pellagra are actually quite different in appearance and distinct in the seasonal nature of their occurence, Fanzago notes. Moreover, in pellagra the sun's rays appear to exacerbate the problem, whereas they have no effect in scurvy. When it comes to the teeth and gums, affected in both, these turn out to be primary symptoms in scurvy, inseparable from it, but 'secondary or non-essential symptoms' in pellagra.[24] Furthermore, pellagra goes on to affect the nervous system and the brain, which is not the case in scurvy. At most scurvy leads to languor, sadness and despondency, as in any long-lasting illness. The madness associated with pellagra is quite different, as Fanzago had observed first-hand:

> The sight of those miserable wretches when they are overcome by madness truly
> moves one to pity. They mostly flee from their domestic abodes; they seek out solitary
> places; they eat earth, grass, and every kind of refuse; they scream, sing and when they
> are taken by fury they threateningly shout abuse at passersby; and they often try to
> throw themselves into water when they can and drown themselves in it.[25]

Other, intermediate symptoms are shared by both scurvy and pellagra: diarrhoea, dysentery, consumption, dropsy, paralysis and contractions. But these
are common to many diseases caused by a 'prevailing acrimony', such as syphilis,
scrofula and gout. Whereas scurvy is amenable to treatment, provided the correct remedies are administered, these same medicines appear to have little or no
effect in treating pellagra. Fanzago gives the example of lemons.[26] The final point
against making too close a parallel between pellagra and scurvy is that none of
the 'Milanese authors' (meaning Frapolli and Strambio) mention it. Rather they
point to pellagra's distinct nature, the fact that it 'observes a periodic order, following the cycle of the seasons; affects women much more than men; is based
more prevalently amongst country inhabitants, although on some rare occasions
striking city dwellers'.[27] The Milanese get the last word.

Fanzago dedicates another substantial discussion to the second parallel, that
between pellagra and leprosy (elephantiasis). Leprosy is classed amongst the
'cutaneous diseases' and, more broadly, amongst the 'affections' that 'concern the
exterior surface of the body', to the extent that it actually resides in the skin.[28]
In pellagra, however, the skin is only affected periodically: 'the skin affliction
appears, goes away, comes back and then disappears altogether'.[29] Moreover, in
its later stages the effects of leprosy are absolutely horrendous, whereas at the latter stages of pellagra the skin is unblemished.[30] Fanzago noted that fortunately,
at least, pellagra would not appear to be 'spread by contagion', unlike leprosy,
which had been seen to be so from the time of the ancients.[31]

Thus when it came to 'their characteristic signs' the differences between
pellagra and leprosy outweighed the similarities.[32] What about causation? Temperament and environment do not seem to be factors in pellagra, unlike leprosy,
which is closely associated with damp conditions and urban settings. Poor diet,
however, would seem to be a factor behind both diseases. Increased poverty,
with its deleterious effects on 'healthy and strict nutrition', has to be acknowledged as the main 'remote' or indirect cause of pellagra.[33] Fanzago suggests that
in this pellagra is similar to leprosy, also a disease of poverty – although the same
could be said of many other diseases, as famine routinely showed.

The main limitation in identifying pellagra with leprosy is that the latter is
a disease of the past, at least in Italy. Some physicians made the same mistake
with syphilis when it first appeared (in the late fifteenth century): 'not being
accustomed to thinking or reasoning beyond the confines established for them
by the ancients, [they] sought to demonstrate that syphilis had very ancient

origins, and they confused it with many other diseases as a result, especially leprosy'.[34] But Fanzago notes that the most striking and convincing argument for diversity of leprosy and pellagra lies in their treatments. When it came to leprosy, ancient physicians recommended frequent and abundant bloodletting, drastic purges (using hellebore, colocynthus or scamony), scarification, unguents and medicated baths – if one can call a bath in a mixture of sulphur, nitro and alum 'medicated'! For pellagra, however, bloodletting and purges are positively harmful, and because the skin affection goes away by itself, no scarification or corrosive plasters are necessary.[35]

Fanzago's third 'parallel', that between pellagra and hypochondria (hypochondriasis), means a departure from considering pellagra as 'a simple skin affliction' and seeing it instead as 'an affliction mainly of the nervous system'.[36] However, the 'highly-strung feeling' and 'frailty and sensitivity' of hypochondriacs bears little resemblance to the insanity of pellagrins, not to mention the fact that most hypochondriacs are 'well-off and well-nourished men', whereas it is precisely 'abundant and nutritious food' that turns out to be an 'excellent remedy' for pellagra.[37] If centuries have passed and we still do not know the exact nature of *acrimonia* like syphilis, gout and scrophula, we are fortunate in having identified the causes and symptoms of pellagra, as well as its treatment. At the same time, Fanzago was quite aware that implementing this cure was far from easy: the peasants (especially the hired farm hands) had no choice but to work hard, were conservative in their habits and had little regard for their health, 'taking a thousand times more care over the health of their animals than their own'.[38]

Padua and Treviso, 1809–10

Diet was a central concern in Fanzago's next major foray into pellagra, a lengthy paper delivered before Padua's Academy of Sciences, Letters and Arts in 1807 and published two years later.[39] By this time Fanzago had been professor of practical medicine at the University of Padua and, following university reforms, was now professor of both pathology and legal medicine there. Fanzago's paper focused on pellagra's causes and would attract the ire of another illustrious physician active in the Veneto, Giambattista Marzari (1755–1827). It also takes us into the final phase of early explorations of pellagra, the aetiological, where questions about causation predominated. Pellagra's aetiology would prove even more controversial than its nosology.

The two men had much in common. Marzari, nine years older than Fanzago, had, like the latter, taken his degree at Padua, and had gone on to become professor of physic and eventually regent of Treviso's Real Liceo, later the Ateneo (founded by Napoleon in 1810). Like Fanzago, Marzari was also a medical author, having written a treatise refuting the 'medical system' of the Scottish physician John Brown, with its notion of 'excitability' (a basic quality present in living matter) and the need to balance this with outside stimulation in order to maintain health.[40] Marzari's reforming zeal found expression in Treviso's first newspaper, *Il Monitor di Treviso*, which he founded in 1807, and in his own medical practice, 'assisting the sick poor free of charge'. 'When he [Marzari] went to visit the sick', the physician Jacopo Pellizzari would write years later, 'by means of his cheerful disposition, his plain speaking and his suitable treatments he [Marzari] provided comfort and succour to those suffering families'. For Pellizzari, this included pellagra sufferers, cured as a result of Marzari's contribution to understanding the disease's causes.[41] Marzari published his 'medico-political essay' on pellagra in 1810, as well as two other works on the subject several years later.[42] Marzari's 1810 *Saggio* would later be described as a 'learned and philanthropic work' by the German physician and botanist Kurt Sprengel, which is an accurate characterization, as we shall see. But Sprengel's real praise would be for Fanzago, whose 1809 *Memoria* is described as 'the best work that has happened to come out so far on this subject'.[43]

Despite their geographical proximity, shared reforming outlook, approaches to medical investigation, and – as we shall see – conclusions, the close contemporaries Marzari and Fanzago are conspicuous in their absence from one another's works. In fact what we have is a classic priority dispute, only the first of a series in the small field of what would become known as Italian pellagrology.

Accordingly, Marzari went to great lengths to antedate his 1810 *Saggio*. He stated that he had first been requested to write it by the Austrian government in 1805, based on ideas he expressed in a pro-memoria sent to several Parisian doctors in 1804; and he reproduced his 1806 dedication to Eugène Napoleon, by this time viceroy of the kingdom of Italy (on behalf of his stepfather, Napoleon Bonaparte), and his original preface. And in the conclusion to his *Saggio* one hundred pages later, Marzari devoted ten pages to a refutation of Fanzago's ideas, despite not having much to refute, since the two works are much alike in both structure and content. Here Marzari claimed to have written his *Saggio* a year before Fanzago presented his 1807 paper, although unidentified 'unforeseeable circumstances' had prevented Marzari from publishing it until 1810. His newspaper explained his absence with reference to an unnamed 'illness'. (In fact Marzari had been arrested by the Napoleonic government for comments made in the December 1807 issues of *Il Monitor*.) Mazari thus exclaimed, 'I think that for these reasons I can maintain *a priority right* on this aspect of the pathological doctrine [of pellagra]'.[44]

Fanzago did not let this go unanswered. In his 1815 re-edition of all of his own pellagra studies, Fanzago affirmed that his earlier publication date (1807) gave him evident priority over Marzari, not to mention that he had been lecturing on the subject since 1803 from his chair in practical medicine, a fact to which his many students from Treviso, Marzari's hometown, could testify. In any case

Fanzago did not wish readers to think that their points of view were identical, given that what for Fanzago was an explanation 'put forth with a few reservations', for Marzari was doctrine.[45] Having made his point, Fanzago attempted to occupy the moral, and medical, high ground: 'I willingly grant all the priority rights to Mr Marzari, desiring only that my opinion ... be examined and discussed impartially for the consequences of public usefulness that might result'.[46]

What 'doctrine' was the source of dispute between the two medics? Let us begin with what they disagreed on. These areas turn out to be minor points. Fanzago was quite satisfied with the now well-established term 'pellagra', whilst Marzari would have preferred to go on using Pujati's label of 'Italic scurvy' (*scorbuto italico*), given that pellagra was not only a disease of the skin and worse symptoms followed, as in scurvy. Whilst Fanzago discounted the parallel between pellagra and scurvy, Marzari was happy to see pellagra as one of a category of diseases labelled scurvy.[47] The problem with using 'pellagra' to designate the illness, according to Marzari, was that 'the skin affliction that is expressed in that word, and that is the standard and sometimes only symptom appearing in the first stage, either does not appear in the second [stage] or, if it does, does not form an observable element of the morbid state'.[48]

They also disagreed on the number of pellagra's stages. Whilst both concurred that the symptoms and manifestations of the disease could vary widely from sufferer to sufferer, Marzari believed that this variety was a reflection of individual temperament, sex and age, as well as climate. Climate was important for Fanzago too, but none of the other factors were.[49] Fanzago also still thought the sun might act as a trigger on the 'cutaneous organ' of people with a certain predisposition, causing what was popularly known as *salso* on exposed areas. By contrast Marzari excluded the sun as a factor, noting the 'infinity of people' who are more exposed to it than peasants but who never get pellagra, and the pellagrins who begin to suffer as a result of nothing more than the warmth of spring.[50]

Turning to what Fanzago and Marzari agreed on, both authors discounted environmental factors like air or water, given that the disease affected only certain people within given areas. They agreed that pellagra was a disease of the countryside, but one that was limited to the poor peasantry. As an indication of the state of knowledge about pellagra at the end of the first decade of the nineteenth century, they agreed that it was less than fifty years old; that it started as seasonal; that it progressed by degree; that it was not hereditary, contagious or transmissible by touch; that there were more women pellagrins than men; and that given its cause, further investigations would turn up cases in other parts of Italy and Europe. And, above all, they both believed they had pinpointed the disease's cause, which lay in the diet of the affected peasants. Marzari was adamant that their maize diet 'constitutes the true and certain cause of pellagra', whereas Fanzago was slightly more circumspect. But it was a difference of degree and approach.[51]

Fanzago and Marzari both noted how the diet of peasants in the Veneto had changed during the previous century, a result of the worsening of economic conditions and the introduction of maize.[52] They identified poverty as the predisposing or indirect cause, the direct cause being a maize-based diet, consumed in the form of polenta. Fanzago and Marzari were also of like mind when it came to prevention. If a maize-based diet is the cause, in particular during winter months when little else is available, then prevention is simple: better food. A publicity campaign would be necessary in order to spread the message. Marzari proposed a 'work of popular education, written by order of the government by an author who is both well known and well versed in this subject, and who, with clarity and vigour, knows how to make himself understood everywhere, right down to the most rustic of huts'.[53] Who could Marzari possibly have had in mind? After all, only he had the journalistic panache required. It must have piqued him that this honour would eventually go to Fanzago, who published his *Istruzione catechistica sulla pellagra* in 1816 at the government's behest – and with the same printer Marzari used.[54]

But to return to their duelling essays, Fanzago diverged from Marzari in his conclusion, with a discussion of the physiological causes of pellagra. For Fanzago, what happened on the surface of the body was a manifestation of what was happening inside. It was all about chyle, the fluid formed in the intestines, the quality and quantity of which varied with the foods ingested and which was necessary for the production of healthy blood. The cause of pellagra 'resides primarily in the lower gut and consists in the reduced and depressed excitement of the guts specifically dedicated to the two most important functions of digestion and chylification'.[55] This problem of the lower gut then manifested itself in pellagra's three classes of symptoms: skin burns, bodily weakness and impairment of reason. In terms of the particular link between digestion and the skin, Fanzago cited the old adage: '*mal di pelle, salute di budelle*' (which, to keep the rhyme, could be translated as 'disease of the skin, treat the intestine'). Many diseases of the skin can be cured by treating the lower gut, something 'so clear and evident that it would be useless to want to demonstrate and illustrate it with examples'.[56] And this link is doubtless true when it comes to pellagra: 'when the cutaneous affliction begins, it must be held for certain that the abdominal disorder is already pre-existent, and it is precisely from this disorder that the cutaneous phenomenon consensually originates'.[57] The same disorder of the lower gut likewise affects both the body (leading to weakness) and the brain (leading to insanity).

In his attempt to claim the maize theory for his own, Marzari responded to Fanzago's notions about the gut in an additional section which Marzari claimed to have written in 1810. Just because Fanzago mentioned the external and true cause of pellagra – that is, maize – in the first part of his paper, it did not give him priority rights over the pathological doctrine in all its particulars, Marzari asserted.

Moreover, Fanzago deduced the direct cause of pellagra – the 'reduced excitement of the ventricle' – from a false and arbitrary principle. And finally, Fanzago's explanation of pellagra's 'pathognomonic signs' (distinguishing symptoms) was derived from a hypothetical and improbable principle that cannot be convincing.[58]

Marzari accused Fanzago of 'sophistic arguments', but his are no less so. This is evident in Marzari's own self-proclaimed 'new theory' to account for how pellagra develops in the body, based on three 'principles'. First of all, the blood of pellagrins abounds in those principles contained in vegetable foods, especially *carbonio* (carbon); second, their blood lacks the sufficient 'fibrous substance' necessary to sustain bodily movement; and third, the excess of carbon, which is 'naturally both stimulating and fleeting', exits through the skin, especially where it is exposed to the sun.[59] Together these 'principles' explain the weakness, delirium and skin inflammation experienced by pellagrins. Placing his theory against Fanzago's, Marzari triumphantly concluded: 'Now with a theory this simple, that does not make up either substances or forces, nor defends itself by means of ambiguous words and hazy ideas, all the pellagrous phenomena receive a satisfactory explanation, and the questions hitherto put forward and considered unanswerable by physicians are now happily resolved'.[60]

Conclusion: Florence, 1814

Despite their animosity, Fanzago and Marzari were on the right track, although it would be another hundred years before the solution to pellagra's aetiological puzzle began at last to emerge. In the meantime, physicians continued to investigate and write about the subject as if they were among the very first to do so. The medical representatives of every Italian state had to re-invent the wheel. Thus the first Tuscan to write about pellagra, the Florentine physician Vincenzo Chiarugi in 1814, went through all the same phases – clinical histories, nosology, aetiology – represented by the three investigators surveyed above, Odoardi, Fanzago and Marzari. Chiarugi reformulates the same arguments and evidence as previous authors in his attempt to account for, classify, identify causation, and propose cure and prevention. He devotes a long section to positing a maize-based diet as the most likely cause, evidently unaware that both Fanzago and Marzari had done so, and more convincingly, just a few years earlier.[61]

Chiarugi (1759–1820) was a contemporary of Fanzago and Marzari, although all his academic formation and medical experience was within the Tuscan grand duchy. Two features are new and specific in Chiarugi's pellagra essay. The first is the focus on Tuscany, as the disease spread southwards with the spread of maize cultivation and consumption. Second, Chiarugi devotes more space to the cutaneous symptoms of pellagra than any other author before him. This would seem strange, since by Chiarugi's time the skin rash and desquamation associated with pellagra was seen by all observers as but the primary stage of the disease. Chiarugi's interest in the surface aspect of pellagra is easily explained, for he was the author of an early treatise on skin diseases, based on cases he had observed whilst director of Florence's Bonifazio hospital, a purpose-built asylum for the insane.[62] Moreover, Chiarugi has earned himself the title of the 'first professor of skin diseases' amongst historians of dermatology because of his appointment to teach the subject at Santa Maria Nuova hospital in 1802 (although without stipend until 1805).[63] His stature in the history of psychiatry is just as renowned, being an early proponent of the systematic study of mental illness and the humane treatment of sufferers, both of which he endeavoured to put into practice at the Bonifazio hospital. Given his expertise in both areas, diseases of the skin and diseases of the mind, it is strange that he did little to connect the two when he came to write about pellagra, focusing almost exclusively on the former.

It is in the context of the Bonifazio hospital, as well as his public health role as 'medico delle epidemie', that Chiarugi comes across numerous cases of pellagra in the Mugello region north of Florence. Chiarugi gives detailed descriptions of the skin rash and desquamation that appear in the early stages of the disease, accompanied by illustrations; he is the first to do so in some forty years of study of the subject. Not only is this the result of an ongoing interest on Chiarugi's part in diseases of the skin, it is also to allow his fellow Tuscan physicians to be better able to diagnose the disease and distinguish it from other apparently similar 'cutaneous diseases'.[64] He remembers a case twenty years earlier, in 1794, of an insane man who had peeling skin, which Chiarugi did not then recognize as pellagra. And sure enough, pellagra had no place in Chiarugi's two earlier works on mental illnesses and skin diseases, published in 1793–4 and 1799, respectively.[65] By 1814 Tuscan doctors needed to be made aware of it, especially since they too often did not consider pellagra's skin symptoms worthy of much attention. The disease is not reported to doctors at the skin stage because sufferers can still work; and many physicians would not be able to recognize its true nature in any case.[66] And yet when it comes to classifying pellagra, the skin symptoms are the most characteristic and fundamental elements of the disease, according to Chiarugi.[67] His representation of pellagra as essentially cutaneous may appear to take us back to the earliest reactions to it, as reflected in its very name, but it does so by taking investigations and observations to an entirely new level of detail.

Chiarugi devotes a tenth of his pellagra study to a detailed and vivid discussion of the skin rashes: their appearance, nature and location, the periodic desquamation and reappearance, and how they can vary over the often very long course of the disease.[68] The rash can even disappear entirely for several years: 'So pellagra, right from the very start of its invasion, undermines [the body] with a hidden and deceptive progression, leading towards its destruction'.[69] Chiarugi's descriptions are accompanied by frequent references to the plates at the back of the book, which illustrate different phases of desquamation on the hands, feet and chest. His focus on the cutaneous aspects is also the reason for his lengthy discussion of the role of the sun's rays and heat in triggering the disease in predisposed individuals.[70] And it is the reason why his discussion of treatments and cures deals so much with medicated baths and skin rubs, before he finally turns to the importance of improved regimen.[71]

Chiarugi's lengthy discussion of pellagra's nosology and his comparisons between pellagra and other diseases remind us of the extent to which pellagra was still up for debate, despite the many previous studies. When it comes to classification, Chiarugi follows William Cullen's scheme: he opts for the 'cachexia' class of diseases (weakness and deterioration of the body, without accompanying fever), of the order of impetigo (which chiefly deform the skin and exterior of the body).[72] Chiarugi puts the emphasis on the exterior signs of the disease because they were enough to diagnose pellagra, whereas the gastric and nervous symptoms could easily be confused with other forms of illness. Most other investigators into pellagra, including Fanzago and Marzari, had reversed the emphasis, devoting more attention and placing more (or at least equal) importance on the gastric and nervous symptoms, which after all ran the gamut from diarrhoea and dizziness to dementia. Chiarugi's solution to the pellagra problem, his 'big idea' that concludes the book, is that the authorities encourage landowners and peasants to plant white maize instead of yellow.[73] His proposal was not taken up (it would not have made any difference anyway), nor was his theory that the key to understanding pellagra lay in the skin. Nevertheless studies and proposals like Chiarugi's serve as a sign that the disease was being taken seriously, in all its social and economic implications, even whilst its classification and causation remained matters for dispute. By the early nineteenth century Italian investigators largely agreed on the clinical picture of pellagra, even whilst they continued to debate its nosology, which was much more problematic. As for its aetiology, this would prove the most difficult, continuing to preoccupy what would become the field of pellagrology well into the twentieth century.

5 THE MORAL BIOLOGY OF 'THE ITCH' IN EIGHTEENTH-CENTURY BRITAIN

Kevin Siena

Historians of eighteenth-century institutions, whether jails, workhouses, orphanages or hospitals, are familiar with a disease vaguely termed 'the itch'. Infirmary reports for the workhouse in St Margaret's Westminster identify it as the second most common ailment,[1] while prison records occasionally went further; in 1782 three-quarters of the female patients in Clerkenwell Bridewell's infirmary had it.[2] Hospitals typically refused sufferers for fear of epidemics in the wards.[3] The itch was omnipresent, nagging, disfiguring and heavily moralized, yet few scholars have analysed it.[4]

Debate about what caused the itch colours both its history and historiography. Indeed, the records suggest significant diagnostic confusion. Doctors trying to make sense of it often linked it to diseases like leprosy and the pox, with two important results. Firstly, this enhanced the range of terms and ideas associated with the disease and complicated its interpretation. Secondly, this magnified the opinion that the itch was odious. Since at least the time of medieval leprosy, unsightly skin infections were read to evidence moral failure, a belief still robust in eighteenth-century Britain. The itch thus became a multi-barbed rhetorical weapon put to a range of nasty uses. Moreover, doctors lent credence to some of the period's distasteful prejudices. Although they debated much, physicians discussing the itch agreed that identifiable elements of British society generated it, suggesting physiological distinctions for classes and nations.

To historians of dermatology, the itch was scabies, the infection caused by the parasite *Sarcoptes scabiei*. Medical dictionaries show that the term 'scabies' was used during the Enlightenment: '*Scabies*, a scab, is used sometimes for the itch, and such like cutaneous eruptions'.[5] Nevertheless, identifying the itch as scabies risks anachronism. Cultural historians caution against applying modern diagnostic terms to diseases predating the bacteriological revolution.[6] For example, the 'French disease' was not merely syphilis, but rather referenced a collection of conditions we now separate.[7] Equating the two prevents scholars from understanding pre-modern medical systems according to their own terms.

However, the itch unsettles these critiques. Whigs can make a strong stand on its history. Advances in microscopy produced a radically new – and to the modern eye, surprisingly accurate – vision of the disease. In 1687 microscopist Giovanni Cosimo Bonomo reported tiny animals in itch sores.[8] His illustrations bear striking resemblance to modern photographs of the scabies mite. The suggestion that a microorganism caused disease was undeniably remarkable in the seventeenth century, and is still hailed as a landmark in medicine's march to modernity.[9] The identification of a parasite similar, if not identical, to our scabies mite should convince cultural historians that in this case the modern diagnostic category can help interpret a past disease. It is hard to imagine that many itch sufferers were not harbouring *Sarcoptes scabieii* or a similar parasite.

However, it is equally hard to imagine they all were. Just as many 'venereal' patients were not syphilitic, the records are too vague to presume that all itch patients had scabies. The definition above reveals the diagnostic confusion surrounding eighteenth-century skin diseases. 'Scabies' denoted the itch, as well as numerous 'like cutaneous eruptions'. Moreover, presenting Bonomo's discovery as a scientific revolution risks oversimplifying its history. For example, Daniele Ghesquier skips too quickly over the eighteenth century in her study of the itch, claiming that Bonomo's breakthrough was 'forgotten' in the eighteenth century and rediscovered in the nineteenth.[10]

It was not forgotten. However, though seemingly impressive, Bonomo's discovery met with mixed reception. Some, like royal physician Richard Mead and most microscopists, endorsed it,[11] while others denied that a so-called 'animalcule' caused the itch. Some physicians argued that tiny animals would not stay confined to certain body parts as the itch often did,[12] while others rejected that mites could reproduce fast enough to account for its rapid spread.[13] Still others criticized treatments that parasitology logically suggested: poisonous ointments to kill the tiny bugs.[14] Rather, the vast majority of British doctors presumed that the disease lay much deeper. When they stressed that treatment must address 'the State of the Blood', they did not ignore Bonomo but rather chose different authorities.[15]

After all, developments other than microscopy were afoot. Notably, the late-Stuart physician Thomas Willis and surgeon Richard Wiseman both described the itch in the emerging language of iatrochemistry, emphasizing its deeper systemic roots. Wiseman identified 'a vicious salt in the blood', while Willis cited 'putrefaction' in the blood.[16] They demonstrate a distinctly pre-modern understanding of the skin as a porous membrane connecting the body to the world rather than closing it off from it. They accepted that the itch could *begin* in the skin, but '[as] the Disease groweth more vigorous, [it] spreads father inward, and infects the whole Mass'.[17] The body cast this putrid matter outwardly, where it was thought to corrode the skin. Topical remedies alone were ineffectual and dangerous because they ignored the root cause and forced back inward precisely what the body expelled.[18] If more than Willis's and Wiseman's authority were needed, Europe's leading physician, Herman Boerhaave, lent his: the Dutch professor's chapter on cutaneous diseases made no mention of animalcules and instead attributed the itch to 'purulent matter' in the blood.[19]

Influenced by these ideas, two English authorities emerged in 1714, when Daniel Turner published *De Morbis Cutaneis*[20] and Thomas Spooner published the first English treatise devoted to the itch.[21] Neither supported Bonomo. For Spooner, the itch arose from a corrosive ferment in the blood.[22] Turner accepted that some diseases might be 'vermicular', but never finding the creatures himself, he remained 'dubious'.[23] Both quoted Willis extensively, showing that his influence far overshadowed Bonomo's in England.[24]

Spooner and Turner reveal how doctors connected the itch to other diseases. Spooner said it encapsulated three successive conditions: the itch, scabies and leprosy. 'The itch' and 'scabies' were thus not synonyms. At first the itch remained confined to particular body parts, especially the hands. If untreated, it became more obstinate and morphed into a worse disease, scabies: '[The] Itch ... in length of time, turns to a foul *Scabies* or *Scabbiness*, of the whole body'.[25] The itch was local, scabies universal.[26] However, scabies could arise as a separate entity: 'Sometimes a Scabbiness happens when the *Itch* has not gone before it'.[27] If left, scabies morphed again:

> from the *Itch* it turns to an universal and nauseous *Scabies*, which many times kills the patients unfortunately troubled with it, and if it does not, turns to a loathsome *Leprosy*.[28]

Boerhaave concurred, suggesting that the itch 'is called a leprous psora when it arises at a very great height'.[29] Turner similarly conflated diseases. He presents psora and scabies (terms that he elsewhere uses synonymously with the itch) as *symptoms* of *Lepra Graecorum*.[30] However, the itch then presented itself as a disease worthy of its own chapter, albeit one that 'nearly border[s] on the Scab or *Lepra*'.[31] Spooner and Turner again drew heavily on Wiseman, who had proclaimed a generation earlier: 'I shall understand by *Lepra* the highest degree of the itch'.[32] In 1781 Bartholomew di Dominiceti, a Chelsea physician specializing in medicinal baths, showed how long these links remained: 'The ITCH and LEPROSY proceeding from the same causes, and the latter being frequently produced from the former, I judge it unnecessary to class them under separate heads'.[33] For many in the eighteenth century, then, the itch represented a mild but worrisome form of leprosy, suggesting that this medieval disease mattered more in the Enlightenment than often assumed.

Doctors also connected the itch to scurvy and the pox. These scourges shared with leprosy two essential characteristics: they had nasty skin lesions and they were morally odious. The second point seems less obvious for scurvy, but it was so frequently discussed in tandem with venereal disease that by the later seventeenth century it had inherited some of the pox's cultural taint.[34] Scurvy was associated with lowly characters, especially the poor and sailors, and often linked to immorality. For example, laziness was commonly cited as a predisposing cause. Thomas Trotter proclaimed of sailors that 'the first scorbutics are skulkers', while physician Lewis Mansey still concurred in 1800 that 'a lazy slothful disposition' caused it.[35] Doctors complained that 'scurvy' became a generic name for almost any skin condition.[36] However, they contributed to that confusion when they referenced different *varieties* of the itch, such as 'scorbutick itch',[37] considered an obstinate form of the disease developed from a common itch that had 'degenerated' in blood harbouring scurvy's remnants – what doctors called a 'scorbutic taint'.[38]

Links with the pox were more pronounced. Not acquired by aerial miasma, both pox and itch spread by contact. Doctors of no less import than Boerhaave, Jean Astruc and John Hunter compared the pox's contagion to the itch. Astruc, for example, did it repeatedly:

> What we have observ'd of the multiplication of the Venereal venom or ferment is common to other poisons or ferments ... So one person, that has got the itch, can give it to a great many more by a very little ichor.[39]

By categorizing the itch and the pox in the same 'Class of Diseases', Boerhaave and others forged powerful links.[40] These were reciprocal, and so theories on the itch resonated back to venereology, as in claims that the pox might be caused by minute bugs.[41] One surgical dissertation proclaimed, 'the causes of the Itch and French pox are much the same; and therefore the diseases are nearly allied'.[42]

More than just similar, they were intimately related. First, doctors warned about the obstinate 'venereal itch' that, like scorbutic itch, evolved in blood harbouring a 'venereal taint'.[43] Dominiceti even suggested that the itch grew out of the pox, giving cause to suspect that itch sufferers recently had that disease or scurvy, or both:

> Like the *lepra*, the *itch* is a foul, contagious disorder, the effect of certain sharp, saline humours, generated by a scorbutic, a *venereal*, or a *scorbutico-venereal* taint, whether hereditary or acquired.[44]

That diseases could merge into new ones was an old idea. For example, syphilis was said to be a hybrid outgrowth of leprosy.[45] Physician Gideon Harvey claimed the pox represented the itch fused with, what else, scurvy: 'the Pox is caused by a commixture of a scabby Itch, and an inveterate Scurvy'.[46]

The itch thus emerged as a venereal disease. Arguing that a woman transmitted the pox to one man, but gonorrhoea to another, Andrew Duncan opined: 'Had she also been subject to the itch, a third might have caught that infection'.[47] Considering that the itch spread by casual encounters like handshakes, it was hard to doubt that 'the contagion of itch, though essentially different from [gonorrhoea and pox], has been communicated with either'.[48] Boerhaave was explicit: 'if a man who is free from the *scabies*, has to do with a woman affected in her private parts (& *vice versa*) he will certainly catch this disorder'.[49] Assumptions about sexual transmission coloured numerous issues. For example, the itch threatened patients' marital and reproductive prospects. Spooner was just one of the doctors who, like Dominiceti above, warned about hereditary infection.[50] Francis Spilsbury lamented the threat the itch posed to prospective suitors, boasting of a patient: 'He ventured upon marriage, and has children, without any appearance of the father's distemper'.[51] Connections with the pox also prompted the use of the same medicines for both. Mercury was second only to sulphur as the most common drug for the itch, and patent medicines for the pox, like the well-known *Lisbon Diet Drink*, were also proscribed.[52]

With so much confusion surrounding the itch – was it its own disease? a symptom, relative, progenitor or effect of another disease? – it is nigh upon hopeless to bring perfect order to such rhetorical chaos. David Gentilcore's and Anne Kveim Lie's chapters reveal similar attempts to link pellagra or the Norwegian radesyge to scurvy and leprosy, suggesting that such diagnostic confusion affected many early skin ailments. Because doctors believed the itch spurred the body to purge foul matter, some asserted that it could *cure* other diseases and even suggested inoculation with it![53] However, two things are clear. Linked to such serious diseases, the itch was a significant health concern. The deaths ascribed to it in the *Bills of Mortality* suggested that it was potentially lethal. Secondly, its connections to such odious ailments as leprosy and the pox gave it an especially lowly place among Enlightenment diseases.

That odium also stemmed from perceptions that it was a disease of the immoral poor. Its omnipresence in prisons and workhouses enhanced this assumption, but medical theory contributed significantly. Doctors did not think all people posed similar risks for the itch. What I have elsewhere called a moral biology – the sense that moral action transformed physiology, with particular importance for disease-risk[54] – functioned in discussions of the itch. Spooner made the crucial point:

> Yet some Persons are much more subject to be infected with it than others; for in many there is a certain aptness to receive Diseases of this kind, and such Persons catch it sooner than others, as Experience demonstrates.[55]

Spooner referenced the medical concept of 'predisposition', a fundamental element of eighteenth-century pathology that has been too rarely explored.[56] Although the humoural system – in which fluid imbalances explained disease – was a relic, Enlightenment doctors held on to one of its core components, the individual constitution. Each body had its own constitution, a factor believed to influence health and personality. Importantly it determined how likely a body generated or fell prey to contagious diseases. Diseases could only take root in bodies prepared, or 'predisposed', to receive infection.[57] Doctors explaining the itch frequently suggested that poverty – its diet, filth and vice – rendered bodies uniquely composed to breed and spread the itch.

Spooner again drew from Willis, who theorized on why the immoral poor generated the disease by stressing the physiological effects of idleness, although it was not the only vice:

> Wherefore, not only they that have been long in prison, but also those who being of a sedentary life, are used to nastiness and sluttishness, do live obnoxious to the above-mentioned maladies; inasmuch as the cutaneous humour being not at all eventilated, is corrupted by mere standing, after the manner of putrefying water.[58]

The apothecary who later quoted this very passage made the subsequent claim to which it pointed: 'as *Nastiness* is a great Source of Infection, so *Cleanliness* is the greatest Preservative; which is the true Reason, why the Poor are most obnoxious to Disasters of this Kind'.[59]

The itch was contagious, but it was not *only* contagious. Doctors believed it could be generated with no external source of infection. London physician John Quincy, whose treatises on plague and pestilential diseases made him an authority on contagion, had this to say:

> [M]any cutaneous Foulnesses that are generally propagated by Infection, do sometimes derive their Origin from a Constitution thus disposed to generate the same Humour within itself, without any Infection; as what is ordinarily called the Itch, which is commonly got by Infection; does yet in some scorbutick Habits arise to the Height of that Distemper, so as to be in a Condition of infecting others, tho' it was generated *de Novo* of it self.[60]

By living in filth, leading lives of sluttishness, laziness or 'intemperance' (usually drinking), eating poorly, living in foul air, or having had a lowly disease like scurvy or the pox and harbouring its 'taint', the bodies of the poor were said to undergo transformations that rendered their constitutions 'disposed to generate' a range of diseases, of which the itch was just one.[61] Physicians like Charles Bissett, for example, repeatedly attributed the itch to the poor, stressing their constitutional predisposition and unique susceptibility to the disease:

> The most obstinate species of the scorbutic itch ... is infectious only with regard to predisposed persons ... families among the vulgar are more susceptible than others of both this and the former species of cutaneous scurvy.[62]

Not only did the poor generate it, but once infected the itch could remain in their system as a longstanding, even permanent feature of their essential fluids. William Salmon cited Sydenham when he warned, '[i]f it gets into the whole habit of the Body, it is very rarely cured', while Christopher Packe cautioned that patients' very 'Blood and Juices are Envenom'd with the *itchy Character*'.[63] Thus bestselling physician William Buchan assured his vast readership that the itch was 'banished from every genteel family in Britain', yet it 'prevails among the poorer sort of peasants in Scotland, and among manufacturers in England'.[64]

Of course the itch threatened to break forth from poor bodies. Domestic servants and wet nurses were the most common vectors accused of transporting disease from impoverished zones to elite ones, fears that Matthew Newsom Kerr and Adrien Minard detect elsewhere in this volume. To physician Lewis Mansey, the threat of 'unsound', 'wanton' or 'drunkard' wet nurses was self-evident:

> It is no wonder, then ... that infants are often affected with ulcers, the itch, scald heads and other cutaneous disorders by nurses whose diet is irregular, or if the nurses are afflicted with the venereal disease, that the children contract the same; or are contaminated with pustules and eruptions, and a thousand other infirmities.[65]

Spooner issued a similar warning almost a century earlier.

> the *Itch* is communicated from one Person, or Family to another, by means of lying in strange beds, by children of different Families playing together; or by Servant Maids or Nurses &c. that have had this loathsome Disease, and come into Families before they are perfectly cured of it.[66]

William Ellis's family health manual told the frightening tale of a servant infecting four separate families, and recommended strip-search examinations of prospective employees.[67] Records from the Middlesex Quarter Sessions suggest that doctors were hardly imagining things: in 1712 the itch forced Elizabeth Halham to petition for poor relief, because 'noe body will take her into Service till she be Cured';[68] while the mid-century petitions of apprentices Joshua Jackson and William Johnston both claim that employers cast them out when they became infected.[69]

Wedded strongly to immorality and poverty, the itch was shameful. As cultural theorists have suggested, the skin was a vital text. Eighteenth-century Britons were neither the first nor last to look to the skin for signs of virtue and to read blemished skin harshly.[70] The itch was never simply disfiguring in a purely aesthetic sense. It was that, of course; the contemporary ideal of beauty was marked by pure expanses of white skin, which the use of powder tried to emulate and conditions like the itch foiled.[71] But the itch struck harder because it raised suspicions about sufferers' character. Skin specialist Robert Dickinson quoted Addison when he said, '[a] good appearance is the best letter of recommendation'. His explanation conveys the harsh assumptions that accompanied skin infections, and connects this point to moral biological claims about immorality that rendered the blood hereditarily putrid:

> [A] face and countenance disfigured by those forbidding appearances are usually con-
> sidered either as the consequences of intemperance, drunkenness, and debauchery in
> ourselves, or of the whole mass of blood and juices being corrupted and contaminated
> from the vices of our ancestors.

Dickinson displayed the emerging modern sense of skin as an organ unto itself when he lamented that such criticism was misplaced, because 'the skin is affected by diseases and disorders peculiar to itself, in which the blood and system remain wholly unaffected'. Nevertheless 'these suspicions ... powerfully operate' on the innocent.[72] He captured the psychological impact thus: 'those afflicted with these unwholesome and forbidden appearances, feel, unhappily, so conscious of the disgusting ideas created in the mind of those with whom they converse'.[73] Case studies suggest that this shame was a class issue. It certainly was in Spilsbury's example of a young noblewoman rendered 'so loathsome that she was ashamed to go abroad and converse with others of her quality'.[74] Satirists' pithy advice probably did not help: 'Such, whose fat hands are itchy in the joynt, / When they discourse, let them not use to point'.[75] One understands why sufferers tried to conceal their infection.

The market responded much as it did for the itch's shameful cousin, the pox.[76] Like the poxed, the itch-stricken 'endeavor to conceal it, make use of any Quack Medicine, or empirical Cure, that are advertised as infallible; and the whole Affair is kept to themselves'.[77] Empirics stressed their treatments were inconspicuous. One even camouflaged his bottles: 'The word ITCH is not mentioned on the Paper that is pasted on the Bottle, that you may set it any where, & use it, without any one's knowing what it is for'.[78] Alternative medicines had potential because the most common treatment was sulphur, usually mixed into an ointment with butter.[79] However, sulphur stank and thereby exposed sufferers. Spooner warned, '[I]t is as natural for People to believe that those who use Brimstone, use it for the *Itch*, as it is for them to believe that those that smell of it, use it'.[80] By contrast Christopher Packe's *Aqua Phagadencia* promised to work 'without the least Danger, Dawb or offensive Smell'.[81]

It is worth testing doctors' claims about shame. After all, some stood to gain by *augmenting* patients' anxiety. Regardless, the shame associated with the itch can be gauged because it was literally proven in a court of law. The decision in *Villers vs Monsley* (1769) was precedent setting for libel and routinely cited in textbooks. Villers sued because Monter wrote a letter calling him an 'itchy old toad' who stank of sulphur.

> Old *Villers*, so strong of brimstone you smell,
> As if not long since you had got out of hell,
> But this damnable smell I no longer can bear,
> Therefore I desire you would come no more here;
> You old stinking, old nasty, old *itchy old toad*,

If you come any more you shall pay for your board,
You'll therefore take this as a warning from me,
And never more enter the doors, while they belong to J.P.[82]

The judges' debate demonstrates just how damning the itch was. Monter's lawyers argued that since the itch could be caught innocently, the accusation 'implies no offence'. The justices obliterated that argument: Chief Justice of the Common Pleas, Sir John Eardly Wilmot, staunchly disagreed, defining libel (for generations, as it turned out) as 'any thing in writing concerning another which renders him ridiculous, or tends to hinder mankind from associating or having intercourse with him'. He saw no material difference between the itch and leprosy. Like a leper, 'No one will eat drink or have intercourse with a person who has the *itch* and stinks of brimstone'. A colleague concurred: 'it is a cruel charge, and renders him both ridiculous and miserable, by being kept out of all company'. Notably the justices considered theories on how the itch was communicated, including the possibility of 'animalcula'. But despite how innocently it might be contracted, the itch led sufferers to be anathematized. As far as the judges were concerned, the itch-stricken were treated quite like lepers.[83]

'Itchy' was thus a powerful insult, charging victims with filth and immorality in ways that parallel 'poxy's' insinuations of sexual deviance. Moreover, like the French disease, the itch could smear entire groups. Seventeenth-century propagandist Marchamont Nedham opted to deride the French as 'itchy' rather than the more common 'poxy', while Tory satirist John Shebbeare aimed his barbs at the Welsh.[84] However, anti-Semitic and anti-Scottish slurs were more common.

Perhaps inevitably the itch's links to leprosy transferred the longstanding anti-Semitic associations of the latter to the former.[85] Demonstrating why early parasitologists should be explored more complexly than they have been, Benjamin Marten supported the position by citing Leviticus to suggest that animalcules infected 'not only the Jews, but their Cloathes, and the very Walls of their Houses'.[86] Turner, who we will remember was dubious of parasites, used similar language.[87] Like the poor, the itch was claimed to be rooted in Jews' constitutions; to make the point, a 1705 edition of Ramazzini presented the itch as natural to Jews, again employing the rhetoric of a lasting taint from a previous disease. Moreover he simultaneously invoked class, noting that the itch was so endemic to Jews that even rich ones had it:

> for there are but few, even of the richer Jews, who have not some Tincture of the Itch; so that this Foulness seems to be a natural Disease, and the Remains of the Elephantiasis which was formerly so familiar to their Nation.[88]

When Harcourt de Longville called Jews 'a leprous, itchy Race', he only added one more link to a chain that stretched for centuries in both directions binding Jews to frightening and loathsome disease.[89] As other chapters argue, predilection for skin disease provided a weighty imaginative tool in early constructions of race.

Far more common were claims about the Scots. If the pox was the French disease, the itch was the Scottish disease. Linda Colley has described English vitriol towards Scots following the Act of Union, and central to xenophobia were fears that Scots moved too aggressively into English society, stealing Englishmen's positions in the economy, government and other areas of public life.[90] Characterizing the attitudes he encountered, Scottish physician James Makttrick Adair proclaimed, 'There is nothing rouses the choler of an *Englishman* so much as the idea that an *itchy lousy* Scot should be preferred to him in any instance'.[91]

Such attitudes can be detected early in the century and in an array of genres, as a 1709 (allegedly) pro-Union pamphleteer demonstrates.

> What if the Scots are troubled with the *Itch* sometimes, why should *we* be afraid on't at a *Distance*? Or if the *Infection* should spread among us, where's the mighty *Harm* on't, when we have *Brimstone* and *Milk* enough in ENGLAND to cure the *Distemper* effectually?[92]

The Scribbler's Club, which included Swift, Pope and Gay, give more biting examples in their 1731 demolition of Scottish newspaper publisher Thomas Gordon. Characterizing Scottish influence in England as a kind of itch, they advocated violent purging:

> Really, I think, that as the Scotch Itch, when it is pamper'd and improv'd to the Heighth in England, generally centers and breaks out in the Cod-piece, there is very great occasion for Whipping, Lashing, Scarifying, Drawing the Testicles, Cupping, Blistering, Bleeding, Purging and Brimstone. To lay, quell and punish, not raise, mount and curry the Scotch unruly Devil.[93]

They later cast Gordon as arrogant: 'no sooner, do ye see, has a *lousy, itchy, hircanian Scot* been fill'd with our *Bread*, but he must immediately be acting like an *English Duke*, with a Pox on him!'[94] They finally come to their overt message to defeat Scots politically:

> And if you don't join with us in voting down these Miscreants and all other venomous Beasts, with all their vile, and wicked surfeiting *Paper-trash*, may *Itch, Scab, Louse, Poverty, Slavery, Oatmealness, and Kirkishness,* and all the *Curses and Plagues of Scotland* alight on your Heads![95]

So heated was one politically inspired rant that it is easy to overlook 'itchy' among the *forty-seven* pejorative adjectives describing some 'Scotch Gentlemen Critics', which included pocky, beggarly, dastardly, malignant, blockheaded, bullying, whoring, farting and stinking, to name a few.[96]

Less overtly political genres employed similar rhetoric.[97] In his burlesque version of the *Odyssey*, Thomas Bridges described a soldier borrowing a blanket from a Scot, with predictable infectious results:

> By th' water-side the men all kept,
> And in their buff-skin doublets slept,
> All but poor me; but here I had,
> Borrow'd an itchy lousy plaid,
> Of a Scotch loon, from whom I bought
> A rare good neckcloth for a groat;
> Those plaids are special things to watch in,
> They keep a man so warm with scratching:[98]

Connecting the itch to the Scots was so common that James Thistlethwaite could compare the Devil's burning smell to that of a Scot undergoing sulphur treatment: 'Besides he smelt as if he'd got / The yuck, and brimstone of a Scot.'[99] As Johnson's dictionary explains, 'Yuck' was a term for the itch (based on the Dutch word for itch 'Jocken'), suggesting the need to re-evaluate of the etymology of 'yuck' to express disgust.[100]

Doctors lent theoretical credence to the idea that the Scots, like Jews and the poor, were inherently itchy. Nicholas Robinson was another physician who connected the itch with leprosy, scurvy and the pox. He invoked the same vices of idleness and filth, employing theories of insufficient perspiration and fluid putridity ('scorbutic humours') to argue that skin diseases were natural to northern peoples:

> I observe, that the Leprosy is a Disease, inseparable to all Countries, Climes and Nations, where the people are very indolent and lazy; and their Children foul and nasty in their Manner of living; for whatsoever will occasion an Obstruction of Perspiration in gross Bodies, abounding with scorbutic Humours, will necessarily generate the itch, the Scab, and very often Leprosy: And for this Reason, we perceive, that the foregoing Affections are very rife in *Westmoreland, Cumberland, Northumberland*, and some Parts of *Scotland*, where the generality of People where their Linen foul for a long Time, and do not shift themselves above once a Week at most: And, by this means, the cutaneous Emunctories are stuffed with a greasy, clammy Sweat, continuously impressed upon the Skin from a foul shirt: And this, I take to be the Reason, why the Northern People, of all others, are so subject to the foregoing cuticular Affections.[101]

Other doctors blamed Scottish diets, heavy in smoked meats and salted fish, for the high incidence of the itch in Scotland.[102] Proponents of northern spas even perpetuated the idea of endemic itch to promote Scottish spring waters as strong medicines.[103] One of the most powerful ways that doctors associated the itch with Scotland was through discussions of a related disease called Sibbens that has connections to both the St Paul's Bay disease and the Norwegian radesyge analysed elsewhere in this volume. Sibbens deserves its own study, but a brief analysis shows how theories about it recycled many of the claims we have already seen and served further to pathologize the Scots.

As with the itch, doctors debated Sibbens's origins. A Scottish theory blamed Cromwell's soldiers – full of pox of course – for laying the seeds of the disease in the 1640s. Some, like surgeon James Hill, thought Sibbens was syphilis, but others, like the Edinburgh medical student he paraphrased, insisted that it was a unique disease endemic to Scotland, a mutant hybrid of pox and itch.

> [T]he sibbens is a mixture of distempers, from a mongrel breed between the venereal animalcula and those of the itch; A *pocky* cock with a *scabbed* hen producing a *yaw* chick.[104]

Regardless, Hill conveys the leper-like treatment that sufferers experienced: 'servants, on this account, have been turned out of their places ... begging that I would procure them rooms to be cured in, being refused admittance by all their relations'. He relates a case of an infected family turned into the street by their landlady.[105]

When Scottish doctors like Buchan or Benjamin Bell addressed Sibbens, they unsurprisingly omitted anti-Scottish slurs. Instead they emphasized poverty, deploying the moral biology of the poor to redirect blame from nation back to class. Bell made the crucial point that Sibbens,

> prevail[s] among the common people, who, from want of cleanliness, frequently labour under the itch; and so much is sibbens confined to this set of people, that, excepting children, who are more particularly exposed to receive infection from servants, those in the higher ranks of life are scarcely ever attacked with it.[106]

Buchan added the points that nurses and servants provided 'almost the only way by which it has found access to families of rank'; that Sibbens was hereditary; and that in some parishes 'above three fourths of the inhabitants were infected'.[107]

Conclusion

The itch was both real and imagined in eighteenth-century Britain. Places like London, bulging with a million inhabitants by 1800, witnessed major health and hygiene problems related to overcrowding. Infectious diseases, including opportunistic infections like scabies, were common and presented major challenges for institutions like workhouses and jails. Yet institutional epidemics only seemed to prove that the itch resulted from moral failure, as paupers' skin was read to broadcast their ethical deficiencies. Importantly, the sense that the itch was a manifestation of depravity also resulted from its connections to the pox and leprosy. These two diseases cast enormous shadows over dermatology in the eighteenth century, begging a chicken-and-egg question: were skin diseases odious thanks to the legacies of the pox and leprosy, or were the pox and leprosy themselves odious because of their horrible skin lesions? Centuries of tradition suggested that outward appearances gave signals about inner qualities. Health, beauty and morality implied one another, as did homeliness, sickness and wickedness, making it hard not to see *any* skin disease in moral terms. Regardless, the idea that the itch was a foul disease of foul people rendered it a powerful rhetorical device put to a range of vicious uses. If Claudia Benthien is correct in noting that blemished skin assumed more powerful psychological and cultural force in the later Enlightenment, then the impact of the itch may have only deepened as time went on.[108] Masking cosmetics that might have once helped cover its sores went out of fashion, yielding to more natural-looking ones born of a new age that was more critical of attempts to conceal the true self.[109] The skin had long been a text, but as the nineteenth century approached, the inner failure suggested by blemished skin may have been more damning than ever. Finally, it is crucial to note physicians' roles in these endeavours; for it was not just satirists or politicians making claims about the itchy poor, itchy Jews or itchy Scots. Physicians supported these claims with scientific theories on why certain groups were predisposed to this disease. If ideal skin was unblemished, it stands to reason that predilection for a skin disease offered an immediately visible, often grotesque, way of arranging taxonomies of difference. In their theories on the itch, doctors presented nation and class as biological categories not unlike gender and race. Over the longer term neither class nor nation retained this essentialism quite as strongly as race and gender would. But in the eighteenth-century classes and nations had physiological distinctions, one of the most important and dangerous of which was predisposition to diseases like the itch. In that way, this largely forgotten skin disease contributed to much larger Enlightenment debates.

6 SYPHILIS, BACKWARDNESS AND INDIGENOUS SKIN LESIONS THROUGH FRENCH PHYSICIANS' EYES IN THE COLONIAL MAGHREB, 1830–1930

Adrien Minard

In 1858 Jules Arnould, a young military physician aged twenty-eight, was appointed to the hospitals of the Algiers division. Ten years after the end of the war of conquest waged by French troops, he was sent to Dellys, a small coastal town in the region of Kabylia, where he was put in charge of the medical services of the Arab Bureau (*Bureau arabe*). This local administrative structure, established throughout Algeria since 1844, was placed under the authority of the army and was composed of an Arab secretary, an interpreter, officers and a doctor. At a time when the French military and teachers faced strong resistance,[1] it was frequently up to doctors to establish contact with the indigenous population and to win their confidence by fulfilling the 'civilizing mission of France' in the medical field. For many young military doctors Algeria appeared not only as a training ground, but also as an enormous field of observation, suitable to further their doctoral thesis or publications, which were more likely to be noticed insofar as they contributed new knowledge of still poorly understood spaces, populations and diseases.[2]

Taking advantage of his eight months of practice in the Dellys hospital, Arnould decided to render an account of his observations of the indigenous patients who came to see him. In 1862 he published his study, which quickly became a sensation within the metropolitan medical field. His study described in detail 'one of the most hideous spectacles that dermatological museums could offer'.[3] They were 'monstrous poxes of which the Middle Ages had left a souvenir – these hideously deformed beings, living ulcers that make even the physician shudder'. He added, 'I never could have thought that the human skin could suffer such ravages'.[4] These lesions, which affected many of the indigenes, were so disturbing that the doctor was embarrassed to deliver his diagnosis. Their form, their colours and their progression unquestionably suggested syphilis, but their dimension, like their sequelae, made them an unusual variety. A 'scientific rarity', declared Arnould, who referred to the similarities with the *pustula* mentioned in the *Vulgate*, so that even as he recognized the syphilitic character of these skin conditions, he called the sickness 'Kabyle leprosy'.

This chapter seeks to illuminate how, following Jules Arnould, French physicians conceived of the French North African colonies as a field of experience and experimentation that offered the opportunity to observe a form of syphilis that was unknown in France. Its ambition is to demonstrate how these physicians, fascinated by the vision of exotic skin lesions, defined a new pathology in such a way that revitalized syphilology, while also developing a representation of the indigene as a being who was simultaneously both repulsive and vulnerable. In this respect the making of 'Kabyle leprosy', also called 'Arab syphilis', had a double function in legitimating the colonial order. Namely, by being part of a dialectic of inclusion and exclusion, it allowed the categorization of the indigene as radically other, while designating him as a being that French medicine must take charge of and transform into human appearance.

A Voyage in Space and Time: The Discovery of an Unknown Dermatosis

From the beginning of the conquest of Algeria in 1830, military doctors accompanying French troops endeavoured, in addition to caring for the wounded, to draw up an inventory of the colony's health. Following quickly in the wake of the armies, their investigations translated into a multitude of articles, books, reports and theses, constituting a kind of scriptural and scientific dimension of the appropriation of the territory.[5] If at first their attention was mostly drawn to the gunshot wounds, sunstroke and stomach upsets affecting the soldiers, they did not delay in cataloguing the most widespread diseases that could hinder a lasting French presence. In the newly conquered towns, they observed without great surprise epidemics of fever and cholera. They studied topography and sewage systems. But the illness that most often impressed these young physicians was syphilis.[6]

In 1833 Foucqueron, surgeon *sous-aide-major*, described the 'ravages' of venereal diseases in Algiers: 'In the hospitals I have seen many examples of these illnesses that end in the most horrible deaths; many ulcers that had invaded the soft palate, the soft parts of the face, sometimes even the scalp; gnawing chancres that had attacked the abdominal integuments and spread in a dreadful manner.'[7] In Constantine, where a civil hospital was established after the siege of the city, Dr Deleau did not hide his horror either: 'I do not believe that in any hospital of Europe there exist more dreadful examples than those that I have seen daily. I have seen wretched infants at the breast, often blind, covered in pustules and growths.'[8] Fascination, pity and terror are the principal emotions that show through a reading of these writings, traditionally dominated by the cold rationality of the scientific exposé.

The discovery of these disturbing characteristics of syphilis in North Africa progressed as the army's columns subdued new regions and penetrated into the interior. Doctors did not have the sole vocation of treating the troops or of collecting information. Their mission equally consisted of providing medical assistance to the indigenous population, in order to demonstrate to them the benefits of French colonization. This was the message that Salvandy, minister of public education, delivered in his visit to Algiers in 1846: 'Without a doubt, the government wants you to know its gratitude for your dedication to the soldiers, but you have another mission that is just as important to fulfil. It is to take a large part in furthering the penetration of our civilization among the Arab and Kabyle tribes. Your proselytism is perhaps the only one that could succeed within the next several years'.[9] The following year a circular created a health service with the 'Arab Bureaus'. These local administrative structures created by the French, which played a policing role and functioned as an intelligence service and liaison between the military authorities and indigenes, thus allowed some military doctors to meet rural populations, despite the tremendous difficulties of travel. From 1857 army doctors were officially assigned by the Ministry of War to the finally subdued mountainous regions of Kabylia to treat cases of syphilis.

It was there that they became familiar with this new, especially visible, form of syphilis with almost exclusively cutaneous symptoms. Nonetheless these deformities corresponded so little to those that physicians normally observed in the metropole that they had to refer to a distant past to find an equivalent to what they had before their eyes. Dr Vincent, for example, recalled the elephantiasis of the Greeks and the leprosy of the Middle Ages.[10] The lesions that afflicted the syphilitic indigenes so resembled those of leprosy that there could be confusion in the diagnosis.[11] In western medical thought the analogy was often made between these skin diseases since the modern period, when they were associated with sin and lechery.[12] But in the 1860s it was also deployed to attract attention to the syphilis of Kabyles at a time when leprosy elicited keen interest in the medical world. Leprosy was then perceived as an illness linked with backwardness and destitution which had nearly disappeared in the metropole, but which had fearfully been rediscovered in the colonies and reconceptualized as a tropical disease.[13]

If the meeting of military doctors with Kabyle tribes required long trips, they considered this travel in space as a journey through time that permitted them to contemplate not so much a form of highly advanced syphilis, but *the* syphilis, untreated, given free reign, and thus in a pure state. As Dr Lacapère stated later in the 1920s, 'The syphilis that we observe among the Arabs is thus the French syphilis of the Middle Ages, that which existed before the spread of therapeutic methods introduced in Europe around the end of the fifteenth century, a syphilis that very few documents allow us to suspect'.[14] Desiring to relate their observations to a known precedent, but disoriented by the severity of the lesions, these colonial physicians of the Maghreb spontaneously recalled the famous epidemic of the 'Naples disease' that struck the troops of King Charles VIII in Italy. The ravages caused by these bodily and facial lesions had at that time strongly impressed Renaissance physicians such as Fracastoro and Ulrich von Hutten.[15]

An Embodiment of Degeneration: The Clinical Examination of Indigenous Syphilis Lesions

Once they got closer to the rural populations of the interior, the physicians should have proceeded to the clinical examination of the sick. However, despite the free care, they had to take into account the latter's reluctance to be examined and extreme modesty. Often located in an adjoining department of the hospital or in a makeshift infirmary, doctors attracted many men who balked at stripping naked and who absolutely opposed the examination of women. With the help of interpreters who were often recruited from among the colonial troops, doctors had to develop elaborate strategies of persuasion so that the patients would take off their garments and show their genitals. The questioning was not any easier, for if the indigenes did not hesitate to name the illness from which they suffered (*alou* or *meurd-el-kébir*, which is to say the 'great sickness'), they often proved unable to date their infection and the progression of the symptoms. The difficulty of diagnosis was compounded by local therapeutic methods, as the sick often placed various dressings on their wounds. These frequently altered their appearance completely, and obliged the physicians to clean the lesions in order 'to restore their normal appearance and to allow them to be placed within the known classifications'.[16]

Once these obstacles were overcome, French physicians devoted the bulk of their publications to presenting the indigenes' skin lesions in order to complete the clinical picture of the disease and to provide a morphological study. In its nuances and precisions, these studies appear modelled on the geographic descriptions of the newly conquered lands. Since the end of the nineteenth century, thanks to the use of light and easy-to-use cameras, doctors increasingly illustrated their descriptions with plates, permitting extremely realistic images of the indigenes' skin diseases. This recourse to photography corresponded to a desire to facilitate diagnosis. However, it was part of a broader revival of colonial doctors' attention to the ways of perceiving the indigenous population, moving from topographic maps to portraits of the sick.[17]

The physicians who examined the skin of infected indigenes encountered difficulties related to its pigmentation, which quite often called into question the division of peoples into racial categories. During their studies, they barely received sufficient training to recognize the cutaneous symptoms of syphilis on the white skin of metropolitan patients. In the Maghreb, they were confronted with epidermises representing a wide spectrum of colours, even within the same family, which they attributed to polygamy and mixing between Blacks and Arabs.[18] Consequently the characteristic lesions of syphilis lost their usual appearance and took on a strange aspect. 'The closer to black the skin is, the more the syphilids lose the red coloration that they have on the white epidermis ... taking on a dark tint, which can even be pure black.'[19] The skin colour of the indigenes rendered their lesions even more dramatic insofar as they often led to de-pigmentation and to large scars, so that even those healed bore the conspicuous marks of previous symptoms (see Figure 6.1). Hardly confined to certain organs, these syphilitic lesions frequently extended to all bodily surfaces. Physicians described large and deep ulcerations covered with thick crusts (see Figure 6.2). The chancres and mucous patches were characterized by phagedenism, which is to highlight their hypertrophy, or abnormal growth. This was linked to an 'exaggeration of the ulcerative process, radiating outwards from its original source when it is a superficial phagedenism. When it is a burrowing phagedenism, it is piercing, digging, destroying, and mutilating deep down'.[20] The most common skin conditions were diagnosed as resulting from a crusted ulcerative syphilis, which in some cases when left untreated, resulted in an ulceration of the centre of the face causing the loss of the nose, leaving only a gaping hole and totally disfiguring the patient.

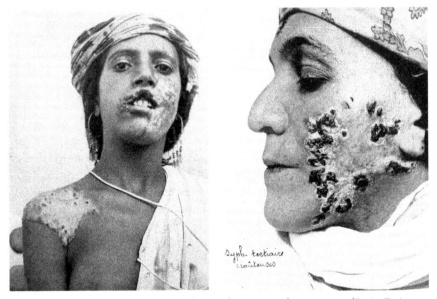

Figure 6.1 (left): G. Lacapère, *La syphilis arabe: Maroc, Algérie, Tunisie* (Paris: Doin, 1923), plate 20. Image © BIU Santé (Paris).

Figure 6.2 (right): G. Lacapère, *La syphilis arabe: Maroc, Algérie, Tunisie* (Paris: Doin, 1923), plate 11. Image © BIU Santé (Paris).

Through the use of terms such as 'phagedenism', 'mutilating syphilis' and 'ulcerative crusted plaques' in their clinical descriptions, physicians were able to render an account of the lesions they confronted. However, they had great difficulty in linking their observations to the syphilis that was known in the metropole. Alibert, the well-known pioneer of French dermatology, had already described syphilitic lesions covering the whole body; but such cases were rare exceptions, and the first military physicians of Algeria, who were generally not specialized in skin diseases, had probably never heard about them.[21] They were more accustomed to the clinical progression of the disease in three distinct stages, which was the object of growing consensus in France and contributed to the establishment of syphilology as a recognized medical specialty, thanks to the teachings of Philippe Ricord and Alfred Fournier. In the Maghreb, indigenous syphilis called into question the threefold progression of the disease, as the initial chancre was very uncommon. More frequently the disease began with the sudden manifestation of secondary syphilis, which seamlessly turned into the most destructive forms of tertiary syphilis. Insofar as it immediately presented in its malign form and knew no interlude, the syphilis of North Africa presented a challenge to colonial physicians.

Climate, Sexuality or Hygiene? An Etiology of Backwardness

The first attempts to establish the etiology of these skin symptoms were largely inspired by the theory of climates. In the mid-nineteenth century one did not yet speak of 'tropical diseases' but rather of 'diseases in the tropics', whose particular traits had less to do with their own specificities and more to do with the geography and climates where they developed.[22] Many physicians affirmed that a hot climate was beneficial for the skin. By promoting sweating, high temperatures would lead skin pathologies to heal more quickly. Cold climates would be particularly fearsome, as the writings of Wilhelm Boeck showed regarding the many cases of leprosy and tertiary syphilis in Norway during the first half of the century.[23] How then to explain the severity of syphilis observed in the Maghreb? At first French doctors remained faithful to climatological explanations, attempting to invert its assumptions. Several of them insisted on the functional hyperactivity of the skin, which in hot countries made it more susceptible to syphilitic infections. The indigenes' dermises, constantly exposed to the heat of the sun, would be characterized by an early ageing, and aggravating syphilitic lesions. Fairly quickly, however, given the frequency of the disease among young people in the mountainous regions, climatological theories were abandoned in favour of explanations relating to the milieu and mores.[24]

The investigation of the causes of the disease then settled on a comparison of the forms that syphilis assumed among the different populations then present in

North Africa. Since their arrival, military physicians took care to note the extreme rarity of visceral or nervous symptoms among indigenous Muslims, whereas they were frequent among Europeans and Jews living in cities, often taking the form of general paresis or dementia. The nearly total absence of Muslims suffering from tertiarism, the third stage of syphilis, among the lunatics confined in local hospices or asylums thus appeared as proof of the specificity of their disease.[25]

Because syphilis was considered to be a venereal disease, physicians at first suspected the indigenes' dissolute sexuality and taste for debauchery. Their remarks thus freely reprised the main clichés of an erotic imaginary of a fantasized Orient, which certain travelogues in particular disseminated, describing the lasciviousness of Orientals and the intrigues of the harem.[26] Many French doctors noted the pervasiveness of prostitution and its affinities with local customs, citing for example the courtesanerie of women of the Ouled Naïl tribe. In contrast the endogamy and continence of Jews allowed them to avoid the 'dangerous contact with Muslims', so that syphilis was less widespread among them and presented as it did in Europeans. Moreover, Jews more frequently associated with the latter, especially in Algeria, where they obtained French citizenship in 1870.[27] Nonetheless, despite the saturation of their discourse with these stereotypes about the debauchery of the indigenes, French doctors had to acknowledge the evidence: many patients persisted during questioning to deny any sexual misconduct. Above all the disease often touched children, who also bore large skin lesions, but whom could not be suspected of vice.

The sight of these very young patients led French physicians to revise their conception of the disease's etiology and look to a method of contagion, considered relatively uncommon in the metropole, induced by the lack of hygiene and close living quarters. The matter in question was non-venereal contagion, which fuelled much speculation among syphilis experts. Since the 1830s many inoculation experiments had shown the contagiousness of secondary syphilis's cutaneous symptoms, but Ricord, who dominated the specialty until the 1880s, rejected this hypothesis for a long time, until it won full acceptance thanks to Alfred Fournier at the end of the century. In contrast the transmission of syphilis through the intermediary of an object, called 'mediate contagion', won consensus, particularly due to studies of cases of infection among the glassblowers' guild.[28] For physicians of the colonies, the specificity of indigenous syphilis was that the proportion of patients affected by these diverse modes of contagion was the inverse of those of European populations – Arabs and Kabyles of rural regions were only rarely infected during sexual relations, which was the most frequent mode of infection in metropolitan cities.

Regardless of the non-venereal nature of the contagion, the doctors thus continued to diagnose syphilis. Even after the end of the military regime in 1870, and despite the gradual replacement of army surgeons with civil physicians, none of them referred to yaws, a disease with similar symptoms, which is transmitted by cutaneous contacts and which had been described by Alibert as specific to the black populations of Africa.[29] They also did not make the connection with other resembling skin diseases that had been observed in the eighteenth and nineteenth centuries in Norway or in Canada (see Lie's and Moran's chapters in this volume), as if the supposed origin of syphilis in the colonial world made the disease totally different from its manifestations in the West.[30]

This characteristic led French doctors to suspect the deplorable conditions in which the Muslims lived, particularly the Berber populations of the interior. They painted a portrait of the indigene as a backward person, totally ignorant of hygienic practices. 'Dressed in a *gandoura*, which he does not wash until the colour is indistinguishable, and a *burnous*, which he does not change until it becomes ragged, he is ignorant of cleanliness,'[31] wrote an indignant physician in his medical thesis. 'It is proven', added Dr Raynaud, 'that the indigene is dirty, often repulsively so, incredibly negligent of his body. Many have numerous parasites on their body or on their clothes, and consequently they have pruriginous dermatoses ... They do nothing to rid themselves of their vermin'.[32]

Some practitioners paid close attention to the housing conditions of the indigenes, in keeping with hygienic preoccupations and theories of infection that then held sway in the metropole. It was a rare description that did not insist on the squalor that reigned in the tents and *gourbis* (huts), where large families lived in alarmingly close contact. Closely echoing the rhetoric of metropolitan reformers, who denounced the unhealthy lodgings for workers in industrial cities, physicians practising in North Africa situated the source of the infection in the intimacy of the domestic sphere. There people were confined to small and unhealthy spaces, forced to sleep skin against skin, one against another. Besides direct physical contact, contagion was associated with the soiling of their clothes, which vermin could only worsen and transmit the infection to nearby persons.[33] Similarly the collective use of certain objects, such as a pipe or utensils, was considered a privileged vector of the disease, explaining its familial character. While Europeans were supposed to be able to impose salutary norms of distance and hygiene on their own social relations, it was the local populations' primitive and communal way of life, characterized by the exchange of everyday objects and the proximity of bodies, that condemned them to syphilitic infections and to the worst skin diseases.[34]

This cultural indictment of indigenous habits often alluded to the poverty of the patients who presented for consultation, as it was often a determining factor in the severity of the illness. Some doctors pointed out the fact that phagedenism affected the poorest of the *fellah*, those who, living in destitution, could not obtain the least remedy and thus left syphilis to develop its most frightening consequences. However, the vast majority insisted instead on the individual responsibility of the sick. References to the ignorance and religious beliefs of the Muslims fed this image of a totally passive and improvident patient, incapable of dating his infection and trusting God for his recovery. Faced with the silence of patients unable to furnish information that could guide diagnoses, many physicians focused on this passivity that was hindering their practice. 'Can we do anything other than practice veterinary medicine when not the slightest recollection comes to complete the examination of the lesions we see?', lamented Dr Raux, assigned to the military hospital of Miliana.[35] Following this point of view, the fatalism of the sick was explained less by the absence of effective treatment and more by the inability of the indigenes to look ahead and take their destiny in their hands by relying on French science.

Ultimately French physicians associated the specificities of indigenous syphilis not to climatic conditions, but to the primitive customs of the local peoples.[36] It was Dr Lacapère, physician at the syphilis clinic in Fez, Morocco, who in his 1923 book *La Syphilis arabe*, besides popularizing this new name, theorized this correlation between the various forms of syphilis and the degree of civilization of the peoples it afflicted.[37] For the indigenes, early tertiary syphilis, mutilating injuries, ulcers and giant crusts inscribed on their flesh their radical strangeness and fundamental backwardness. For the Europeans, it was neurosyphilis, less expressive, that attacked the internal organs. As Rod Edmond finely observed about leprosy, as European medicine developed in the colonies, the distinction between the cleanliness of the white man and the unhealthy negligence of the indigene defined this sort of 'grammar of difference' that tropical medicine cultivated on its path to institutionalization, and which implicitly helped naturalize colonial hierarchies.[38] What did it matter if the illness was foremost due to socio-economic factors? It appeared in their descriptions and representations as a symbol of the indigenes' inferiority and biological otherness.

Following Nancy Stepan, Edmond has shown how the photographic staging of the character disfigured by diseases like elephantiasis or leprosy helped construct an image of the indigene as a being set apart, monstrous and primitive, whose deformities showed that he belonged to a corrupted species. This was likewise the role played by the many images of tertiary syphilis of the face that French doctors took and circulated to attest to the ravages of 'Arab' syphilis.

Syphilis of the face was the most dramatic form of the disease among North African indigenes. It was also the form that most struck French doctors upon their arrival. It constituted an obligatory passage in their descriptions, and with regards to its symptoms alone, they shared their emotions of surprise, horror and pity in their scientific writings. Manifested by a facial ulcer that gnawed at the centre of the face, it gave a particularly repulsive appearance to the individuals it struck (see Figure 6.3).

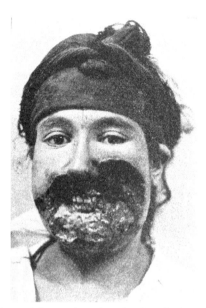

**Figure 6.3: J. Brault, 'La syphilis en Algérie', *Archiv für Schiffs- und Tropen-Hygiene*,
12:20 (1908), pp. 647–60, on p. 651. Image © BIU Santé (Paris).**

Most frequently it was women who posed for the camera, even though few went
to the examinations, probably because they were more subject to the authority of
the doctor who directed the shooting. The repetition and dissemination of such
photographs illustrate that this was not solely about refining documentary tools
for diagnosis. They show a mix of horror and fascination that, in the doctor, reveal
something other than simple, medical curiosity. As in contemporary depictions of
lepers,[39] this focus on facial deformities embodied eugenic theories then in vogue
in the metropole concerning the role of social ills on the quality of the population.[40] The indigenes' tertiary syphilis thus furnished a living representation of the
idea of degeneration, projecting on a face the fears of the time. Many physicians
further affirmed that it was hereditary syphilis, affecting children from their earliest years and doomed to perpetuate itself from generation to generation.

These monstrous forms of syphilis thus helped to define the contours of a
suffering sub-humanity living on the margins of civilization and of progress.
However, at the same time they appeared as obstacles to the ideal of assimilation
and to the use of the colonies' labour force. Accordingly, in 1875 Dr Bernard
deplored that many Europeans avoided associating with the indigenous population. 'The symptoms are so bad, sometimes so horrible, that the indigenes are
excluded from society, despite the services they could very advantageously render it. Thus an Arab or Kabyle woman is rarely accepted as a wet-nurse.'[41] It was
precisely against this de facto segregation, which harmed the colonial order, that
French physicians intended to mobilize their therapeutic skills. In rendering a
human figure to the sick, metropolitan science should regenerate the indigenous
population and demonstrate the benefits of colonization.

Restoring a Human Face to the Indigene: The Treatment of Native Syphilis

One of the most common clichés of the mission accounts published by colonial physicians concerned the regression of Arab medicine from its medieval golden age. In fact many practitioners associated the severity of indigenous syphilis with the inefficacy of local treatments. The remedies utilized by the Arab and Berber tribes, made from traditional plants and natural substances, contrasted with the new chemical medicines developed by the French. 'The Arabs dress their chancres with a small decoction of henna, and their syphilitic wounds like their ordinary wounds. That is, they cover them with a mixture of coarse wool and honey, sometimes moulded with clay. The whole is held in place as well as possible with rags and bits of string.'[42] Local medicine appeared equally impotent, as it seemed to colonial physicians to be inextricably linked to religious superstitions used for healing. 'For many, Arab medicine included amulets placed on the diseased parts, verses of the Koran written on the limbs or especially on the head, or ink written on an old shard, then dissolved in water and swallowed. When they got to the infusion of rockrose, anis, or mallow, they were at the height of their therapy.'[43] Cow or camel faeces, lemon juice, cauterization with a knife, dressings of goat hair or dried herbs – many medical theses only reported on the variety of indigenous treatments in order to attest to their complete inability to check an ill that they frequently only worsened.[44] However, doctors who practiced there longer demonstrated a better knowledge of local therapeutic methods and mentioned the efficacy of a strict treatment followed by those who withdrew into total darkness for forty days, consuming only unleavened bread and sarsaparilla infusions.[45] One variant included mercury fumigation, a method comparable to that practiced in the metropole, where mercury was the basis of all syphilis medicines until the early twentieth century. It was also used in tablet form under the name of 'Paris pills' (*habb-el-Baris*), sold by hawkers.[46] Nonetheless there was a significant gap between the cities, where these products were relatively cheap and accessible, and isolated rural regions, where they were nearly absent. It was there, as we have seen, that the most severe syphilis developed and where the sick depended most on colonial doctors.

Their taking charge of treatment, however, touched upon the inadequacy of facilities for treating syphilis. Throughout the nineteenth century, only the prostitutes of the large cities' red-light districts were sent to specific facilities, whether a health clinic for periodic medical visits or hospital wards that welcomed the infected. The rest of the population theoretically had access to military hospitals, but the indigenes were often reluctant to go to these enclosed places fully administered by the settler *colons*. For their part, the presiding practitioners did not fail to indicate their disgust at the destitute syphilitics and their dreadful procession of skin lesions, as well as the high costs they incurred.[47] These mutual reluctances led the few physicians dedicated to caring for these patients to fulfil their mission in connection with the Arab Bureaus and to establish themselves in the makeshift location of a field infirmary near an outpost garrison in the interior.

It was within this context of travelling medicine with limited means that, beginning in the late 1840s, army physicians used mercury and silver nitrate and tested the effects of potassium iodide. From the outset they observed the formidable efficacy of this imported product on the seemingly most recalcitrant lesions. The extreme responsiveness of the indigenes to these treatments was largely explained by their 'virginity' in this domain. The speed of their healing, given the malignancy of their symptoms, was hence considered a miracle of colonial science. 'We have restored to his tribe, to his family, an unfortunate man who had suffered under the disgust of the public and of himself', enthused Jules Arnould. 'We have sent back to the midst of the indigenes a living example of the relief that French medicine can bring to their miseries.'[48]

Several practitioners insisted on the inability of patients to follow their prescribed doses and thus the need to avoid giving them medication in pill form. Nonetheless potassium iodide spread well beyond medical consultations and quickly became a therapeutic aid, like quinine, essential for the colonial order. Some *colons*, for example, took the initiative in freely distributing it to the indigenes in exchange for hens, milk or honey, even if on the big farms where several hundred agricultural labourers worked, potassium iodide was replaced with tincture of iodine to save money.[49] That is why the government sent a circular to the prefects in May 1898 to regulate its usage, requesting they establish permanent stores of potassium iodide in the *communes mixtes* of Algeria, available for free distribution, but on the prescription of public or settler physicians.[50] After 1906 the problem of diversity in hospital departments and access to care was in the process of being solved, thanks to the establishment of infirmaries reserved for indigenes. In the aftermath of the Great War, serological tests were still used infrequently, due to the lack of laboratories. In contrast arsenic compounds – especially the 'magic bullet' of Paul Ehrlich, arsphenamine (also known as Salvarsan) – established itself in the colonial therapeutic arsenal. Clinics specially dedicated to the treatment of venereal diseases were opened, as in Tunis, where the first was inaugurated in 1930 by the French League of Tunisia against Venereal Disease.[51]

From 'Arab Syphilis' to 'Bejel'

Nearly eighty years after the first missions of military doctors in Algeria, the initial disease was considerably altered by contact with the *colons*, until it could no longer be observed except in Morocco. Its geographic location receded with the growth of European influence in North Africa. Thus in the large cities of the coast it was replaced by the disease of the Europeans, as understood in the metropole, which was sexually transmitted and quite frequently led to symptoms of neurosyphilis – locomotor ataxia and general paralysis – although these had been unknown in the interior previously.[52] This transformation was marked by the increasing rarity of the more dramatic skin conditions. However, to physicians this did not constitute progress, as the 'pure' syphilis of the rural inhabitants, though it revealed their backwardness, was equally the token of a simplicity and innocence that were quickly dissolved in urban centres, 'where the indigene, in contact with the European population, is more subject to the habits of intemperance, intoxication with wine, and the appeals of industrial and intellectual activities'.[53]

The tone of medical discourses regarding the indigenes had evolved as the disease transformed, normalizing its etiology and symptoms. From a terrible skin disease interpreted as a sign of backwardness, it had become that venereal disease that was the symbol of urban civilization, with mostly internal symptoms. This bio-geographic transformation was accompanied by a change of discourses that had predominated until then, as colonial optimism that metropolitan science would save the indigenes gave way to a more pessimistic vision, according to which they had been saved from their own vices only to indulge in European ones.

During the Great War, several mobilized doctors lamented the absence of health control on the borders and the risk of an inflow of migrants affected by syphilis in France. In the summer of 1916 Dr Pautrier warned the Military Health Service after the discovery of fifty North African colonial workers suffering from 'enormous lesions' in a war factory in Bourges. As a consequence, in January 1917 a ministerial circular ordered that all colonial workers be subjected to compulsory medical examination.[54] Then, between the two wars, physicians continued warning against the importation of 'exotic' syphilis.[55] Once conceptualized as radically different from European syphilis, the syphilis of colonial peoples became a new danger for the metropole because, having lost its unique characteristics, it was distinguished only by its prevalence, which was judged greater than that in metropolitan France. The project of assimilating colonized populations was unexpectedly fulfilled in this respect: If indigenous syphilis became identical to that of Europeans, its mode of infection was also the same and it became all the more dangerous insofar as the carriers of the disease, often rid of their most miserable lesions, were less conspicuous.[56]

Paradoxically, it was also precisely when 'Arab' syphilis seemed to be increasingly rare in French North Africa that it was rediscovered elsewhere, resulting in its enduring recognition under a new label in medical knowledge. At the end of the 1920s, Ellis Herndon Hudson, a young American doctor and founder of a medical mission and hospital in Deir-ez-Zor in the Syrian mandate under the auspices of the Presbyterian Church, observed the disease among the Bedouin tribes of the desert.[57] Characterized by large lesions of the skin, transmitted within families living in cramped quarters with poor hygiene, it corresponded exactly to the syphilis that French doctors had discovered nearly a century earlier in the Maghreb. The nomads of the Euphrates valley called it *bejel*. The term was taken up by Hudson, who in numerous articles published in the specialist Anglophone press equally invoked an 'endemic' or 'non-venereal' syphilis,[58] which could only be a variation of a broader disease group, treponematosis, spread on a global scale by the African slave trade and taking various forms (yaws, bejel, venereal syphilis) according to the climates and mores of the populations. Since then Hudson's name remains linked with this 'unitary theory' and the disputation of the 'Columbian theory', the famous account of the American origins of syphilis and its importation to Europe by Christopher Columbus.[59]

Thus, reclassified and later integrated into a new global history of the disease, 'Arab' syphilis ceased to be a monstrous defect of the indigenous peoples of North Africa. Reconsidered outside of a colonial context, from the 1950s it became a simple dermatosis, characteristic of remote regions of the Third World.

7 DISCOVERING THE 'LEPER': SHIFTING ATTITUDES TOWARDS LEPROSY IN TWENTIETH-CENTURY UGANDA

Kathleen Vongsathorn

Some assume it is in humanity's nature to be disturbed by difference and to stigmatize signs of difference upon the skin.[1] Leprosy, in particular, has long been regarded as the ultimate manifestation of stigma growing from a disfigured external appearance.[2] Belief in the universal stigmatization of leprosy has become so entrenched in the modern Western world that it has become a myth in itself.[3] Yet in reality there is no universal idea of what constitutes a 'normal' human, and as such no universal response to the disfiguring symptoms that mark a 'leper'.[4]

This chapter draws upon missionary and government archival materials, anthropological texts and patient interviews in order to understand why leprosy sufferers were feared or accepted in twentieth-century Uganda. It traces ideas of leprosy in Britain and Uganda and explores how they interacted to shape attitudes towards the 'leper' among each of the four Ugandan ethnic groups whose districts contained large-scale leprosy settlements. These settlements were founded by Christian missionaries in the early 1930s and housed primarily the Bakiga of south-western Uganda, the Baganda of central Uganda and the Basoga and Iteso of eastern Uganda.

It was during the nineteenth and twentieth centuries that the British middle class acquired the ideas about leprosy that influenced the missionaries who founded Ugandan leprosy settlements, and who later shaped policies and influenced Ugandan concepts of the disease. The Bakiga saw their concept of leprosy shift most radically with missionary intervention, from an initial acceptance of leprosy sufferers in the 1920s to a deep fear of leprosy by the 1960s. This change was wrought by decades of missionary excursions throughout the region, during which missionaries emphasized the contagion of leprosy, singled out individual leprosy sufferers and pressured them to leave their homes for a segregated island leprosy settlement. The exploration of ideas about leprosy among the Baganda, Basoga and Iteso further demonstrates that attitudes towards leprosy differed among each of Uganda's ethnic groups, and that these attitudes changed in response to interactions with European missionaries.

In the Western world, stigma has attended visible difference, something leprosy sufferers have experienced particularly acutely. Yet attitudes towards leprosy are culturally conditioned according to shifting standards of normality. Whereas in twentieth-century Britain normality was premised in part upon unblemished skin, among the Bakiga this mattered less than other factors, such as the ability to be economically productive. Thus leprosy patients in south-western Uganda were only stigmatized when the disease crippled them so severely that they were unable to provide for themselves. This minimal stigma towards leprosy patients continued until the Bakiga came to associate ugliness and contagion with the symptoms of leprosy, thus increasing local fears of the disease. Reactions towards leprosy sufferers were not universally dependent upon visible disfiguration, but rather upon the symptoms of disease that deviated most from the culturally accepted norms of the whole and healthy human.

The Founding of Ugandan Leprosy Settlements

Uganda's first sizeable in-patient leprosy settlements were conceived, created and maintained by missionaries from the Church Missionary Society (CMS), an Anglican mission based in Britain. Missions were often the earliest and most extensive providers of biomedicine in Africa.[5] Even after European colonial governments became involved in African public health programmes in the early twentieth century, missionaries remained the primary providers of biomedicine to leprosy patients, mothers and infants.[6] When Dr Clare Wiggins initiated CMS leprosy settlements in 1927 at Kumi and Ongino, in Teso, eastern Uganda, he was one of many missionaries opening leprosy settlements in the colonial world.[7] Following suit, Drs Leonard Sharp and Algie Stanley Smith began plans for another CMS leprosy settlement on Bwama Island in Lake Bunyonyi, south-west Uganda, which opened in 1931.[8] All three missionaries had similar motivations in founding leprosy settlements: evangelization; medical and palliative care for leprosy patients; a decrease in leprosy through the 'protection of the general population from infected people'; and saving leprosy sufferers from neglect and stigmatization.[9] These motivations were based on an assumption of universal stigmatization of leprosy, biomedical ideas about leprosy and its control and years of experience serving as doctors in Uganda.

While Mother Kevin, the Catholic missionary who followed the CMS example in founding two smaller leprosy settlements in south-eastern Uganda, did not share the same biomedical training as the CMS settlement founders, she had been pursuing medical work in Uganda since 1906.[10] Acting in conjunction with the British Catholic Mill Hill Mission and the Franciscan Missionary

Sisters for Africa, Mother Kevin founded leprosy settlements at Nyenga in Buganda in 1932 and at Buluba in Busoga in 1934. Mother Kevin shared not only the CMS doctors' preconceptions about leprosy, but also their motivations for the founding of leprosy settlements, albeit with the added desire to compete with the Protestants for 'leper' converts.[11]

A Missionary's Knowledge of Leprosy in Early Twentieth-Century Britain

When the four missionaries who founded Uganda's leprosy settlements left England for East Africa between 1901 and 1916, they brought with them preconceptions about leprosy that shaped the formation of leprosy control policy within Uganda. Leprosy had appeared sporadically in British newspapers from the 1850s, when contact with leprosy in the colonial world brought the threat of leprosy back into the public mind after the disease's centuries-long absence from Britain. Media interest in leprosy peaked after Belgian missionary Father Damien's death from leprosy in Hawaii, catapulting Europe and America into the 'leper scare of 1889'.[12] During their youth in England, Wiggins, Sharp and Smith would have been exposed to London *Times* articles asserting that 'homeless, religionless, friendless, the poor leper ... went out into the world with the constant dread of violent death lurking around him', and consequently calling 'on every civilized community to make such laws as shall effectually stamp out this curse from off the face of the earth'.[13] Responses towards leprosy *within* Britain were characterized by paranoia. A London butcher, Edward Yoxall, had been two years under the care of a physician for leprosy, and people assumed that he had lost his fingers in an accident or was suffering from a skin disease.[14] However, when the public discovered that Yoxall had *leprosy*, fear of contagion and 'the feelings of repugnance which [a leper's] appearance would naturally excite' led to Yoxall's immediate segregation.[15] Father Damien's death had fixed leprosy in the minds of the public, and fear, 'excitement' and the impetus to eliminate leprosy globally became the hallmark of the popular press's response to leprosy.

By the twentieth century, when Uganda's leprosy pioneers were leaving England, media coverage of leprosy was shifting in its focus from sensationalism to the advocacy of leprosy charities abroad. Fears of leprosy spreading to Britain were assuaged, if not banished entirely, by a growing medical consensus that leprosy could not spread on British soil due to Britain's temperate climate and the superior 'personal habits and ... general hygiene' of the 'civilized' British.[16] Leprosy in Europe was deemed to be a relic of the Middle Ages and 'a consequence of the filthiness of our ancestors'.[17] The unfortunate plight of the stigmatized and suffering 'leper' was more likely to be assumed than investigated, and thus while press coverage of leprosy faded, the mythologies of contagion and stigma that were produced during the 'leper scare' remained.

The popular press's ideas about leprosy drew on four sources: the Bible, history, attitudes towards disfigurement and biomedical debates. Many have attributed the stigma of leprosy to the Bible, a trend in scholarship that has continued from the nineteenth century and into the twenty-first.[18] In 1911 Doctor Ernest McEwen wrote that:

> There are many reasons for believing that the extraordinary fear of leprosy, which is so universally present today and which has worked hardship and misery to so many unfortunate victims of the disease, is a result, in part at least, of the influence of the biblical references to 'leprosy'. These accounts, when interpreted literally, depict the condition as most terrible, and belief in them is widespread since the Bible, accepted by millions as a revelation of the divine, is the most read book in the world.[19]

In 1916 a London lawyer defending clients charged with bringing a leprosy patient to a lodging house and conspiring to conceal his disease stated that 'one's horror of leprosy arose at the earliest age, for as children they learned from the Bible to regard a leper as a horrible person; and there was, therefore, a danger of prejudice against the defendants'.[20] At a time when leprosy was extremely rare in Great Britain, the Bible provided many people's first point of reference for the disease.

British beliefs about leprosy were also influenced by the prevailing notion that disfigurement necessarily resulted in stigma. As the medical missionary Stanley Browne wrote:

> It would be quite wrong, and historically unjustifiable, to attribute wholly to the influence of biblical and Christian teaching the widespread stigma attached to leprosy ... The victim of leprosy often does present a repulsive, even nauseating appearance, a travesty of the human form. In many non-Christian lands and non-Christian civilizations, there exist an innate dread and fear of true leprosy.[21]

In writing on the history of skin, literary scholar Claudia Benthien posits that 'the individual's skin is burdened with shame in a special way when it is experienced as afflicted with blemishes and flaws'.[22] The missionaries expected Ugandan leprosy sufferers to exhibit the same bodily shame as British sufferers of skin diseases, who often took night jobs and visited the doctor only in the evenings.[23] CMS nurse Rosa Langley wrote from Uganda that leprosy sufferers were 'perhaps the most repulsive of all men'.[24] The physical disfiguration that could accompany leprosy was severe enough to form an assumption of universal stigma.

The doctors and nurses who were involved in the treatment of leprosy patients in Uganda were informed by a body of medical and scientific research on leprosy that became increasingly united through the early twentieth century. By the 1920s, when Uganda's first large-scale leprosy settlements were being planned, the medically recommended course for the elimination of leprosy was compulsory notification of all cases in the first instance; the immediate isolation of leprous patients; and finally the separation of healthy spouses and children from leprosy sufferers.[25] Leprosy was thought to be only mildly contagious but difficult to prevent, as patients in the early stages of the disease could easily hide themselves if compulsory segregation measures were introduced. As leprosy was believed to be spread by prolonged physical contact among people of 'a low stage of civilization, with the accompanying grave hygienic deficiencies', education about hygiene and contagion was another means of prophylaxis.[26] Thus when Uganda's leprosy pioneers were leaving England to found settlements, they negotiated between ideas gained from the popular press and religious study and ongoing medical research, with which they would become increasingly familiar while working in East Africa.

In removing and isolating Ugandan leprosy patients, missionaries believed that they were both saving healthy Ugandans from leprosy, and saving leprous Ugandans from the stigma and neglect that they must be facing at home. If leprosy patients did not face this stigma and neglect, then it was thought to be the result of the ignorance of a 'primitive people brought very low by suffering and disease'.[27] Leprosy ought to be feared, and by educating Ugandans about the contagion of leprosy, missionaries believed they were doing Ugandans a biomedical and moral service. However the missionaries' preconceptions did not hold true in all parts of Uganda, and leprosy education and segregation did not necessarily fulfil their lofty goals.

Bakiga Attitudes towards Leprosy in the Early Years of Medical Mission, *c.* 1920–40

The first thing that would have concerned missionaries educating Ugandans about biomedical ideas of leprosy was Ugandans' own formulations of leprosy, health and healing. The British did not consider Ugandans a blank slate upon which to be written, and both missionaries and local government officials wrote about local concepts of leprosy. The interpretation of these local beliefs, however, depended upon both British preconceptions and individual familiarity with Ugandans of a particular ethnic group. Of the four groups of Ugandans targeted for large-scale leprosy work, the Bakiga of Kigezi in south-western Uganda were the subject of the earliest and most extensive studies by British missionaries and government officials. After ten years of medical work among the Bakiga, Dr Smith wrote that:

> The native knowledge of the disease is surprisingly exact ... I have had cases brought to me as leprosy in the earliest stages which I would have hesitated to accept as such, until a positive scraping from the nose revealed the bacillus leprae, and proved these primitive diagnosticians correct.[28]

Yet visiting doctor James Ross Innes reported of the Bakiga nineteen years later by stating: 'They did not segregate lepers in the past, nor ostracize them very much. Formerly they did not know much about leprosy'.[29] Innes's drastically different interpretation was most likely based on an assumption that knowledge of leprosy necessarily generated fear of leprosy: in his reports on attitudes towards leprosy in other parts of Uganda, he only recognized knowledge about leprosy when it was accompanied by the fear and segregation of its sufferers.[30] Thus preconceptions about Africans and leprosy influenced not only the ways that the British pursued policies of leprosy treatment and care, but also their perceptions of Ugandan beliefs.

Leprosy patients in Bakiga were accepted or neglected based on their physical condition, which meant Bakiga attitudes towards leprosy were disputed among the British. Smith wrote that it was 'difficult to give a true statement of their views on segregation', but posited overall that segregation was an exceptional response to leprosy.[31] He believed there were occasional 'leper colonies' and 'leper hut[s]' where patients were isolated, but overall individuals with leprosy were 'allowed the freest intercourse with the rest of the community', and the marriage of leprous men and 'untainted' women was common.[32] A 1950 survey of Kigezi leprosy patients living outside of the leprosy settlement indicated that only 4 per cent of leprosy patients lived alone, proving that the segregation of 'lepers' in Kigezi was unusual.[33]

Smith explains Bakiga attitudes towards leprosy with the hypothesis that the Bakiga believed leprosy to be 'an act of God' rather than contagion.[34] The 'ignorance' of the Bakiga in failing to recognize and fear leprosy's contagion was well documented by CMS missionaries.[35] In 1933 an anthropologist wrote that for the Bakiga, illness and misfortune could come through a malevolent spirit; through the High God, who ordered the universe; or through a human intermediary, generally a witch or sorcerer calling upon a spirit.[36] Leprosy in particular was regarded as a supernatural penalty for breaking a ritual proscription or taboo.[37] The absence of any discussion linking leprosy to witchcraft in Kigezi indicates that leprosy was most likely attributed directly to the spite of spirits or a deity.[38] Malevolent spirits, usually ghosts, generally directed their rancour towards their living relatives on a whim, without reference to their behaviour or character. Thus leprosy would not be considered contagious if caused by the breaking of a ritual or by the random act of a spirit.

British missionaries believed that the Bakiga's acceptance of leprosy, despite the selective segregation, was primarily due to their conviction that the disease was not contagious. In searching for causes for stigma, the aspect of leprosy that most occupied the CMS missionaries in Kigezi's leprosy settlement was not its mild contagion, but rather its physical disfigurement. CMS nurse Langley wrote of the 'lepers' of Kigezi that she had 'never seen such a collection of maimed ... and disfigured humanity ... even I who love them for His sake shuddered, handless, footless, featureless and yet His children'.[39] Similarly preoccupied with leprosy's visible symptoms, Smith speculated that segregation was only practiced when 'their condition is so repulsive as to become an offence to society'.[40] Another CMS missionary speculated that leprosy was not feared because the disease's progress was so slow; it was the more innocuous signs of leprosy upon the skin – discoloured patches – that would have dominated the Bakiga's experience of the disease, rather than horrible disfiguration.[41] However it does not necessarily follow that difference and disfigurement would always be a cause for stigma, as Langley insightfully recognizes:

> The leper in Africa is not an outcast *because* he is a leper, but rather as a result of his inability to care for himself in the later terrible stages of the fell disease. For who is going to make time or spend hard-earned cents on feeding or caring for the leper? He must struggle on as best he can until his strength fails him entirely, and he is pushed in to some dark corner and forgotten. It is often from such misery and suffering that these people are saved.[42]

Langley's description of the Bakiga attitude towards leprosy patients makes sense of the apparent contradictions in the selective stigmatization of leprosy sufferers. Leprosy patients were neglected when their physical disability meant they could no longer be economically productive. The Bakiga cared for the elderly or temporarily ill with support and respect, but when faced with the sufferer of a chronic illness that was disabling but not deadly, the response was neglect, a hallmark of attitudes towards those with other physical disabilities.[43] The Bakiga, therefore, did not stigmatize the visible symptoms of leprosy, as the British missionaries expected, but rather its physically crippling symptoms.

The missionaries' disproportionate accounts of isolated Bakiga leprosy patients, all stressing physical appearance, can be explained through a preoccupation with leprosy's visible manifestations, and a need to solicit funding, which depended upon sympathy for leprosy patients as especially vulnerable. In order to attract charitable donations from Britain and government funds from the Ugandan Protectorate, consciously or unconsciously, missionaries overemphasized the stigma and physical deprivation that faced Bakiga leprosy patients. The emphasis on advanced cases of leprosy can be partially explained by the population of the settlements, as those suffering real neglect were more likely to leave their communities. Ultimately, however, the plight of people 'leading the lives of outcasts, uncared for, neglected and the very epitome of misery' was a far more successful plea for humanitarian aid.[44]

From Acceptance to Fear: Changing Perceptions of Leprosy among the Bakiga, *c.* 1931–67

When CMS doctors Sharp and Smith arrived in Kigezi in 1921 and opened the area's first hospital, they found leprosy sufferers to be widely accepted. When the Lake Bunyonyi Leprosy Settlement closed its doors in 1967, leprosy was feared across Kigezi. With the intention of bringing the gift of Christianity to the Bakiga, alleviating the suffering of leprosy patients and eliminating leprosy in Kigezi, these missionaries sought out and segregated leprosy patients and educated the Bakiga about the contagion of leprosy. The result was the religious conversion of hundreds of leprosy patients, the relief and healing of many more, and a gradual shift in Bakiga perceptions of leprosy from acceptance to fear.

The founding of the Lake Bunyonyi Leprosy Settlement in 1931 was professedly due to the over-abundance of leprosy patients that arrived at the nearby CMS hospital.[45] The resistance of most of the district's government and medical officials to this plan (on grounds that the incidence of leprosy in Kigezi did not warrant a large in-patient settlement), and the emphasis on the treatment of leprosy before other more widely occurring skin diseases, does indicate that the motivation for the settlement was not strictly public health.[46] Nevertheless, the desire to prevent leprosy and to heal those who had the disease was a strong component of the mission. In order to enact this plan, the missionaries had to find the district's infectious leprosy patients and convince the Bakiga that leprosy was contagious and therefore necessitated segregation, endeavours which, over time, affected the response of the Bakiga towards leprosy patients.

Missionaries saw education as vital to the elimination of the unhygienic habits and lack of dread that they perceived as responsible for the spread of leprosy among the Bakiga.[47] Nurse Langley wrote in 1931 that:

> The Bakiga ... are only a few years removed from cannibalism ... Civilisation and education is doing much for them, but it will take years before they will in any way resemble their more civilised brethren.[48]

The Bakiga were never cannibals, but this statement is an example of the perceived 'primitiveness' that propelled the missionaries' civilizing mission. Another CMS nurse wrote that 'the difference between health and disease does not seem to have penetrated into the depth of their understanding'.[49] To address this problem, the missionaries went on 'medical safaris' around Kigezi, asking the chiefs to gather villagers together. In addition to preaching, they discussed contagion and the threat that leprous patients posed to families and community. Dr Sharp also wrote a small book about leprosy in the local language, so that literate Bakiga would be able to disseminate relevant biomedical information.

The most important aspect of mission medical safaris in the early 1930s was locating Kigezi's leprosy patients and ensuring that they left their families to live in the relative isolation of the settlement. Since leprosy was well understood by the Bakiga, and heretofore leprosy patients had no reason to hide the disease, many were known by their chiefs and therefore brought to the missionaries. Sharp, who led these medical safaris, provided villagers with basic biomedical care and inspected them for signs of leprosy. Once a case was located, Sharp took them aside and talked to them 'in their own language about the Island and what the advantages are and what it means to them and the future generation.'[50] Sharp's daughter reported that a leading reason that leprosy patients chose to enter the settlement was the concern that they might infect their families and neighbours.[51] While a single conversation with a missionary was not likely to persuade someone to accept leprosy as contagious and leave home potentially permanently, evidence indicates that Sharp emphasized the personal responsibility of a leprosy patient for his or her disease and its spread. Linking leprosy with ideas of personal responsibility and contagion may have influenced members of the patient's family or community to exert pressure upon them to join the settlement.[52]

Until the late 1940s, there were never more than three CMS missionaries working at the Lake Bunyonyi leprosy settlement, and thus the mission relied upon the readily available help of local Bakiga authorities and colonial government officials to convince leprosy patients to enter the settlement.[53] Few leprosy patients immediately travelled to the Lake Bunyonyi settlement with the missionaries; rather, most travelled there separately, often shortly after the missionaries' visit.[54] While this could indicate that the leprosy patients needed time to consider what course to follow, the increased difficulty and expense of travelling separately, particularly for the disabled, and '*the natural fear* and reluctance of the native to leaving his old home' more likely suggests that the decision to enter the settlement was not a personal one, but rather the result of pressure from kin or authority figures within the community.[55] Oral evidence and records from a government resettlement scheme begun in Kigezi in 1946 indicate that many people relocated under pressure from kin who had stronger claims to the family land, or from chiefs who would gain political or economic benefit from their resettlement.[56] Furthermore, one CMS nurse reported that from at least 1957 few leprosy patients wanted to enter the settlement, most who left the settlement did so without discharge, and violence was perpetrated only on leprosy patients who returned home and aggressively sought to reclaim their land.[57] By singling leprosy out and encouraging government officials to remove leprosy patients from communities, missionaries created an environment that made discrimination towards leprosy patients potentially beneficial, not necessarily for reasons of public health, as they intended, but for political, economic or social gain.

As the CMS missionaries pursued a gradual campaign to decrease leprosy in Kigezi, Bakiga attitudes towards leprosy changed rapidly, unlike the slower shifts in general Bakiga conceptions of health, hygiene and other diseases. Dr Sharp wrote that 'the little book that has been written for the natives to read for themselves explaining the dangers of untreated leprosy is beginning to influence the people and make them anxious for their afflicted friends to be treated'.[58] Nurse Langley exulted: 'One of the greatest sources of cheer and encouragement is the fact that the lepers themselves are realising that the disease is contagious, especially among blood relations [and] with their children'.[59] Not all aspects of the mission's campaign against leprosy and the 'backwardness' of the Bakiga were successful, but in spreading an awareness of the contagion of leprosy, they accounted themselves triumphant.

Throughout the leprosy settlement's existence from 1931 to 1967, the Bakiga's fear of leprosy grew, though not necessarily due to an acceptance of the biomedical conception of leprosy, which was alien to their previous understanding of the disease. It was more likely an unintended consequence of the missionaries' efforts: taking leprosy patients aside or away; having community and government authorities exert pressure on leprosy patients to leave home; and settling them on an island in a large lake. One interview suggested that regardless of the degree of visible symptoms or disability caused by leprosy, only the patients who had lived in the leprosy settlement were subject to stigma.[60] Even in the late 1930s a fear of leprosy was growing among the Bakiga, and the missionaries complained frequently of the difficulties in recruiting and maintaining healthy staff, because of a fear of contagion.[61] People started hiding their leprosy from visiting missionaries and doctors in the 1940s, and by 1967 they concealed signs of leprosy from other Bakiga. 'They wore long sleeves, they put scarves down over their heads, they put bandages on their hand pretending they'd hurt their hands, they did all sorts of things to try and hide it – the fact they'd got leprosy – for as long as they could.'[62] Ugliness was now expressed through comparison with leprosy, and in the 1970s leprophobia was rampant in Kigezi.[63] Fear of the 'leper's' contagion was so extreme that Ugandan medical staff would not touch patient records that had been in the pocket of a leprosy patient, workers refused to build a road near a leprosy hospital, and a wandering old woman with leprosy was incarcerated in a cattle shed at a prison until a hospital worker came to collect her.[64] Whereas missionaries reported in the early 1930s that there was little or no dread of leprosy, by the late 1960s there had been a tangible shift in Bakiga attitudes towards leprosy, from acceptance to fear.

While the creation of stigma was surely not the intention of the missionaries, their assumptions about leprosy, medicine, Christianity and Africa influenced the policies of singling out and segregating patients, thus gradually increasing the stigma towards leprosy. Anthropologists Zachary Gussow and George Tracy point to isolation as a critical mechanism in the Western myth of leprosy as a universally stigmatized disease. They write: 'Segregation in special communities, *and the presumed necessity for it*, has engendered a labeling [of leprosy patients] that is difficult to counteract'.[65] CMS missionaries presumed the necessity for segregation, brought it into Kigezi and reinforced the myth of universal stigmatization. Their medical safaris emphasized the uniqueness of leprosy, and their education campaign exaggerated the prevalence of the disease and created an anxiety that was disproportionate to the morbidity threat that leprosy actually posed.

Alternate Concepts of Leprosy in Uganda

The trajectory of Bakiga beliefs about leprosy from acceptance to fear was not uniform across Uganda, for each of the ethnic groups among whom leprosy settlements were started had a unique perspective on the disease. Among the Iteso of eastern Uganda, leprosy was not recognized as a distinct disease, but went by multiple names depending on discernible symptoms.[66] A 1979 survey done in Teso indicated that many locals believed that leprosy was first brought to the region by missionaries.[67] In the 1930s the Iteso accordingly had a 'complete indifference to leprosy'.[68] Interviews with elderly leprosy patients completed in 1979 and 2010 indicate that people initially believed leprosy spread through heredity, sorcery undertaken by other leprosy patients, or the breaking of a ritual.[69] Yet Iteso patients reminiscing on the 1940s and 1950s all emphasized the terrible loneliness they felt when they realized they had leprosy, and their village began to fear them and make them eat and drink separately.[70] Given that CMS missionaries in Kumi undertook a campaign of medical safaris, education and segregation similar to that in Kigezi, it may be that stigma towards the disease grew by way of a similar dynamic, albeit shifting from the starting point of indifference rather than acceptance.

In Busoga, of south-eastern Uganda, the trajectory of change, though difficult to chart, differs again, shifting from a mild and ambiguous stigma to a more serious one. Prior to the involvement of Europeans in leprosy treatment, the Basoga recognized and feared leprosy, and while it is unclear whether segregation was part of the traditional Basoga response to leprosy, they cooperated when segregation measures were introduced in the early twentieth century.[71]

> It [segregation] was only brought in very gradually and was entirely a voluntary system but being so it 'took root' and is now almost universally adopted in Busoga. When a person is found to have leprosy, a hut is built outside the village ... to which the leper goes ... Food is taken to the leper, who is visited by the 'conjugal partner' during the early stages or first period of the disease only.[72]

It seems that leprosy was already feared by the Basoga, but until the involvement of Europeans, there was no universal stigma towards the disease strong enough to induce families and communities to eject leprosy sufferers from their midst. If isolation went on, it was probably within family units, as an elderly Musoga man who contracted leprosy in the 1940s described: 'You no longer fit in society, you no longer share a meal with others. You are isolated and fed elsewhere ... [but] I did not experience many problems since I was a child and would not traverse the village'.[73] Within families leprosy was accepted, but outside the family it was feared because it was contagious, people did not like those without fingers and toes and there was no good medicine for the disease.[74] Yet all of the Basoga leprosy patients interviewed stressed that they did not know how they had caught leprosy, even though they had relatives with the disease, and that they had always interacted freely with people living near the leprosy settlement who seemed not to fear them. So while government officials and missionaries stressed that the Busoga already feared the disease and patients' recollections confirm this point, it is difficult to pinpoint the extent of that fear or explain its causes for the period preceding Europeans' involvement.

The Baganda of central Uganda were regarded by the British as the most 'civilized' and intelligent ethnic group in Uganda, and as proof of this civilization, missionaries and doctors were gratified to discover that the Baganda had an appropriate fear and stigma of leprosy. As visiting Dr Innes wrote in 1947: 'They know leprosy well, are afraid of it, and extend the usual social ostracism to lepers'.[75] Leprosy was one of the most feared illnesses in Buganda, and it carried a stigma so extreme that sufferers were reportedly driven from their villages, a fact that is speculatively borne out by the drastically low incidence of leprosy in Buganda.[76] A comprehensive survey of the disease in Uganda in the late 1940s showed that approximately 0.27 per cent of Bagandans had leprosy, whereas 2 to 15 per cent of the people examined in most other parts of Uganda had leprosy.[77] The segregation of various misfits was unusually common in Buganda, where a 1960s survey showed that 10 per cent of all Bagandan homesteads housed individuals rejected by their communities because of old age, epilepsy, mental illness, leprosy or tuberculosis.[78] Leprosy patients were quite literally cast out of their families, losing their second names when expelled; no one would inherit from a 'leper', or bury a 'leper' near a homestead, for fear of catching leprosy.[79] Luganda proverbs concerning leprosy show a preoccupation with the physical appearance of leprosy patients: of seven proverbs, four concern the loss of fingers, one the effects of leprosy on the skin, and another the overall disfigured appearance of a 'leper'.[80] Furthermore, anyone suffering from a skin disease was feared as a possible leprosy sufferer, indicating that, as the British missionaries expected, leprosy was feared for its contagion and its disfiguring signs upon the skin.

Considering the harsh stigmatization of leprosy patients in Buganda, the foundation of a leprosy settlement was not likely to appreciably change attitudes towards leprosy in the early twentieth century. Nevertheless, despite reports of fear and stigma from missionaries and doctors, spanning most of the twentieth century, interviews with Baganda leprosy patients at the Nyenga leprosy hospital told another story. Contracting leprosy was not always followed by expulsion from the family: 'Whether those neighbours loved me or not, for us we were in our home and I was not going to their homes. My people loved me, I was their child'.[81] Further, Dr Innes reported that although the Baganda feared leprosy, he had 'not found strict village segregation anywhere' in Uganda. More recently, elderly leprosy patients at Nyenga said that they never had difficulties with the people who lived around the leprosy settlement. While these memories may be coloured by the increasing acceptance of leprosy over the last two decades, it is evident that even in the most extreme cases, stigma and isolation were never universally applied.

Conclusion

Although the British missionaries treating leprosy in Uganda began with the assumption that leprosy carried a universal stigma, and therefore that their care would be of unmitigated value in saving leprosy patients from social ostracism, in reality attitudes towards leprosy differed vastly across Uganda. As a result, missionaries' ideas about the Bible, history, disfigurement, biomedicine and Africa interacted differently with pre-existent concepts of leprosy among Uganda's various ethnic groups. The shifting concepts of leprosy among the Bakiga show that attitudes towards leprosy were not based solely on visible disfigurement and contagion, as contemporary popular culture suggested they should be. For the Bakiga, the danger of leprosy was in the rare cases of debility that threatened the productivity of an agriculturally dependent society. While Europeans and some other ethnic groups in Uganda were more preoccupied with leprosy's visibility and cultural history, the Bakiga stigma towards leprosy patients grew in response to the labelling and segregation of leprosy patients. It was not necessarily signs of leprosy upon the skin that shaped attitudes towards the disease, but rather physical and social deviations from the culturally accepted norm of the healthy human.

8 SEX AND SKIN CANCER: KAPOSI'S SARCOMA BECOMES THE 'STIGMATA OF AIDS', 1979–83

Richard A. McKay

[November 1982]
CLUB BATHS,
SAN FRANCISCO

Back in the bathhouse, when the moaning stopped, the young man rolled over on his back for a cigarette. Gaetan Dugas reached up for the lights, turning up the rheostat slowly so his partner's eyes would have time to adjust. He then made a point of eyeing the purple lesions on his chest. 'Gay cancer,' he said, almost as if he were talking to himself. 'Maybe you'll get it too.'[1]

For most of the twentieth century, the soft-tissue sarcoma first described in 1872 by Hungarian dermatologist Moritz Kaposi was widely understood to be a rare and relatively benign form of skin cancer. Though a separate, more aggressive type of Kaposi's sarcoma (KS) would become more commonly diagnosed among young African patients in the 1950s, most European and North American physicians familiar with the cancer would have viewed it as a comparatively mild affliction mainly affecting elderly men of Mediterranean and Eastern European Jewish backgrounds.[2] According to Kaposi's initial description, the cancer's lesions ranged from 'corn kernel- to pea- to hazelnut in size' and from 'brownish red to bluish red' in colour; they would appear in isolation or in clusters, often on the feet. Those treating the cancer in the second half of the twentieth century noted that the tumour typically responded well to chemotherapy, a factor which allowed patients, on average, to live for about a decade after diagnosis.[3]

Beginning in 1979, however, dermatologists began noticing uncommonly aggressive and often fatal cases of KS presenting in younger men in New York and California, men whose most readily noted shared characteristic was their homosexual identity. During the next five years, KS would become firmly linked with the emerging Acquired Immune Deficiency Syndrome (AIDS) epidemic. Indeed, over a short period of time this skin cancer became inscribed with a new meaning: that of a sexually transmitted disease (STD). By the end of 1983 most people would agree that a sexually transmitted agent was the cause of AIDS, a deadly immune disorder that manifested itself in a number of opportunistic infections, including KS. But what was it like to be diagnosed with KS at the beginning of this five-year period, as the skin cancer underwent this significant change in its identity?

Of the opportunistic infections associated with the new syndrome, KS was the most readily visible and would become the most easily mobilized for symbolic and often stigmatizing representations of the condition. Many readers will be familiar with the film *Philadelphia* (1993), in which the lesions of KS fulfil an important narrative function. They signal the growing impact of the Human Immunodeficiency Virus (HIV) on the immune system of the main character, a corporate lawyer played by actor Tom Hanks.[4] The makers of a film released well into the epidemic's second decade could rely on audiences to be familiar with the significance of these marks: a visual shorthand for disordered immune function.

'HIV', the cultural theorist Cindy Patton has observed,

> cannot be rendered as a surface phenomenon, although the insistent portrayal of the KS-lesioned body pervades medical conferences and enlivens Randy Shilts's novel about Patient Zero. Culturally, we want a stigmata of AIDS – if it cannot plausibly be KS, the wasting figure of the person with AIDS will do.[5]

Patton's words offer a useful place to begin this chapter. They rehearse the link to one of the best-known popular histories of the American AIDS epidemic – *And the Band Played On*, written by the San Francisco-based journalist Randy Shilts (1951–94). By referring to Shilts's history as a 'novel about Patient Zero', Patton signals her disdain for the reporter's dramatizing approach, which highlighted the actions of a KS patient previously identified in the medical literature as 'patient 0'.[6] Shilts revealed that 'patient 0' was French-Canadian flight attendant Gaétan Dugas (1952–84), and suggested that he may have introduced HIV to North America.[7] The media pounced upon the story. A nationally broadcast *60 Minutes* news feature on AIDS entitled 'Patient Zero' focussed on the actions of this single KS patient; *People Magazine* named Dugas one of their most intriguing people of 1987.[8]

The tale of 'Patient Zero' was compelling, not only for its simplified explanation of the origin of the North American AIDS epidemic, but also for its description of Dugas's many sexual encounters and his alleged malice. In passages like the one at the beginning of this chapter, Shilts related tales of how Dugas resisted medical interventions and visited gay bathhouses to deliberately infect other men. During these visits, he reportedly showed his partners his skin lesions after sex, telling them that they might catch 'gay cancer' too. By the close of 1987 the story had saturated the media landscape. 'I've got gay cancer. I'm going to die and so are you', was a quote-of-the-week featured by *U.S. News &*

World Report within weeks of the book's release; this lurid focus symbolized much of the media's response.[9]

To North American readers of Shilts's book in 1987, the link between unprotected sex and AIDS went largely unquestioned, a 'fact' built upon a rapidly growing foundation of scientific and medical knowledge that had emerged since 1981 when the first cases were reported. This included important epidemiological work conducted between 1981 and 1983; the discovery of a causative virus in 1983 by French scientists and, more vocally, in 1984 by American researchers; the development and distribution of antibody-sensitive blood tests in 1984; and the official naming of the virus as 'HIV' in 1986.[10] Readers horrified by Dugas's actions, and his alleged attempts to deliberately 'spread AIDS', based their interpretation on the by-then readily accepted fact that KS was a manifestation of AIDS, and that the syndrome was caused by HIV, a virus that could be transmitted sexually. Readers in 1987 were staring across a gulf in time towards the actions of a man in 1982, a time when the state of accepted knowledge was markedly different.

I draw upon oral history interviews, articles from gay newspapers and records of AIDS organizations, among other sources, to argue against this 'deliberate disseminator' characterization.[11] Instead, I emphasize the fluid and unfixed nature of a KS diagnosis during this transitional period of 1979 to 1983, when little was known about the causes, treatment regimens or chances of survival for this aggressive form of skin cancer. Dugas's experience allows exploration of the attempts of young KS patients to make sense of shifting medical and social paradigms in which their skin lesions attracted new aetiologies, rumours and meanings. I argue that Dugas's actions might be better understood as a strong reluctance to concede power over his sexual activity to as-yet unproven medical suppositions. I propose that the visible nature of his lesions marked him out for heightened scrutiny and judgment, two factors that helped to generate a number of historical accounts of his actions. I make use of these varied accounts to suggest that rather than standing out as unusual, Dugas shared much in common with the concerns and challenges faced by other KS patients during this early period of confusion.

I begin with Dugas's diagnosis with skin cancer in that time of transition when KS began to be linked to an epidemic of immune suppression. I then consider the influential role of dermatologists in promoting a response to the epidemic in the gay community, bringing their expertise in reading signs on skin. I also offer a sense of the confusion present among gay men receiving a diagnosis of KS, as well as those in the gay communities surrounding them. In so doing, I hope to raise questions about the usefulness of the concept of 'denial' in a period of such rapid change in information. Often used to suggest a refusal to deal with reality, or more precisely with a reality defined by medical opinion, in this case the charge was often levelled against those who resisted changing their sexual behaviour. The final section considers the personal impact of the cancer's disfigurement on Gaétan Dugas, whose clear complexion had previously been a personal and professional asset. Throughout, I emphasize the social aspects of the disease – the interpretive interplay between patients and their communities in establishing the competing readings of the skin markings. I also hope to bring to light moments of interpretive incommensurability: where the marked individual's reading of their own skin lesions might differ drastically from that of those around them.

Early Signs and 'Patient 0'

Dugas, no doubt like many of the early diagnosed cases of the more aggressive KS, initially interpreted his diagnosis within the typical framework adopted by skin cancer patients. After the shock of a diagnosis of a potentially life-threatening disease, he focussed his attention on seeking treatment and recovery. A friend and former colleague recalled that he came to her in the spring of 1980 when they were both based at the small Air Canada base in Halifax and he had learned that he had skin cancer:

> he was terrified he was gonna die and he was *so* upset over that ... and I mean I know it scared him and it just, it was really sad, he cried when he told me ... he asked me if I remembered the kind of medication and everything my Dad had been given, because my Dad was kind of a guinea pig, they were trying new different things out when my father got this cancer, but I didn't remember because when he died I was only 17 ... and he told me that he was gonna go to New York that he had found a specialist which he thought was a specialist for this type of cancer that he had, he thought he had lymph node cancer.[12]

Many cancer patients report undergoing a change in identity shortly after their diagnosis, with 'the disease itself [becoming] inscribed into their biography'.[13] Dugas, too, appears to have undergone such a transformation after enduring swollen lymph nodes and noticing lesions on his skin in early 1980. He became focused on acquiring a new medical vocabulary, discovering and researching treatment options, and adjusting to the self-perceived role of skin cancer patient.

In early June 1981 the US Centers for Disease Control (CDC) published a brief report about a rare pneumonia reported in five young homosexual men in Los Angeles.[14] Shortly afterwards CDC epidemiologists received a call from Alvin Friedman-Kien, a dermatologist at the New York University Medical Center who had for the previous two years accumulated about thirty gay male patients presenting with KS.[15] Over the next two years CDC investigators remained at the forefront of efforts to determine what factor or factors – genetic, environmental, microbial – seemed to predispose gay men to the pneumonias, KS and other rare diseases, and whether a common loss of immune function linked these disparate conditions.

Ray Redford, a former lover who remained friendly with Dugas, recalled that the flight attendant phoned him in the second half of 1981 to say that he was one of the gay men in New York receiving chemotherapy for 'gay cancer'. Redford was very worried about his ex-lover, despite reassurances from his friends 'that it was not serious as it was "only skin cancer"'.[16] According to Redford, Dugas stayed in contact with other members of this group of early 'gay cancer' patients. Dugas shaved his head in June 1981, in anticipation of the hair loss that chemotherapy would bring.[17]

By that time Dugas had become one of Friedman-Kien's patients in New York. The dermatologist's collaboration with the CDC's efforts enabled that agency's workers to interview Dugas and link him to a number of other early AIDS cases in the Los Angeles area in mid-1982. The Los Angeles cluster study, as this CDC investigation became known, examined the sexual connections between a number of early AIDS patients in the Los Angeles and Orange counties. Interviewers were able to obtain names of sexual contacts from thirteen of the nineteen first reported cases of AIDS there. Of these thirteen, nine reported sexual contact with other AIDS cases over the previous five years, and four named among their contacts a man with KS who was not a resident of California.[18] The study originally abbreviated the man's status – as a resident living 'Outside of California' – as 'patient O'; by the time the study reached publication, this designation had changed to 'patient 0'.

This subtle but crucial shifting of terminology was not questioned at the time, but can be demonstrated to have had important consequences. Later, when members of the media – particularly Randy Shilts – and even other epidemiologists came across the study, they often mistook the role of 'patient 0' as representing the 'source case'. Today the asymptomatic incubation period of HIV infection is known to range from ten to fifteen years, so the significance of the links depicted as important in the cluster study – some of which suggest that symptoms were displayed as soon as nine months after a sexual encounter – is open to question.[19] At the time, however, when the suspected average incubation period was fourteen months, the study appeared to offer convincing evidence to support the theory that AIDS and its opportunistic infections were caused by a sexually transmissible agent.

'Gay Cancer', Dermatologists and Patient Confusion

Flying regularly to New York, Dugas joined a cohort of other cancer patients receiving experimental chemotherapy treatment at New York University. This early therapy was both time-consuming and physically exhausting. One of Friedman-Kien's other KS patients wrote of the significant time devoted 'to receiving chemotherapy (three days a month), weekly blood tests, shots, and an endless battery of other tests'. Early patients were put on a regime of VP-16 (etoposide), a common chemotherapy drug, or interferon, although it appears that there were few standard protocols for either treatment. Accounts left by early patients reveal that they often felt frustrated with the lack of understanding and cooperation displayed by the medical establishment. Patients attending different physicians at different hospitals could receive vastly different treatment regimens.[20]

'Gay cancer' patients faced an additional challenge in a homophobic society when the already negative associations of cancer became amplified by an explicit linkage to homosexual practices. Only three years before the outbreak became widely recognized in 1981, Susan Sontag had written an influential essay about the devastating burdens placed on individuals with cancer. Not least among these was the damaging metaphors taken on by the illness. 'As long as a particular disease is treated as an evil, invincible predator, not just a disease', she wrote, it would be inevitable that most people who were sick would become demoralized when they received their diagnosis. Furthermore, Sontag argued, cancer was seen by many as representing either divine judgment or the consequence of a flawed individual character.[21] Familiar with her writing, one gay health writer in New York added an additional concern for patients with the new, more severe form of KS. 'The gay cancer victim', he wrote, '... suffers three burdens because even though there is so far no proof whatever that promiscuity is a cause of disease, there are background murmurs everywhere that say it is'.[22]

Against a backdrop of ever-shifting scientific hypotheses and increasing media nervousness, North America's urban gay communities gradually became aware of the threat of AIDS in 1982 and 1983. Initially, news of a disease that appeared to target gay men led to disbelief, scepticism and even humour.[23] Soon, however, these responses gave way to deepening alarm. Concern had grown rapidly in New York in 1981 and 1982 and reached an intensity that was initially unmatched in other North American cities, chiefly due to the steadily increasing number of local cases and deaths in the country's largest city. After quiet murmurings of a health problem, San Francisco awoke to the paranoia of AIDS in the summer of 1982. There, efforts to alert the community were led by Friedman-Kien's friend and colleague, dermatologist Marcus Conant, who had founded an interdisciplinary KS research clinic the previous year. Canadian gay communities in Vancouver and then Toronto experienced their own gradual awakenings later, in 1983. This uneven terrain of knowledge, with different groups gaining an appreciation of the severity of the situation at different times, led to a staggered series of responses and disjointed levels of knowledge and experiences across North America.

Typically the alarm was sounded by gay doctors, alerted through their various professional and personal networks to developments in New York City and later in San Francisco. They held community health fairs and information forums, often in concert with other community members interested in sexual health. From these efforts emerged community-based AIDS organizations, which sought to assist the afflicted, raise funds to increase awareness and levels of research, and provide public education.[24]

Dermatologists played a key role in these efforts. KS's rarity (it was estimated that only 600 cases were diagnosed in North America in the first half of the twentieth century) made expert advice invaluable for raising the concern of both patients and physicians and for instructing them on what signs to look for.[25] In some ways the response paralleled the one charted by Jamie Stark in his study of anthrax in this book. Health leaflets featured among the earliest literature distributed in response to the epidemic. These sheets often displayed close-up photographs of KS lesions – in isolation and in clusters – on the (usually white) skin of unidentified patients' upper torsos, legs, ankles and feet.[26] Clinical experience was presented as crucial, since the appearance of KS was 'atypical and may be easily overlooked'; lesions could vary in appearance, ranging from reddish-purple or brown in colour and from 2 millimetres to 2 centimetres in size.[27] Looking back on his work in San Francisco, Conant likened his role to that of Cassandra, foretelling that 'all hell's going to break loose', a message that frequently went unheeded in the early months.[28]

Many early efforts focused on helping physicians identify patients with KS, as well as other AIDS-related diseases, and to warn sexually active gay men to be careful about the partners they slept with, in case the condition was sexually transmissible. With most efforts focused on prevention, very little practical information was provided initially to those diagnosed with AIDS. In the absence of effective treatment, or even certainty about whether the condition was rooted in a genetic or infectious cause, the easiest guidance to provide – refrain from sex – was the most difficult for many AIDS patients to put into practice.

Denial and Scepticism

Stuart Nichols, a New York-based gay psychiatrist, wrote in the fall of 1982 about the urgent needs of those who had been diagnosed with AIDS:

> This illness is especially terrifying because there is little medical understanding of AIDS and no presently effective treatment for it. The emotional adjustment to such an illness goes beyond what has been described for other life-threatening diseases ... in that it frequently necessitates an immediate disruption in one's lifestyle with a loss of supportive relationships and a reliable social network.

He described a support group that he ran for AIDS patients and articulated the 'enormous needs for reassurance and information' new patients felt. 'They should be given straight answers, without hedging, from the medical doctors', he stated, 'and if questions are not answerable, they should be told so clearly'. Nichols warned that '[m]isleading information, even slight differences of opinion among doctors, has dramatic impact among patients, intensifying panic, inflaming suspicions, and diverting valuable energy into unnecessary panic'.[29]

The lack of consensus and expertise was noted, particularly by some of the first individuals diagnosed with AIDS. Philip Lanzaratta, an early KS patient, wrote about the discontinuities in treatment in New York, expressing the serious concerns he and other patients felt 'with all the establishments and people involved'. He opined that:

> My feeling is that patients must ask all the questions that occur to them: What? Why? How long? Are there *alternatives*? Certainly all KS patients should realize that, along with the AID (acquired immunodeficiency) and GRID (gay-related immunodeficiency) patients, we are all white rats in one laboratory being tested, probed, and monitored.[30]

Lanzaratta's comments, which categorized KS, AID and GRID patients separately, suggest that the patients themselves were not convinced that their different conditions were linked. They point to a brief window of time before an agreed-upon definition of AIDS had solidified, when patient identities were still constructed around the external manifestations of their diseases, not by a shared underlying cause.

'AIDS is a new syndrome and there are no authorities', declared the Gay Men With AIDS group in a November 1982 advertisement in the *New York Native*. '[W]e believe that it is crucial for us to begin to share with others like ourselves our personal experiences in getting treatment.' They urged sick men to educate themselves 'by going outside the gay press. Get as broad a view and as many different opinions as possible'. The advertisement also stated, in block capital letters, that 'SOME IMMUNOSUPPRESSED GAY MEN WHO HAVE STOPPED INDISCRIMINATE SEX ARE BEGINNING TO SHOW SIGNS THAT THEIR IMMUNE SYSTEM IS HEALING'.[31] This advertisement and its claims were illustrative of an alternative view of causation, one which was endorsed by many others in opposition to the emerging medical consensus. The 'immune overload' theory suggested that the immune suppression was not caused by a new virus, but by the frequent and ongoing exposure of many gay men to STDs, and particularly their repeated reinfection with cytomegalovirus, a herpesvirus excreted in bodily fluids and most concentrated in sperm and urine.[32] Part of the concept's appeal for patients was its practicality: it offered them the prospect of regaining their weakened immune function if they reduced their exposure to external infections.

In an article summarizing a New York University conference on KS that took place in mid-March 1983, a journalist for the *Medical Post* reported the results of dermatologist Bijan Safai, who was treating KS patients with 'total skin electron beam radiation'. Seventeen of his twenty patients so treated had enjoyed complete remission for forty-eight months (the other three died within four months). 'Despite the ugly purple-colored tumors and extensive treatments', the journalist quoted Safai as saying, 'plus a large loss in patient self-esteem once the diagnosis [had] been made', half of his KS patients went 'back to their previous promiscuous lifestyle and acquire[d] a new lesion'.[33] One can draw two conclusions from this summary. First, a number of men with KS in New York continued to have sex following their diagnoses.[34] Second, and more intriguingly, it would appear that 'going back' to 'promiscuity' was seen as representing a sufficient cause for a recurrence of cancer. By resting and recuperating, and by decreasing the number of sexual contacts, an immunosuppressed patient might hope to regain his damaged immune function. Following this logic, one might imagine a KS patient of the time, like Dugas, finding in such work the evidence to support the immune overload theory, which in turn could support his view that his skin cancer was not contagious.

Both Friedman-Kien and Conant appeared to struggle with Dugas's reluctance to abstain from sex in their respective cities in 1982. The flight attendant's popular reputation as a deliberate disseminator of disease owes a great deal to their recollections. Conant assisted Shilts when the journalist was writing his history of the epidemic in 1985 and 1986, providing access to his personal collection of notes and records compiled since 1981. Numerous interviews with the physician resulted in Conant being featured as a central character in the book. At one point, Shilts writes: 'As far as Conant was concerned, however, Gaetan Dugas was a sociopath, driven by self-hatred and inner turmoil'.[35] Friedman-Kien offered a similar interpretation. In a collection of oral history interviews with AIDS physicians published in 2000, the New York dermatologist recalled:

> While he was in New York, he would go to gay bathhouses and have unprotected sex with a variety of people despite the fact that we warned him against it. I once caught him coming out of a gay bathhouse, and I stopped the car and said, 'What are you doing there?' And he said, 'In the dark nobody sees my spots.' He was a real sociopath. At which point I told a colleague [Linda Laubenstein] the story. She was enchanted with him, as most people were. I stopped seeing him. I refused to see him, I was just so angry.[36]

It is apparent that the dermatologists' reading of Dugas's lesions and their cause left no room for moral ambiguity in their interpretation of his actions. Nor did Friedman-Kien allow for the possibility that in seeking the low-visibility environment of a bathhouse, Dugas may have been seeking to minimize the impact of a spoiled complexion, regardless of the new meanings that were becoming attached to his 'spots'. Furthermore, the speed with which the establishment view of the cancer changed deserves mention. Friedman-Kien informed a medical reporter in August of 1981 that the idea that KS and other immune-system disorders might be caused by communicable 'disease-producing organisms' was 'not given much credibility at this time'.[37] Evidently, from his condemnation of Dugas's bathhouse activities, the dermatologist found that the knowledge generated over the following twelve months was compelling enough for him to change his mind. He seems to have had little tolerance or understanding, however, for those patients – whose initial understanding of their illness was no doubt shaped by the initial non-contagious framework – who took longer to change their own minds and behaviours than he did.

When Shilts described Gaétan Dugas's confrontation with a panel of speakers at a public meeting organized by AIDS Vancouver in March 1983, he dismissed the flight attendant's heated interrogation of the assembled medical experts as 'a textbook case of denial and anger'.[38] This view seems to stem from Bob Tivey, one of Dugas's friends and an AIDS Vancouver support worker, who was interviewed by Shilts in 1986. Shilts's interview notes show that Tivey recalled Dugas's 1983 lament: 'I have skin cancer but it hasn't been proven it's anything else'.[39] Marcus Conant, in a recent interview, also suggested that this resistance to doctors' advice was denial.[40] Yet denial, a notoriously imprecise concept, does not seem to capture the complexity of this response. It fails to allow for extremely rapid changes in knowledge and differences in medical opinion, and it does not account for the politicized lenses through which this knowledge is invariably interpreted, a point to which I turn in the next section.[41]

Discrimination and Hostility

Regardless of the possibility that KS might be caused by an immune overload, the emerging climate would prove hostile to those who were outwardly identifiable as a 'threat' – in other words, those whose KS lesions rendered them visible to the community. In San Francisco, an early AIDS organization's hotline had apparently received calls about a man with a French accent having sex in the city's bathhouses and then telling his partners that he had gay cancer. According to Shilts, Dr Selma Dritz – an official at the city's public health department and another of his key interviewees – felt that 'it was one of the most repulsive things [she] had heard in her nearly forty years in public health'.[42] In a 1992 oral history interview, Dritz recalled an encounter with Dugas that Shilts would date to November 1982.

> I knew that Gaetan Dugas was still in town. I couldn't get to him, but I put word out, 'If you see Gaetan Dugas, let him know I want to see him'. He came up. I told him, 'Look, we've got proof now'. I didn't tell him how scientifically accurate the information was. It wasn't inaccurate, but it wasn't actually scientifically proven. I said, 'We've got proof that you've been infecting these other people. You've got AIDS, you know. We know it's transmissible now, because you're transmitting it'.

Dugas did not believe Dritz, and told her to mind her own business, and that he could do what he wanted with his body. She continued: "'Yes, but you're infecting other people". "I got it. Let them get it". I said, "You've got to cut it out!" "Screw you". He walked out. I never saw him again'. Dritz conceded that Dugas was only 'presumptive proof' that AIDS was 'transmissible from an infected person directly to the uninfected person'.[43]

Dugas thus reacted strongly to Dritz's attempts to overstate the current evidence for transmission. In addition, he was almost certainly influenced by the defiant articles published by gay activists in a number of periodicals. That month's issue of the left-wing periodical, *The Body Politic*, produced in Dugas's home base (at that time) of Toronto, contained articles cautioning against medical policing of sexuality, calling it 'a major setback' to the cause of gay liberation.[44] 'We must', wrote Michael Lynch, 'challenge the medical profession whenever it attempts to regain its power to define us, or to cloak a moral programme in medical terms'.[45] A friend of Dugas who knew him from Toronto and Vancouver emphasized this theme in a recent interview:

> I'm sure Gaétan heard it as ... telling him to stop being queer, okay, because at that time that's how most fags saw themselves, sucking dick and getting fucked is what made you queer and if you stopped doing that you might as well be a straight boy ... if he threw it back in their face that was what he was throwing back in their face, you know, 'No, I'm not going back in the closet for you, not for nothing'.[46]

Shilts writes of a 'stranger' threatening Dugas with violence on the streets of San Francisco in the fall of 1982, if he did not leave town, since he knew what Dugas was doing.[47] By this, it was implied that Dugas was the rumoured individual deliberately infecting others with his 'gay cancer' in the bathhouses. But how could a stranger know this, since he would be relying on – at best – second-hand information? It is difficult to determine how much, if any, Dugas's activities contributed to these rumours, or whether rumours simply stuck to Dugas more securely because of his visible KS.

It is also conceivable that the rumours in San Francisco were directly linked to the increased public education efforts in that city. In late July 1982 the Kaposi's Sarcoma Research and Education Foundation set up a telephone hotline and began printing informational brochures; by November it had distributed nearly 25,000 copies of the brochure, and the office continued to be 'barraged by phone calls and information requests'.[48] That month Conant praised the foundation's hotline and community forums, noting that these had 'met with excellent success and have been responsible for identifying patients with Kaposi's sarcoma'.[49] Of the approximately 450 callers to the hotline in October 1982, for example, approximately a quarter were referred on for medical screening; through this process, twelve patients with 'KS/AIDS' were identified in the first four months of the foundation's operations.[50] Conant may have been mistaken, however, when he added that the foundation's efforts had succeeded in 'allaying the fears and hysteria that is occurring in New York and which could so easily have occurred in San Francisco'.[51] The aggregation of the hotline's statistics into monthly totals, as well as a complete absence of any reference to problematic patients with KS in the organization's records from that period, prevent the interrogation of Conant's claim that the phones would ring whenever Dugas was in town.[52] It seems quite plausible that Dugas, not believing his KS to be contagious, would have been calm if asked by a sexual partner about one of his skin lesions. To someone in Dritz's or Conant's position at that time and convinced of the existence of a sexually transmissible agent causing AIDS and its opportunistic infections, such calmness might easily be interpreted as a cold-blooded act of malice.

Complexion and Disfigurement

In addition to the personal difficulties that visible lesions posed for a sexually active man like Dugas, professional challenges could also accompany a blemished complexion. The word 'complexion' has a long history, tracing its roots to ancient western ideas of humoralism and the balancing or mixture of constituent qualities within individuals. This balance of qualities determined their health and was intimately tied to their personal comportment, or temperament.[53] Over time the meaning of 'complexion' settled onto the skin, as this organ was seen to allow the most readily visible reading of the internal balance.[54] In a sense, then, the emphasis placed by airlines on the need for well-poised candidates to exhibit a clear complexion bears the trace of the time-worn connection between internal qualities and external appearance. Air Canada, like other airlines in an era of glamorized air travel, put considerable importance on flight attendants' appearances.[55] Applicants for the airline in 1977, for example, were meant to be 'attractive, natural, and spontaneous'.[56] In training programmes new employees were taught, among other skills, how to properly apply make-up and attend to personal grooming.[57] A contemporaneous guide for would-be applicants even suggested that for most employers skin problems would disqualify a candidate from consideration.[58] Another guidebook noted the imperative for healthy looking skin, informing the reader that interviewers for the airlines would value:

> *A clean, clear complexion.* Blemishes, heavy make-up, pock marks, or scars on face and neck are carefully noted by the interviewer. (Passengers may think that scars were the result of an air accident.) Excessive hair on arms and legs is also detrimental. On the other hand, a few freckles may actually enhance an applicant's appearance. Most important is a clean, natural-looking complexion.[59]

It is interesting to note how keenly the interviewers were attuned to the idea of 'reading' the skin, and particularly to the dangers of a false reading: that alarmed passengers might attribute marks on a flight attendant's skin to the dangers of air travel. Regardless of whether this was simply a weak justification to exclude candidates who did not meet an idealized standard of attractiveness, the importance placed on a healthy complexion is evident.

By Redford's recollection, Dugas had since his early twenties possessed 'shelves of creams and cosmetics'; even before his diagnosis with KS, Dugas placed considerable importance of the appearance of his skin.[60] Though he worked in an environment that placed a premium on youthful, healthy features, the quality of his complexion still stood out to his colleagues in a strikingly androgynous way. One female former co-worker recalled that Dugas was 'breathtakingly beautiful, not male-wise, not female-wise, but just the most gorgeous head of hair, [and] beautiful skin'.[61] Once sick, the appearance of a pigmented KS lesion on his face would no doubt have caused him distress. While Shilts wrote dismissively that Dugas had the lesion removed for vanity, the role of professional pressures for physical conformity ought not to be overlooked.

After he was dropped from Friedman-Kien's patient roster, Dugas continued to receive care from the dermatologist's colleague, Linda Laubenstein, an oncologist and haematologist. His obvious appreciation for her efforts in helping him to deal with his skin troubles was preserved in a small marble statue he had designed for her and which emerged in an auction over two decades after his death. The engraved message on the front of the smoothly rendered sculpture reads, 'Linda J. Laubenstein, M.D., Thank You, Gaetan Dugas, 1982'.[62] Notwithstanding the gratitude of patients like Dugas, physicians eventually realized that chemotherapy's benefits for KS were outweighed by the toll that the medication took on an already weakened immune system. Patients' skin would clear of lesions, but they would often die soon after from a more serious infection.[63]

Dugas's friend and Air Canada colleague, Richard Bisson, recalled that Dugas made an effort to put on a brave face:

> I knew what his situation was, he never looked, um, *ill* really, whenever I saw him, but I remember helping him with his make-up at one point and that was a funny kind of, um, encounter as well, I just said, you know, 'Your rouge is just a little too much here', so I, you know, brushed it off and saw that he was dealing with, what it would, what, what he needed to d-, deal with, with respect to how he looked once this had kind of taken over, and, ah, I didn't blame him at all for that, I thought, I mean everybody wants to present their best face.[64]

Indeed, by 1983 concealing make-up would be more widely promoted in the gay press for individuals with KS and other disfigurements, a practice that continued throughout the 1980s.[65] Noah Stewart, one of the men responsible for the community support efforts of AIDS Vancouver – the first Canadian group to organize in response to the disease – recalled the rumours that surrounded Dugas in Vancouver at the time that the flight attendant took up residence in that city:

that Gaétan was lurking in Stanley Park infecting people, uh, that Gaétan was dis-
guising himself, ... that Gaétan was teaching people how to disguise themselves, ...
ridiculous things ... it was a bunch of scared people making up stories. And I think
even they realized it.[66]

It would appear that Dugas's efforts to use make-up to mask facial lesions – a cop-
ing response adopted by many KS patients and later reproduced exactly in the film
Philadelphia – contributed to these rumours. The example suggests that when the
marks became publicly visible, some people felt strongly that masking them in
any way would constitute an act of lying, denying others valuable information for
establishing personal health risks. Contemporary health recommendations but-
tressed this position, recommending that gay men have sexual contact with fewer
partners and only 'healthy people'.[67] Determining the health status of prospective partners was, of course, a highly imprecise and ultimately unreliable process;
nonetheless, attempting to do so required vigilance for all possible signs of disease. While Dugas may have relied on applying concealer to put forward his 'best
face', many would have viewed this act as one of suspicious duplicity, one which
interfered with their ability to protect themselves from sickness.

Conclusion

The period between 1979 and 1983 was a highly uncertain time for gay men
diagnosed with Kaposi's sarcoma. These early patients faced much confusion as their condition, initially understood as 'only skin cancer', gradually
became absorbed within and overlain by the emerging diagnosis of AIDS and
its attached social meanings. Furthermore, their often highly visible lesions
allowed others in the gay community – and those outside – to mark them out
as dangerous, leaving them vulnerable to discrimination and intolerance. Their
sexual behaviour fell under intensified scrutiny and they found themselves
viewed fearfully as sources of disease.

Gaétan Dugas's experiences as a KS patient have also received a great deal of
scrutiny, particularly as a result of Randy Shilts's popular history of the American
epidemic and the media coverage it generated. Dugas resisted medical attempts
to restrain his sexual activity during the period when KS underwent its rapid
transformation from an indolent disease affecting old men to an aggressive, sexually transmissible infection. In doing so, he garnered accusations of sociopathy
and self-denial.

Rather than treat Dugas as an isolated case, a wilful spreader of disease, it has
been my argument that his experience can be more usefully seen as representative of the fear, uncertainty and confusion of a rapidly changing medical and
social landscape. His story suggests the limitations of denial as an explanatory
concept for such times of rapid change. It also demonstrates the multiple ways

in which skin markings – and attempts to reveal or conceal them – can be interpreted by sick individuals and those around them. As Dugas and others learned only too well during this period, KS increasingly became a visual metaphor for sexually transmitted disease. From this time onward, the condition's colourful lesions would be read more and more as stigmata, giving rise to competing efforts to see, diagnose and interpret the signs on the skin, while at the same time raising questions as to the processes – physiological and psychological – taking place beneath its surface.

9 'AN ALTERATION IN THE HUMAN COUNTENANCE': INOCULATION, VACCINATION AND THE FACE OF SMALLPOX IN THE AGE OF JENNER

Matthew L. Newsom Kerr

While rarely considered a 'skin' disease per se, smallpox has nearly always been seen as an imprintation of the skin. The story of smallpox contains two figures who visibly exhibited the disease: the pustuled sufferer and the pitted survivor. Its terrible symptoms and sequela were undeniably unique and practically universally recognizable. Robert John Thornton's description of smallpox in 1805 maintained that 'no disease ... presents a more melancholy scene'. Following the earliest symptoms of backache, intense fever and delirium, an eruption of pimples mature into pustules, which then ooze pus before sinking into depressions on the skin. These distinctive 'pocks' cluster on the face, neck and arms, and mark an individual as a smallpox sufferer. In severe cases, the 'human face divine, bereft of every human feature, then exhibits the most distressing sight, being one mass of corruption'. Often permanent, these seams and scars also identify the smallpox survivor. Fortunately, a single attack conferred immunity to the disease; if it had not, Thornton believed, 'the human race would have presented a frightful spectacle of corroded scars and mangled deformity, or, what is more probable, would have become extinct'.[1]

The competition between two medical responses to smallpox – inoculation and vaccination – underlines the complex interstices of skin and visuality. More than practically any other affliction, smallpox was consistently associated with the terrifying ability to see disease and to visualize infection. Its social meaning resided within practices of displaying the body and, in particular, the skin. It represented contagion inscribed in the flesh of the dangerous sufferer and immune survivor; written across the face, smallpox was shockingly and necessarily spectacular. Similarly, the medical and popular meanings of inoculation and vaccination also rested in large measure upon their visible imprint. Both procedures drew upon the perceived character of smallpox's inscription and its ability to transform skin into text. Yet the contest between inoculation and vaccination in the years around 1800 produced a potent representational dynamic: how the skin was displayed offers important clues to the ways medicine could construct the meaning of disease. Skin in this context provided a canvas of medical and body politics. The scope of this chapter is the intense debates that accompanied the brisk adoption of vaccination following Edward Jenner's publication of his cowpox experiments in 1798. The first section sketches how inoculation promoted an ocular tolerance for smallpox: an ambience of pustules and pits in which Britons found safety, normality and even comfort. This is followed by an exploration of how vaccination challenged and ultimately disrupted inoculation's visual regime of prevalence and display. Vaccine promoters prophesized that the cowpox would bestow a new face for Britain and humanity. Seeking to normalize the discrete visibility of the vaccine mark, the Jennerian movement proposed a new public face for smallpox as well. Not only was the introduction of vaccination a contentious episode in the history of medicine, it was also a decisive turning point in visual culture and representation of the body. Part of a larger polemical assault on inoculation and advocacy of vaccination, Thornton's terrifying vision of smallpox was just one position staked in a debate over the visual meaning of the disease, and one which would have been untenable just a few years earlier. Seeing smallpox, therefore, has a history – one inseparable from the practices of showing skin.

Smallpox once contributed heavily to the 'epidemic ambience' of everyday life. Early modern literature and letters frequently reference the appearance of smallpox sufferers in the streets of London and other towns. Samuel Pepys put a note upon this not entirely unusual event in his diary entry for 9 February 1688: 'hardly ever was remembered for such a season for the small-pox as these last two months have been, people being seen all up and down the streets newly come out after the small-pox'. By contrast, in 1751 Dr John Fothergill observed in the *Gentleman's Magazine* the prevailing mildness of that year's smallpox: 'Crowds of such whom we see daily in the streets without any other vestige than the remaining redness of a distinct pock'.[2] Smallpox was a most noticeable contribution to the popular phenomenology of epidemics. While symptoms of fevers and plague could prove murky, Fothergill maintained that smallpox was 'a disease which the most ignorant cannot easily mistake for another'.[3] The ease of detecting the smallpox sufferer was nearly matched by the ability to identify smallpox survivors. Seventeenth- and eighteenth-century journals regularly ran announcements concerning persons (often runaway slaves or wanted criminals) described as 'pock-marked', 'pock-pitted', 'pock-fretted', 'pock-holed', 'pit-marked' or 'full of pock-holes', as well as significantly suggestive ones securing a likeness by the lack of smallpox scars.[4] While admittedly anecdotal and impressionistic, these descriptions are valuable for revealing the rough contours of smallpox's public visibility. The immediacy and legacy of smallpox resided on the skin of Britons of all ranks and locales. Probably one-fourth to one-half of the population was visibly marked in some way by smallpox prior to 1800.

Smallpox's public profile was solidified upon the introduction of inoculation. Long practiced in Southwest Asia and India, this involved taking pus from the sores of a mild case and inserting it into a scratch in the skin of the inoculatee (usually on the upper arm). Subjected in this way to the *variola* virus, the patient suffered a bout of smallpox, but usually a much less serious and deadly one than if contracted 'naturally'. The story most often known in the West is that of Lady Mary Wortley Montagu introducing a variety of this 'variolization' to English high society from Constantinople in 1721. Smallpox via inoculation was occasionally fatal, and it was rarely inconsequential for the skin. Religious and moral objections arose for precisely these reasons, but they also reflect discomfort about deliberately injecting disease matter into the human body or opposing the providential allotment of disease.[5] Incredulous physicians warned that 'Inoculated Small Pox often leaves bad Consequences, as Consumptions, Boils, and Blotches, weak Eyes, etc. ... [and] may communicate other Distempers'.[6] Local practice varied, but inoculation gradually overcame these fears and became fairly widely performed after the mid-century among the well-to-do. Founded in 1746, the London Smallpox and Inoculation Hospital (LSIH) also provided the procedure gratis to the poor.[7] Meanwhile, using an improved regimen for those able to afford it, Robert Sutton claimed to have immunized 2,500 people between 1757 and 1768 without a single death; the Sutton family franchise of inoculators supposedly inoculated 55,000 people in 1767 alone, with only six deaths.[8] The 'Suttonian method' and its imitators solidified the assumption that inoculation must be far safer than the accidental and unplanned contraction of 'natural' smallpox.

Inoculation entered popular understanding as a technique whereby human ingenuity *domesticated* a natural scourge. Yet it was by no means a mild procedure, and could not be absent from the tell-tale signs of smallpox – inoculation *was* smallpox itself, after all. Around the conventional site of insertion in the upper arm, a cluster of pustules broke out. In even the best outcomes, inoculatees would usually have at least a few pockmarks on the face. Some unfortunate patients had pustules spread across their body and their lives imperilled. Nonetheless, while assuring stigmata of some sort, inoculation possessed much less chance of becoming visually stigmatizing than 'wild-caught' smallpox. Still, instead of erasing bodily marks altogether, inoculation etched them on skin that (with luck) may have otherwise avoided pockmarks altogether. Artificial implantation effectively ensured the sight of smallpox, although it was hailed as a more discrete bodily display. One pamphleteer wrote in 1779 that the inoculatee coming into society for air and recuperation and 'abroad in the street, obvious to the approach of every passenger', would be identifiable only by 'close examination'. The sufferer of natural smallpox whose 'miserable body ... is covered with indistinguishable millions', however, would emerge from the sickroom to 'walk the streets ... imprinted with alarming tokens of his dangerous condition, so visible and peculiar as to not be mistaken'.[9] Most believed that fewer pocks denoted reduced infectiousness.

Advertisements of successful 'pocky doctors' invariably praised inoculation's victory for beauty, often with sanguine assurances that smallpox via inoculation 'rarely leaves any ugly marks or scars'.[10] In contrast to these dubious claims, Daniel Sutton perhaps more honestly publicized that his patients had 'upon an Average, not more than twenty Pustules each'. He went on to emphasize that this was noteworthy 'particularly to the Fair Sex; as by this Method the Face is effectually prevented from being disfigured'.[11] At the very least, inoculation contributed to the perception of a general reduction in facial scarring. In his very popular play 'She Stoops to Conquer' (1773), Oliver Goldsmith has a hard-driving matron exclaim: 'I vow, since Inoculation began, there is no such thing to be seen as a plain woman. So one must dress a little particular, or one may escape in the crowd'. His was perhaps nothing more than an ironic poke at pronouncements like those of the poet William Lipscombe, in whose 'The Beneficial Effects of Inoculation' (1772) the procedure figures as a heavenly nymph conquering a trolling, ravishing monster. Montagu, in Lipscombe's hands, had been fired with 'Pure patriot zeal' to deliver this divine medicine, for 'Full well she knew when Beauty's charms decay'd / Britannia's drooping laurels soon would fade'.[12] As this suggests, the fanfare behind inoculation was intensely gendered. As Isobel Grundy notes, 'referring to men, [smallpox] spoke of the danger to life; referring to women, of the danger to beauty'.[13]

Over the course of the eighteenth century, smallpox assumed an air of inevitability. Otherwise, one might suppose, Britons would scarcely have countenanced an operation that deliberately fostered it. '[T]hough it may seem paradoxical', reasoned William Buchan, 'the artificial method of communicating the disease, could it be rendered universal, would amount to nearly the same thing as rooting it out'.[14] And so the most ardent inoculators dreamed of enthroning varioloid smallpox as the normative affliction imprinted upon *everyone*. Indeed, inoculation also indirectly actualized a new visual ambience. The procedure often took place with little effort to isolate patients during their active sickness and while they were still infectious.[15] Inoculatees could convey the smallpox in its worst forms until all scabs had fallen off. This was well known, yet Buchan remarked that he regularly saw begging parents conducting children covered with pustules and 'exposing them to public view' by the roadsides. He also noted it was 'very common in the environs of great towns to meet patients in the small-pox on the public walks' – a practice he suggested was calculated to suiting the purposes of 'boasting inoculators' (i.e. showing off the mild pocks of their practice).[16]

Negative commentaries remarked on this potential to make smallpox a common spectacle. When peddled amongst the wealthy, inoculation encouraged a callous disregard for the safety of others; smallpox was also dangerously distributed to the poor, who lacked the means to protect against its further spread. Scholars still debate whether inoculation lessened Britain's overall number of deaths from smallpox, but in making the disease more widespread, inoculation seems to have shifted the mortality burden to younger ages.[17] Toward the end of the century, urban children rarely escaped it. Sir Gilbert Blane contended that 'an adult person who has not had small-pox is scarcely to be met with or heard of'.[18] This manufactured ubiquity, however, also threatened to make inoculation a victim of its own success. John Haygarth, the influential Chester physician, despaired in 1793 that general inoculations by that time had met resistance from 'the lower classes of people [who] have no fear of the casual smallpox. Many more examples occurred of their wishes and endeavour to catch the infection, than to avoid it'.[19] Whether endemic in the cities or epidemic in the countryside, smallpox was no longer an unexpected intruder. This may help explain both why some persons gravitated toward inoculation and its guaranteed imprintation of the skin and also why many others increasingly shrugged off this 'medicine' and opted for the natural variety.

Inoculation thus moderated the visceral fear of the disease and helped to initiate a specific practice of bodily exhibitionism. Where inoculation was commonly resorted to and smallpox prevalent, remarked one physician at the end of the century, smallpox was 'scarcely so much dreaded, as the measles or scarlet fever'[20] (which is to say, not terribly dreaded). Inoculation's 'victory for beauty' really meant a heightened tolerance for relatively inconspicuous pustules and pockmarks. Indeed, the disease's scars had already become, in some respects and some circles, a desirable feature that served certain identifying functions. 'Unmarked' servants apparently had difficulty securing situations. Although this visible archive of disease history was disproportionally demanded of the working classes, it was probably similarly expected of physicians and surgeons.[21] Buchan most likely did not exaggerate much (although it was certainly in his interest as an inoculator to do so) when he stated that 'such as have not had the small-pox in the early period of life are not only rendered unhappy, but likewise in a great measure unfit for sustaining many of the most useful and important offices'.[22] Imperfect skin, then, stood as surety of one's innocuousness. The random (and hopefully slight) pattern of pockmarks could be a badge of immunity, an emblem that many people went through a rather arduous procedure to secure. So many sources remark upon inoculation's ability to make smallpox a common and courted spectacle that we should not assume that the disease held the same terrors at the end of the eighteenth century as it had earlier, or as it would once again possess in the age of vaccination.

Edward Jenner humbly admitted that his groundbreaking experiments with vaccination were inspired by a folk tradition about the renowned pretty skin of country milkmaids. They owed their ruddy complexions, so the saying went, to their accidental exposure to cowpox – a painful local infection that nonetheless somehow provided protection against the much more serious smallpox. In his famous 1798 pamphlet, Jenner contended that 'cowpox' sores indeed conferred the same immunity as a bout of smallpox itself, and that inoculation with cowpox matter (or *vaccinia*, hence 'vaccination') would therefore be a preferable alternative to inoculation with actual smallpox. Cowpox's peculiar merit over inoculation was that it was a mild infection that communicated no contagion, making it ideal for rapid, outpatient use. The first vaccinators were also struck by its clinical simplicity. Jenner's now iconic illustrations of *vaccinia* on his first subjects highlight the single sore which, unlike the smallpox, did not progress to an eruption (see Figure 9.1). The vaccine mark refigured inoculation's claims of universal prevention, and restated the means of smallpox's wholesale extermination. The *Edinburgh Review* observed: 'In inoculation, we only hunt the wild tygers with the tame ones, and therefore never can exterminate the breed. In vaccination, we run them down with other animals, and, with due exertions, may clear the country of them entirely'.[23] Cowpox suddenly challenged the permissiveness of smallpox and, by implication, the entire inoculating trade. It started by revolutionizing the way epidemics were displayed and read on the skin.

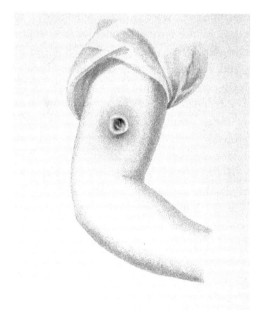

Figure 9.1: E. Jenner, *An Inquiry into the Causes and Effects of Variolae Vaccinae* (London, 1798), plate 2. Image reproduced courtesy of the Wellcome Library, London.

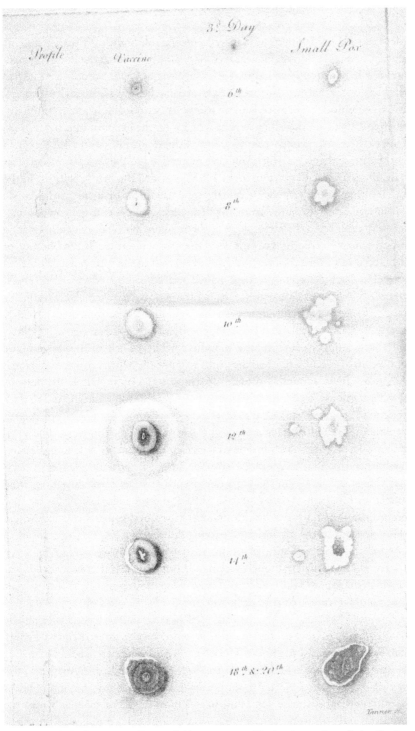

Figure 9.2: J. Redman Coxe, *Practical Observations on Vaccination: or Inoculation for the Cow-Pock* (Philadelphia, 1802), frontispiece. Image reproduced courtesy of the Stanford Medical History Center , at http://lane.stanford.edu/med-history/index.html.

Medical and popular illustration played a pivotal role in the early years of vaccine and the first repetitions of Jenner's method.[24] Dr Woodville at the London Smallpox and Inoculation Hospital started vaccinating in 1799, but only after he had tracked down a rare case of cowpox at a local dairy. Jenner's associates had nothing else to consult but a copy of Jenner's pamphlet, with its illustrations of the distinctive cowpox pustules they were to look for on the hands of infected milkers. One of these, Woodville wrote to Jenner, 'exhibited a more beautiful specimen of the disease than that which you have represented in the first plate'.[25] Incidentally, these trials with cowpox at the LSIH provided the first serious rift in the vaccine community. Woodville casually inoculated some patients with cowpox in one arm, smallpox in the other. Even patients who only received cowpox matter were exposed to the atmosphere of the smallpox hospital, evidently creating mixed cases with eruptions of pustules at the sites of insertion. The publication of detailed plates in the *Medical and Physical Journal* in the spring of 1799 fuelled suspicion that the hospital vaccinations had been contaminated with actual smallpox.[26] Apart from close experience, Jenner warned, 'we view our object through a mist'.[27] To combat any mis-impression the London cases had fomented, he widely distributed a set of coloured engravings demonstrating the proper visual difference between his vaccine and the 'spurious cowpock'. Dr Benjamin Waterhouse of Boston, Massachusetts, used the prints to guide the first vaccinations in North America. 'These admirably colored drawings, transcending all verbal description', Waterhouse wrote, 'have been highly serviceable to physicians and to their patients'. They 'demonstrated the *identity* of the distemper to the *eye* by pictures ... beyond the faintest shade of ambiguity'[28] (see Figure 9.2). This was a time when things were moving quickly for the young vaccine movement. Dr George Pearson established the London Vaccine Institution in 1799. Separately, Jenner's associates forged crucial ties in the most important networks of patronage, securing Jenner his first Parliamentary grant in 1802 and royal endorsement for the new procedure. The next year saw the founding of the Royal Jennerian Society, which was dedicated to the expansion of vaccination through several free stations in London and the distribution of vaccine virus worldwide.[29]

Almost immediately, though, vaccination occasioned a bitter propaganda war in which the skin was the loudest and most contentious broadsheet. Intransigent inoculators resented the rival technique and published cases of supposed failed immunity. Most memorably, the early anti-vaccinationists devised emotionally powerful tales of how deliberate infection with cowpox threatened the distinction between humans and brutes. Dr Benjamin Moseley, physician to the Chelsea Hospital, originated an effective trope of grotesque bodily disfigurement, suggesting that persons subjected to the bovine disease would grow fur, sprout horns or otherwise approximate 'John Bull' in an almost too literal manner. Under the delusions and transformations of the 'cow-mania', Moseley prophesied, an associated 'brood of minotaurs would overspread the land' and 'the british [*sic*] ladies *might* wander in the fields to receive the embraces of the bull'.[30] Vaccinations were opposed in some localities upon reports that cowpoxed persons 'bellowed like bulls'.[31] Anti-vaccine sentiment of a similar and stereotyped sort was expressed through sermons, public debate, graphic satires, plays and poems that prominently featured 'disgusting caricatures of mangy girls and oxfaced boys'.[32] Dr William Rowley of London, for example, infamously displayed specimens of 'beastly diseases' that had supposedly proliferated since the introduction of vaccination. In its first and momentous endorsement of vaccination in 1807, the Royal College of Physicians deprecated insinuations that vaccine matter 'produced various new diseases of frightful and monstrous appearances ... Representations of some of these have been exhibited in prints in a way to alarm the feelings of parents, and to infuse dread and apprehension into the minds of the uninformed'.[33] Jenner's London associate, William Blair, similarly denounced the prevalence of 'hand-bills, newspaper paragraphs, and degrading placards upon the dead walls of London' that mischievously depicted 'cow-manged' maidens and 'cornuted' old women.[34] The best-known fragment of this debate is undoubtedly James Gillray's 1802 graphic satire of vaccinations at the LSIH, which presents Jenner's followers in a less than favourable light, but also evidently delights in pouring comic ridicule upon fanciful warnings of cowpox-addled human monstrosities.[35] Vaccinators warned against the power of imagination, which was nearly the same thing as popular prejudice and optical illusion. John Coakley Lettsom insisted that skin itself would speak for vaccine; with the exhibition of cowpox, 'baseless vision will be dissolved, and the thick mists which exhibit frightful spectres will be dissipated by truth and plain sense'.[36]

This early contest over vaccination produced a spectacle of skin in which the meanings of illustration and inscription were desperately contested. The vaccine mark permanently marked skin with the unmistakable and verifiable sign of medical intervention. Jenner himself declared that the keenest arguments for or against the practice of vaccination would be '*those which are engraved with the point of the lancet*'[37] – a phrase in great use amongst the early vaccine supporters, and one pointing to the complex textual possibilities of skin at this time. Proof ultimately would be written in the pages of medical discourse, but truth would first be etched on skin. Discussions of smallpox had long been infused with printing metaphors. The disease 'imprinted' itself upon the sufferer, making skin the living, historical parchment of sickness. But vaccination was clearly a radical new inscription device. Vaccine matter, so to say, was the indelible ink which, imparted through a scratch, would testify to the artistry of the vaccinator. The skin consequently becomes the engraving plate by which medicine imprints the vaccinated subject. Smallpox inoculators, on the other hand, remained part of an older discourse in which nature was the engraver – disease imprinted itself upon the body, not the inoculator. Smallpox took a different form in each person, and the random and unpredictable pattern of the inoculation eruption signified the fundamentally unruly body. In inoculation, disease could be tamed by medicine (as in animal husbandry), but not redrawn or eliminated in its essence. The anti-vaccinator Rowley, for instance, attacked vaccine's innovations as 'artifice' that confounded the design of nature and presumed to place the 'vain conceits' of man against God's will. Vaccination was carried on by 'infatuated visionists and daring projectors'.[38]

Increasingly fierce and personal disputes between vaccinators and inocula-tors prompted allegations of bodily disfigurement and mischievous illusions. Vaccinators rushed to the representational technologies available. Their texts were obsessed with differential diagnosis, and meticulous descriptions and illustrations were more important than ever.[39] Almost without exception, every early treatise supportive of vaccination contained at least several pages filled with minute detail as to how to distinguish cowpox marks from smallpox. The contest with inoculation produced a quick proliferation of engravings, etchings and lithographs, some in relatively cheap editions that afforded a vivid con-trast between multiplicity of smallpox and the circumspectness of cowpox.[40] Such illustrations signify a protracted discourse upon the nature, meaning and appearance of pustules. Under different circumstances, they might warrant men-tion simply as visual aids in a dispute within clinical medicine. But given the extraordinary political importance of vaccination, the images themselves were heavy artillery in the battle taking place over skin. Vaccinators especially were keen to accentuate the legibility and representation of competing pustules. These second-order texts of skin were called upon to display evidence of suc-cess or failure and, equally important, clinical superiority. Followers of Jenner insisted that the cowpox only ever left one mark: a singular, highly characteristic pustule and resulting solitary scar on the upper arm (the conventional site of insertion continued from smallpox inoculation).

Detailed clinical observations by John Fisher are typical of the unblush-ing admiration for the skin's exhibition of *vaccinia*. The lancet insertion mark was 'distinguished by its beautifully circumscribed form' that was maintained throughout its progression, even after a central digression rose into a nearly geometrically perfect cone. Fisher was most impressed by its 'regularly circum-scribed form and rounded margin'; the smallpox inoculation, on the other hand, kept an 'irregular and angullated margin' with a 'globular' surface.[41] The cowpox pustule was sumptuously predictable: its singular mark characteristically rose to a peak resembling a nipple, after which the apex descended and a blushing, beau-tiful areola spread around the pulpy, concave, hardening cicatrix. Vaccinators' descriptive language coloured the vaccine's manner as erect and proud, com-pared to the shameful, slinking, blubbery nature of smallpox. Soon, they were arguing that cowpox never properly produced a 'pustule' at all. The description that eventually stuck was a vaccine 'vesicle'. Scabs too held a particular significance. That of the vaccine was again circular in form, thick and 'of a mahogany color'; the smallpox irregular and angulated, thin and 'a dark color throughout'. The scar left by vaccine was 'round and perfectly circumscribed'; those of smallpox asymmetrical, crooked and of course numerous.[42] Cowpox's attraction lay in its disciplined regularity, simplicity and predictable confinement to a single point on the skin (see Figure 9.3). Illustrations of this era typically place the succession of appearances in a straight line, implying an unvarying linear and sequential destiny from infancy, to maturity, to decline. The patient disappears, while the abstract notion of skin is further abstracted – it is temporally stretched to exhibit the archetypal life history of the vesicle. The ripening vaccine mark was visually enchanting. One commentator in 1805, observing its progression on successive days, remarked that 'the pustule looks charmingly'.[43]

The aesthetic superiority of cowpox was an important theme for the first vaccinators, but one that arose specifically out of the bitter contest with inoculation. Almost immediately this assessment of beautifully adorned skin started to stand on its own. In an anecdote appropriate to Jenner's Romantic age, Whig leader Charles Fox asks him, 'what is cowpox?' – to which Jenner reputedly replies: why it is nothing more than a section of pearl resting upon a rose petal.[44] Floral imagery had long held a place in smallpox imagery.[45] Vaccination called upon a more up-to-date language of natural beauty and the sublime. Jenner patronized the working-class poet, Robert Bloomfield, already famous in literary circles for his pastoral verse, and commissioned a work extolling the medical breakthrough. 'Good Tidings; or, News from the Farm' hails this medical breakthrough as the rustic salvation of the modern world:

> In ev'ry land, on beauty's lily arm,
> On infant softness, like a magic charm,
> Appear'd the gift that conquers as it goes;
> The dairy's boast, the simple, saving *Rose*![46]

The vaccination movement could in this way revisit the older gendered discourse on beauty and smallpox. Expressing again a patriotic concern for feminine attractiveness, Bloomfield predicted that under vaccination, 'Our boast, old Time himself shall not impair, / Of British maids pre-eminently fair'. He considered it a great 'conquest to insure / Our lilies spotless and our roses pure'.[47] Vaccine matter was thus drawn into the popular lexicon of flowers, medical botany and (by association) a specific appreciation of botanical illustration that stressed aesthetic wonder infused with sexual connotations. The vaccinating physician Robert John Thornton (already a well-known botanical illustrator with a taste for lavish depictions of pistils and stamens) insisted that 'female charms [were]

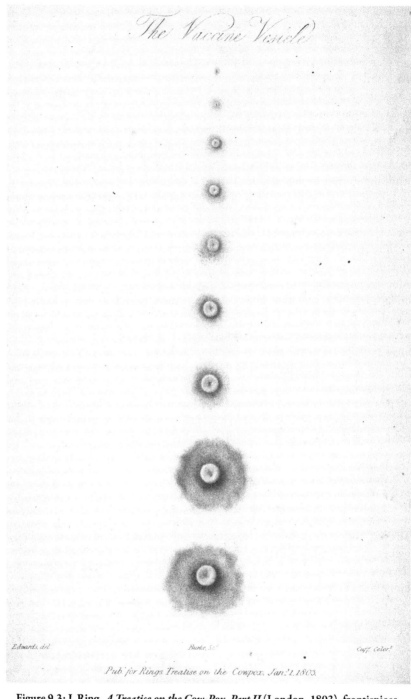

The Vaccine Vesicle

Edwards. del.   Burke. Sc.   Cuff. Color.

Pub: for Rings Treatise on the Cowpox, Jan.ʳ 1. 1803.

Figure 9.3: J. Ring, *A Treatise on the Cow-Pox, Part II* (London, 1803), frontispiece.
Image reproduced courtesy of the Wellcome Library, London.

destined by the ALMIGHTY as the zest of otherwise a vapid existence', and, therefore, all men must praise the *'Jennerian discovery*, which is never known to disfigure (as does the natural and inoculated small-pox) "the human face divine"'. His was a fulsome anti-Malthusian celebration of the passions that guarantee the continuation of the human race:

> [O]ften, at the very first glance, the soul takes fire, and soon after joins in holy bands of wedlock the two sexes, destined by PROVIDENCE to make each other happy. But, when the features are all changed, the nose drawn inward, a speck perhaps in both eyes, and horrid seams pervade the pallid cheek – the mind of sensibility revolts at the ruins of fair nature, and marriage is prevented, unless for the sake of sordid pelf![48]

One of Jenner's associates in London penned 'Vaccinia: Or, the Triumph of Beauty' in 1806.

> Behold creation yet more fair appear,
> The charming sex more lovely and more dear!
> And O! may Virtue yet conspicuous shine,
> Unite with Beauty, and enrich the mine!
> The feature varied, and the varied grace,
> Nought else distinct amongst the human race;
> The pleasing Lily and the glowing Rose,
> Shall rise victorious o'er its worst of foes!
>
> ... A world unspotted! what can be more great!
> Nothing, if crime is banish'd from each state.[49]

In striking contrast to the tolerance of pustules and scars fostered by inoculation, the early vaccinators now unleashed a surge of abhorrence at the least manifestation of smallpox. Moseley, who had warned of vaccine-derived 'bovine diseases', pleaded that 'Inoculation has disarmed the small-pox of its terrors'. Jenner's bulldog in London, John Ring, barked back that 'no care, no skill ever did, or ever can, tame that dreadful hydra – the small-pox!'[50] In the hands of vaccinators, clinical descriptions of smallpox assumed a tone of absolute hideousness, expressing a clear desire to cement a moral equivalence between the natural disease and the inoculated variety. For Ring, inoculated smallpox was invariably 'loathsome, infectious, painful, and sometimes fatal', but most importantly, its deformations were 'more deplorable as they were brought on by a voluntary act'. Vaccination, of course, was a 'blessing', 'scarcely deserv[ing] the name of a disease'.[51] Jenner now called the smallpox the 'speckled monster', and his followers ceased drawing contrasts between vaccination and inoculation – henceforth always simply comparing vaccine to smallpox. The visual nature of this invigorated intolerance is captured by the anonymous author of an 1807 pamphlet who identifies the practitioners of inoculation as 'the worshipers of the Small-Pox'. They were devotees to the Pethox Parvus, 'an idol or fiend, of great malignity'.

Only one thing moderated the fetish's fury: those who impulsively invited him were usually treated with less severity than those he casually encountered. Significantly, this fetish extended a nefarious visual enchantment over its acolytes: '[T]he multitude, habituated to the grim visage of Pethox Parvus, no longer fear him', while the demi-god vaccine 'though of the gentlest disposition startles by the novelty of his appearance'.[52] In this same vein, Bloomfield implores his countrymen to allow smallpox no quarter (clearly a condemnation of inoculation):

> Give not a foe dominion o'er your blood,
> Plant not a poison, e'en to bring forth good;
> For, woo the pest discreetly as you will,
> Deadly infection must attend him still.[53]

The success of vaccination, its supporters insisted, relied upon the complete rejection of the tolerant public ambience of smallpox that had been fostered by inoculation. Eruptive rashes had to become unsightly, and inoculators dishonourable. Early in the contest, vaccinators had argued that inoculation ultimately killed more Britons in the previous century than otherwise would have been struck down. Now, by keeping smallpox in constant public circulation, inoculators continued to impede the beneficial effects of vaccination.[54] William Wilberforce first petitioned Parliament in 1806 for an outright abolition of the procedure – less than a decade after Jenner's initial announcement and at a time when inoculation was still one of the most widely performed medical procedures in the country. Noticing that the Smallpox Hospital continued to perform inoculations on an outpatient basis for the poor, physicians at the forefront of the London vaccine movement burned with indignation that the law allowed 'loathsome masses of living corruption to be carried daily through the streets of London!!! So horrid an exercise of British liberty, in spreading a destructive plague at noon-day ... calls loudly indeed for legislative interference and restriction!!!'[55] (One should remember that these patients were ones that inoculators claimed were impregnated with only the mildest and most unnoticeable disease.)

After failing twice to advance a bill setting criminal penalties for reckless inoculation, the National Vaccine Establishment orchestrated a third, more ambitious proposal in 1813, citing 'the constant open exposure of those inoculated with the small-pox' as causing infection of great numbers. This too failed to persuade Parliament to impede a long-standing medical procedure, but the Commons debate did result in the suggestion that such exposure might be dealt with under common law prosecution.[56] In 1815 the National Vaccine Establishment brought charges before the King's Bench against a woman who exposed her child, covered with pustules, in the London streets after its inoculation. She was accused in the indictment of presenting a public nuisance (allegedly fostering the infection of eleven further individuals, of which eight died and another lost an eye). Significantly, the judges sustained the prosecution on an analogy to the ancient writ of *de leproso amovendo*, by which they cited precedent applying only to those 'who appeared to the sight of all men by their voice and *sores* to be lepers, and not for those infected with the disease, but not outwardly in their bodies'.[57] It had been illegal for lepers to mix in society, but only if the affliction was palpable on their skin. And so criminal 'exposure' was of a specifically visual sort. The case allowed the vaccination movement to draw a clear line of association between smallpox and leprosy (long redolent of ostracism), as well as between smallpox and plague (Stuart-era measures for quarantine and shutting-up of houses had also drawn upon *de leproso amovendo*). Another trial that year resulted in the conviction of a London apothecary who performed inoculations and sent his patients into the public highways. Inoculation itself was not ruled a nuisance, but responsibility for dangerous public exposure was laid firmly at the feet of the inoculating trade.[58] Significantly, for close to a century patients routinely neglected taking precautions directly after inoculation, and yet the first successful prosecutions for visible exposure appeared only in 1815. Law was called upon to sanction the newly emerging visual intolerance of the smallpox pustule. Vaccination had successfully rendered the public exhibition of small-poxed skin unwarranted and suddenly unlawful as well.

While the gathering consensus in favour of vaccination in elite medical circles generated a push to reshape the visual meaning of smallpox, it also aimed to establish the vaccine mark as an icon of health and purity. Thornton was just one among many in exuberantly predicting that in 'a few years, most probably', smallpox would be annihilated by vaccination – an accomplishment that would enshrine 'the cow-pox, like St. George and the Dragon, [as] the proudest emblazonment in the British heraldry'.[59] Although not literally figuring on coats of arms, vaccination was often popularly represented in the rhetoric of taking and bearing arms. Jenner's young friend, John Dawes Worgan, poetically deployed this imagery in a celebration of his patron; the spirit of 'Compassion' equips the great man with a weapon to pacify the demon:

> Straight in his hand a steely point she plac'd,
> With matchless pow'rs and guardian virtues grac'd,
> And said: 'With THIS yon SPECKLED FIEND disarm
> With THIS, Contagion's rav'nous fury charm...'

Worgan and others found extensive play on 'arms' irresistible, especially in vaccination's great contrast to the devastation of the Napoleonic Wars:

> ... smiling Peace her olive-branch displays,
> And faltering infants lisp their Guardian's praise,
> As on their arms the sov'reign shield they show,
> Whose heav'nly powers repel th' ERUPTIVE FOE

With mystic charm extend the fleeting breath,
And blunt the direst of the shafts of death.

... And future ages, wondering as they read
Of woes, which once the SPECKLED FIEND decreed,
Shall bless that arm by gracious Heav'n design'd
T' avert the deadly scourge of human kind.[60]

Jenner's peaceful arm, in short, armed the lancet; children too are armed once their arms bear the talisman that will disarm the enemy. In this pacifist rhetoric of martial prowess, the vaccine was both lance and shield.

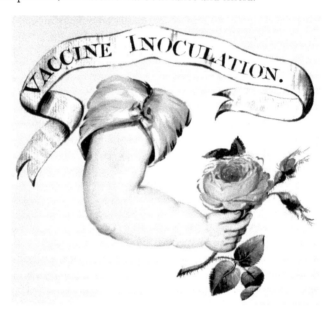

Figure 9.4: Watercolour inserted in Benjamin Waterhouse's copy of E. Jenner, *The Origin of the Vaccine Inoculation* (London, 1801). Image reproduced courtesy of the Harvard Medical Library in the Francis A. Countway Library of Medicine.

The fashionable icon of the bared vaccinated arm represents an early example of the expansion of medical illustration into the realm of popular health propaganda and contains unambiguous references to the place of vaccination within a restructured landscape of clinical aesthetics (see Figure 9.4). Skin bears (bares) a crucial symbol, verifies the bill of immunity and openly flaunts the vaccine scar (or cicatrix), which was comparatively no display of a blemish at all. Further, this vaccine iconography reverses the visual economy of inoculation: one mark is more valuable than many. Partially undressed, it suggests that the exhibition of the vaccination mark must be a deliberate act; vaccinated skin exhibits a 'proud emblazonment'. The anonymous subject is genderless and characterless, and so it stands in for all (white) humanity. The inclusion of a rose bloom is certainly no incidental embellishment, either, but stands for 'vaccine' itself. Plus, the flower doubles the vaccine mark's characterization as 'ornament'. The icon served another role, too. The bared arm was a means of imagining and imaging the absence of smallpox. The rest of the arm's skin is a blank space, a meaningful lack of scars: an embedded criticism of inoculation, to be sure. Crucially, it is a picture of what is and what is to remain; and so the inscribed, vaccinated skin also sketches an imminent history of what everyone will have lost.

Early vaccine proponents' discourse regarding the skin of arms ultimately directed attention toward facial skin. In the medical economics of the body, the small token on the upper arm purchased a body free of 'poxy' blemishes. Faces were thereby 'armed' against smallpox. And indeed, early vaccine enthusiasm involved picturing what the face of humanity would look like upon the banishment of the disease's pustules and pits. Jenner's achievement was therefore at its heart an epic story of universal facial reconstruction. The Reverend Dr Booker, addressing the Third Festival of the Royal Jennerian Society (held each year on Jenner's birthday) in 1805, toasted 'the greatest of human benefactors':

> surrounded whenever he walks on the peopled globe, with monuments to his fame, far more valuable than those of marble or gold, – *living* monuments, fashioned by 'The Divine Hand,' – with manly vigour unimpaired, – with female loveliness undespoiled of those charms which a desolating pest has so long made its prey, – with a race of beings now but little lower than the Angels, and enabled, through the aids of Revelation, to rise to an equality with those exalted intelligences in the regions of immortality and glory![61]

The disease's purported disappearance immediately emerged as a popular trope that anticipated a new visual regime. Vaccine was to annul the epidemic ambiance that had structured smallpox's optical meaning in the era of pervasive inoculation. For example, the National Vaccine Establishment's report for 1822 appealed 'confidently to all who frequent the theatres and crowded assemblies, to admit that they do not discover in the rising generation any longer that disfigurement of the human face, which was obvious every where some years since'.[62] Subsequent reports were hardly less enthusiastic.[63] A vicar in the parish of Great Missendon who himself performed the procedure wrote about his village's vaccination in 1824: 'I never saw a set of more clear-skinned and healthy looking people either before or since in any part of the kingdom'.[64] A crucial aspect in smallpox's evolving visual meaning in the vaccination era was, therefore, precisely the disease's purported disappearance, its lapse into public invisibility. While it left its mark, vaccine was also an absence that will have been etched onto the skin of humanity, specifically the facial skin. The vaccine-armed lancet could be conceived as an eraser, inscribing a lack that was going to be perfectly visible, noticeable and beautiful. Whether or not primarily aided by the propaganda of vaccinators, the theme quickly achieved a stereotyped form of expression, fashionably musing upon how vaccine had already propelled 'an alteration ... in the human countenance'.[65] The anonymous author of *The Art of Beauty* instructed readers on how to read the emerging facial environment: '[Vaccination's] triumphs are gloriously emblazoned on the thousands of smooth faces now seen on our streets, that have, within the last twenty years, taken the place of those whose finest features and blooming complexions were marred by the small-pox'.[66] Indeed, vaccination foresaw a glorious spectacle of disappearance laid out across the skin. Its public expression would be smooth faces (defined as both a lack and a presence) that reflected the influence of the discrete vaccine scar on the upper arm. The face was to become the greatest ornament to the vaccinated arm.

This chapter has sketched a part of the visual politics of skin in the era of Jenner. Upon the arrival of vaccination, skin was re-imagined as a text upon which were written entirely new messages about visibility, exhibition, beauty and safety. Medicine abruptly rethought the marks and inscriptions that composed diseased skin. For its early proponents, vaccine shaped expectations of bodily presentation, representation and circulation in the public sphere. Cowpox revolutionized the visuality of smallpox. Vaccinators successfully prompted a greatly changed climate for governing the ambience of epidemics, essentially sponsoring a new regime of visible disease intolerance. Skin after Jenner was to be simultaneously spectacular and discrete, but in both senses carrying a message about medical inscription. Moreover, part of the skin's new burden was to be haunted by an ever more shadowy spectre of smallpox. As distance increased from the inoculation period, smallpox itself and its traces simply became less seen, and smallpox became a much more terrifying disease. Disgust was re-inscribed into smallpox; it became more startling in proportion to its scarcity. That discursive restructuring of smallpox was negotiated in the early years of vaccination and rested upon a rhetoric of affected skin that the vaccinators found crucial to their agenda. Vaccination, therefore, fundamentally changed how smallpox and the skin were seen.

10 PORTRAYING SKIN DISEASE: ROBERT CARSWELL'S DERMATOLOGICAL WATERCOLOURS

Mechthild Fend

One of the more remarkable nineteenth-century images of a pathological condition represents a woman reclining in a half-upright position, supported by pillows and covered in white clothes and a sheet (see Figure 10.1). When we focus on the upper left section of the watercolour, she seems quite comfortable in her bed despite her very visible skin condition. Her emotionless face does not betray signs of pain or itching; as her eyes do not engage with the viewer, she seems absent and self-contained. The draughtsman, on the other hand, must have looked attentively at his object of study. The question is of where exactly this particular draughtsman, Robert Carswell, a Scottish pathologist studying morbid phenomena in Paris, directed his attention, and what precisely was the object of his study: a sick person or the visual manifestations of smallpox?

What the image confronts us with is a face covered with pustules – an uneven pattern of rash in white colour spread over a reddish ground, suggesting inflamed skin. A scarf wound around the head frames the face, laying bare the symptoms. But this garment is not merely a means of directing focus on the skin disease: a curl escapes from underneath the hair-dress, forming an apparently superfluous but healthy decorous element. Furthermore the draughtsman spared no effort, giving the scarf a stripy pattern and carefully rendering the knot with which it is bound. The inclusion of such figurative elements that distract from the focus of a medical illustration can be explained in various ways. One might argue that the minute depiction of the three-dimensional run of the pattern on a folded piece of fabric works as a means to prove the skills of a draughtsman, and serves as a reference of accuracy in a domain where it can be attested even by a laymen or by the specialist who has not seen this particular condition live.

At the same time, the attention to dress and individual facial features can be interpreted as a reality effect, a way of suggesting that we are looking at an actual sick person. The portrait-like representation of the head nourishes our desire to see the image as a manifestation of an emphatic relation between doctor and patient. I certainly assume that Carswell made his watercolours while looking at the phenomena depicted, and this made – in the case of dermatological conditions observed on a living person – the two hours or so of facing the suffering a fairly long and intense interaction, during which draughtsman and patient might have even engaged in conversation. But this is not recorded, and it does not mean that the resulting image brings us today any closer to a historical patient (a term, by the way, that at least the early nineteenth-century dermatologists I am concerned with never used). If we – and I am judging from my own initial responses and from the responses I witnessed when showing such images to others – experience empathy with the diseased figures, it says more about our relationship with images and in particular with depictions of the human face than about any person represented, or, for that matter, about any potential empathy nineteenth-century draughtsmen and doctors might have had for the sick they were observing. This relation to the image of a face is largely determined by conventions of modern portraiture (certainly in place by the time these images were produced), according to which likeness is understood as a means to render an individual's character and personality.

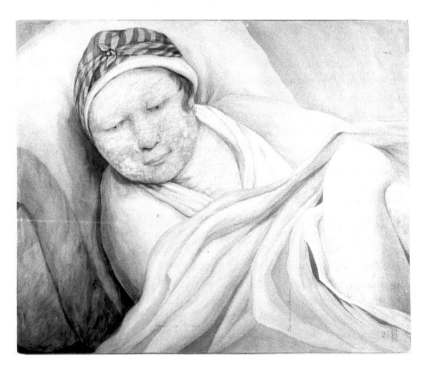

Figure 10.1: R. Carswell, 'Variola and Psoriasis' (1829). University College London Collections, Fd 353; image reproduced by kind permission of UCL Library Special Collections.

There are elements in this image that suggest that we should not see it as a regular portrait in the above sense. First of all, the inscriptions – here as in the other dermatological drawings – name the disease and not the person. And in order to disturb even more the assumption that this might be the portrait of an individual patient tucked in their bed, two conditions are listed: 'variola and psoriasis'. Does the image represent a person with both afflictions, or is it a conflation of two cases? The latter solution is quite unlikely within the conventions of portraiture, but not within those of dermatological illustration. The formal arrangement of the drawing suggests that this might in fact be a composite image, reuniting distinct conditions. The two areas of the body, each featuring a condition, are explicitly separated via the piece of white cloth bundled between trunk and legs. This split is emphasized by the double inscription of the conditions positioned at different angles, which makes it uncertain whether one is supposed to hold and behold the drawing vertically or horizontally. Or are the users invited to turn the picture depending on the body part and symptoms in focus? It seems as if several conflicting tendencies of dermatological illustrations were conflated in this image: a more portrait-like depiction of the head and torso of a woman suffering from smallpox, and the use of a more diagrammatic style in the rendering of the legs, displaying the symptoms of psoriasis.

This ambivalence might be explained by arguing for a simple clash of different cultures of representation – medical illustrations on the one hand and artistic portraiture on the other – or the conflicting representational modes of British and French early nineteenth-century dermatology. While these are important aspects to be further discussed, they are also indications of an uneasy relationship between body and disease in early nineteenth-century dermatological illustrations of both French and British origins. If historians of nineteenth-century French medicine as diverse as Michel Foucault and Erwin Ackerknecht have argued that clinical observation resulted in a focus on the disease and an indifference towards the diseased,[1] then dermatological images complicate that split, as they are precisely within this uneasy relationship. Their purpose is certainly to portray a disease rather than a patient; but the 'carrier of the disease',[2] in the sense of both the body displaying a disease and the sheet of paper on which an image is printed or drawn, does not always remain indifferent.

Collecting Clinical Pictures in France

Robert Carswell, a Scottish physician drawing pathological phenomena in France, bridged the traditions of French and British medicine. Born in 1793 in Paisley, Carswell received his initial medical training in Glasgow, where he was singled out for his drawing skills at an early age. He subsequently moved to Edinburgh to work with John Thomson, a military surgeon and holder of the first Chair of Pathology in Edinburgh, for whom Carswell produced drawings illustrating morbid anatomy. Thomson generally encouraged his students to pursue further studies in France, and eventually sent Carswell, along with one of his sons, to Paris and Lyon. Their mission was not only to study and critically assess clinical practices in French hospitals, such as the Hôtel-Dieu at Lyon (where they stayed between 1823 and 1824), but, most importantly, to record the medical cases they saw by the means of drawings and to collect a set of pathological illustrations that could be used by John Thomson for his teaching back in Edinburgh. Carswell was particularly dedicated to the endeavour and developed a focused interest in pathology, thus also demonstrating the dense interconnection of clinical medicine and pathology during the early nineteenth century.[3]

Carswell remained faithful to the practice of studying and recording pathological formations by drawing them. Even after proposing himself as Chair of Pathological Anatomy at the University of London (from 1836 onwards University College London), a post he finally held between 1831 and 1840, he continued his visual studies of morbid anatomy in Paris, producing a remarkable number of pathological images, mainly between 1827 and 1831; more than a thousand watercolours and ink drawings dating from this period are preserved in UCL Special Collections today.[4] Even if this fund constituted his entire production during the period, he would have produced several drawings a week. In parallel to drawing, Carswell kept notes, which occasionally match the case delineated in watercolour and record some details about a sick person's circumstances. With few exceptions, however (one of which will be considered later on), they remain sparse in comparison with the images, and there are far more drawings than written case notes, suggesting that Carswell's predominant mode of medical observation and documentation was with a pencil or brush in his hand – studying, understanding and defining a phenomenon by drawing it. Only a small portion of the drawings was later used to illustrate his *Pathological Anatomy: Illustrations of the Elementary Forms of Disease*, published in 1838. The predominant purpose for making those images was, therefore, not necessarily the production of a medical atlas. Drawing was to some extent a means in itself, as it was a mode of observation, a tool for studying pathological morphologies. At the same time, it was a way of producing an archive of pathological conditions that would eventually be used for teaching. Signs of usage indicate that the pictures have indeed been extensively handled, and many of them were hole-punched at their upper margins in order to be hung or displayed. In a letter to the University of London Council written in December 1827, Carswell offered himself as a candidate for a future Chair of Pathological Anatomy by advertising the teaching collection he would bring:

For several years my whole time has been spent in the study of Pathological Anatomy. The want of sufficient opportunities at home, induced me to fix my residence abroad, where I have been employed collecting in hospitals the necessary materials for the illustration of a course of lectures in this branch of medicine. I soon found ... that museums formed by great industry and labour and at much expense, fall far short of the object which they were intended to fulfil. A diseased organ kept in spirits loses almost all those characters which enable us to distinguish diseases ...

It is indeed obvious that some other mode of illustrating organic diseases should be adopted, the want of which is strongly felt by the student & the teacher. Such a desideratum I have been endeavouring to supply by coloured delineations, drawn by myself, from recent diseases. Long persuaded that a museum formed of delineations such as I possess, together with diseased organs preserved in spirits, and accurate histories of each individual case, would furnish a collection of materials, without which it would be impossible to teach Pathological Anatomy as it ought to be ... The number of delineations which I have already made is considerable, but by no means sufficient either for the illustration of lectures or publication. To complete my collection, two years at least will be required, during which period it is my intention to remain on the Continent.[5]

Comparing the drawings with preserved specimens, he emphasizes the precision of his images: while diseased organs preserved in fluids tend to fade and even deteriorate, Carswell advertises his 'coloured delineations' as much more apt to retain the characteristics of a disease.

Within the UCL corpus of drawings, there are approximately sixty images focusing on lesions of the skin. Almost all were carried out between 1828 and 1830 in various Parisian hospitals, among these most importantly the Hôpital Saint-Louis, a clinic specializing in the treatment of cutaneous diseases, where twenty-one drawings were made.[6]

It was far from unusual during the period following the end of the Napoleonic Wars that medical practitioners (students as much as professionals) from Britain, other European countries and North America would go on pilgrimages to France. Paris was considered the major medical centre at the time, and the re-organization of hospitals and medical education instituted during the French Revolution and its aftermath had turned the hospitals into sites of clinical observation and teaching. The lure of Paris medicine for foreign students and doctors lay in the prospects of practical experience at both the bedside and the dissecting table, along with access to hospitals with large numbers of patients and the possibilities of conducting autopsies. Furthermore, private clinical instruction complemented the ward rounds by famous professors, and lectures gave additional access to anatomical dissection, surgery and induction to diagnostic techniques.[7] A recently published diary of an Edinburgh medical student, who in 1834–5 spent eight months in the French capital, gives a detailed account of the routine of 'Walking the Paris Hospitals',[8] and so provides some idea of the daily life Carswell might have had as a medical draughtsman. The Edinburgh student typically visited one, sometimes two, of the many Parisian hospitals a day, among them the Hôpital Saint- Louis, which he considers 'an excellent institution'.[9] He followed a physician or surgeon on their ward rounds, and listened to lectures on specialist subjects. As the related entries suggest, the interest was equally not in the patients but in noteworthy cases, the medical attention being focused on the appearance of the disease as visible to the naked eye. Although Carswell was no longer a student when producing the drawings for his future teaching, he toured the same hospitals as the diarist, always in search of new, interesting cases and drawings to be made either of living patients or of morbid organs observed at autopsies. However, as the dating of his watercolours shows (besides including the month of their production, he usually indicated the name of the pathological condition and the hospital), his method was more systematic. There were periods during which he predominantly worked in one hospital, and most of the drawings produced at the Hôpital Saint-Louis, for example, carry the date of June or July 1830.

Besides the sheer number of hospitals and the sick people attending them, the specialization of certain hospitals constituted a further attraction of Paris medicine, and the Hôpital Saint-Louis was a particular case in point. Initially built in the early seventeenth century on the outskirts of Paris for the isolation of the plague-stricken and people with other contagious diseases in periods of epidemics, by the end of the eighteenth century it had become part of one of Paris's newly developed outer districts, the Faubourg du Temple, and was turned into a general hospital. In the aftermath of the French Revolution, it was transformed into the first clinic predominantly dedicated to the cure and study of cutaneous diseases. Jean-Louis Alibert, who worked there since 1801 and founded the dermatological school of the hospital, was well aware of its significance. His first major publication, *Description des maladies de la peau observées à l'hôpital Saint-Louis* (1806), a lavish folio atlas with fifty-two illustrations, highlights within its title the centrality of this particular hospital as a site of dermatological observation. In the volume's preliminary section, Alibert promotes the hospital as the best place to study skin diseases in Europe, stressing the advantages of the clinic for medical study:

> Placed in a theatre where the diseases incessantly show and revolve, I could better than anybody else unravel the confusion introduced in the work of the ancients. I was able to follow the course, the periods, the decline, the recrudescence, the metamorphoses of the diverse exanthemata. It is in the hospitals that their characteristic traits pronounce themselves with more evidence and energy, as one contemplates them in all their periods of existence.[10]

In his later *Monographie des dermatoses* (1832), Alibert makes the hospital's mission even more explicit. A 'note on the hôpital Saint-Louis' is accompanied by a print with a view of the hospital, with 'Urbi et Orbi' written over it. The motto 'for the city and for the universe' not only refers to the pope's Easter and Christmas blessing, but was also an inscription often found in hospitals since the early modern times, or, as Alibert himself recalls, in asylums consecrating themselves to the relief of the poor.[11] With this reference, Alibert makes the claim that the hospital will cure the sick of all ranks and countries as well as to bring dermatological wisdom from Paris to the world, as he praises his hospital as a unique site for dermatological research, attracting physicians from all nationalities.

Alibert describes the hospital as a theatrical space that offers a continuous display of a large variety of morbid appearances in constant transformation.[12] The anonymous Scottish diarist mentioned earlier equally seems to have adopted such a view, for he praises the specialist hospital for 'collecting' all 'forms of psoriasis in the various stages', thus perceiving the clinic as an archive of living specimens. For Alibert, it is as if this physical and performative space in itself transformed the phenomena into images, since the dermatologist moves to using the language of visual representation when speaking of the 'characteristic traits' of diseases 'pronouncing themselves'. The hospital as theatre of maladies is both an architectural and an epistemological space in which diseases become visible as images. The dermatological clinic in particular is a space setting up a specific realm of visibility, rather than inducing a 'medical gaze', a notion that Foucault developed in his *Birth of the Clinic*, but later denounced.[13] It was within this space that Carswell observed, studied and illustrated skin conditions.

Dermatology as Surface Scrutiny and the Education of the Eye

Dermatological illustrations of skin diseases form a special group among images depicting pathological conditions: rather than studying morbid organs after dissection, they mostly result from the visual engagement with living patients, hence the portrait-like appeal of many of them. They represent diseases that are, according to Alibert, themselves still alive and that manifest themselves on the human body's outermost organ.[14] During the first half of the nineteenth century, skin diseases were defined by their appearance on the surface of the body and thus comprised conditions (such as syphilis) no longer classified as such today. Accordingly, diagnosis was predominantly made on the basis of visual observation and surface scrutiny, until the development of bacteriology and virology later in the nineteenth century allowed clinicians and practitioners to contemplate different ways to account for the nature and causes of skin diseases. If there was thus a dominance of visual observation in nineteenth-century medicine, then dermatology seems to be the paradigmatic discipline within that regime of the eye. Images were a medium and instrument intimately linked to these observational practices, and their production and use were indispensable for the formation of dermatology as a discipline. All personalities considered today as the founders of dermatology in Europe distinguished themselves through the production of sumptuous atlases: Robert Willan first published his richly illustrated *Description and Treatment of Cutaneous Diseases* in 1798–1808 in London, and Jean-Louis Alibert produced a series of folio atlases, beginning with his aforementioned 1806 *Description*. All volumes included colour illustrations – at the time hand-coloured engravings – as the subtle and exact use of colour was, in these prints as much as in Carswell's watercolours, crucial for the exact visual definition of symptoms. Visual autopsy was the main instrument for the production of knowledge, and doctors and draughtsmen made their observations mainly with the naked eye rather than with optical instruments (such as microscopes) mediating human vision, since the original size of phenomena was a crucial diagnostic element. Correspondingly, the illustrations were intentionally life-size, allowing Alibert's large-format atlases to represent the head, hand and most other body parts along with the symptoms to be depicted more or less to scale, while the illustrators of Willan's smaller atlas made efforts to represent at least the individual lesions in their typical size.

The significance of visual diagnosis and the use of images provided common ground between the English and French schools of dermatology, despite disagreements in other areas. At the beginning of the nineteenth century, the two schools disaccorded mainly with respect to terminology and to the taxonomy of the skin's lesions, and this despite the fact that both relied on classification systems largely based on those of eighteenth-century natural history.[15] Alibert is especially outspoken about the extent to which he is indebted to Linnaeus and botany in general for the ordering of dermatological phenomena, insisting at the same time that classifications and denominations came to him artlessly, claiming that 'this nomenclature ... formed naturally in my mind to the same degree that the field of observation expanded in front of me'.[16] Moreover, he insisted on the holistic nature of the clinical picture, an entity that accorded to what he called 'natural nosography'.[17]

Despite this alleged natural relationship between words and what they signify, the images in his atlas, although drawing on the portrait genre, do not represent individuals at one moment in time. They do not necessarily refer to a sick individual or even a specific case history, but represent, more generally, a version of a disease discussed in the corresponding chapter. The diseases are mostly represented in what Lorraine Daston and Peter Galison have labelled their 'characteristic' form. Distinguishing between different ways in which medical and natural history atlases of the late eighteenth and early nineteenth century related to the natural phenomena represented and tried to establish what was then mostly called 'truth to nature', they note:

> Atlases of 'characteristic images' can be seen as a hybrid of the idealizing and naturalizing modes: although an individual object (rather than imagined composite or corrected ideal) is depicted, it is made to stand for a whole class of similar objects. It is

no accident that pathological atlases were among the first to use characteristic images, for neither the *Typus* of the 'pure phenomenon' nor the ideal, with its venerable associations with health and normality, could properly encompass the diseased organ.[18]

Dermatological atlases shared this representational problem with all nineteenth-century pathological illustrations that had to abstract to some extent from the infinite variety of pathological appearances in order to produce images that stood for the generic disease, but could be matched with the individual case. Alibert himself addressed this issue in the preliminaries of his 1806 atlas, where he highlights the difficulty of grasping a phenomenon as unstable as a disease in a static image:

> The brush of the painter will trace each of these exanthemata faithfully, the way each of them exists as soon as it reached its perfect state, and it will only have to decline and decrease. I will imitate the exact Botanist who doesn't represent the flower just for our curiosity, but when it is in full bloom and all the parts of the fructification are formed.[19]

The problem faced by the illustrator of botanical or pathological phenomena alike is that he has to capture an object in permanent transformation, and he is meant to solve this problem by representing the object at its peak, thus delivering a characteristic image of a plant or disease. What Alibert wanted his illustrators to capture was a characteristic 'clinical picture'.[20] Although not using this term himself, Alibert adhered to the notion of disease as an entity that gained coherence by being understood as an image.

In contrast to Alibert and the grouping of diseases on the basis of elementary lesions, Willan was less concerned with the perfect clinical picture of a disease in 'full bloom', and more with the accuracy with which the individual symptoms were rendered and named. Neither words nor images seem to come to him naturally, and although he relied on illustrations, Willan did not believe in their self-explanatory value:

> In order to convey distinct ideas of the subject, I shall elucidate every genus by coloured engravings representing some of its most striking varieties. This method is new, and will be attended with many advantages; though at the same time subject to a variety of imperfections. Such drawings cannot sufficiently represent the various degrees of opacity and clearness in Pustules or Vesicles; nor the quantity or quality of the matter discharged from superficial ulcerations: nor can they extend to every minute circumstance in the course of a disease, being usually taken at their acmè. The engravings, as auxiliaries to the verbal description, will, however, be found useful in exhibiting the number, form, size and colour of the Papulae, Pustules, Tubercles, Spots, &c. appearances which cannot always be clearly communicated in words.[21]

Verbal and visual descriptions need to assist each other, and Willan consequently begins with 'definitions' in which he matches words and images.[22] He first defines isolated lesions such as *scurf, scale,* or *papulae* in words that correspond to illustrations represented on a single page filled with small fields, each dedicated to the depiction of one symptom on non-textured, flat beige ground. The *papulae*, for example, are represented in three clusters of reddish dots in various sizes, shaded slightly to indicate an elevation. Despite Willan's claims that images are only auxiliaries and that certain qualities such as the translucency of blisters are hard to render in engravings, in his *Cutaneous Diseases* the descriptions of basic symptoms and those of particular diseases gain their precision through the images. Only names, descriptions and images in conjunction enable visual education, teaching the eye what to look for and how to discriminate phenomena. And only the distribution of images of individual symptoms ascertains, along with the nomenclature, that they are always called by the same name, thus allowing for the standardization of medical language and observation. The subsequent descriptions and delineations of skin conditions (which are general accounts of the characteristics of a disease, rather than deriving from case notes as in Alibert's atlases) take up the initial verbal and visual definitions, and only make sense in relation to them. A page with two images referring to three different types of *Strophulus*, for example, features in the upper section the head and trunk of a baby with the symptoms of what is colloquially called 'tooth rash', and in the lower a small child's arm divided by an abstracted fold into two segments carrying *papulae*. Those on the upper arm closely resemble the *papulae* circumscribed in the definitions, while the lower arm shows what Willan describes as 'circular patches, or clusters of papulae'.[23] A physician using this atlas could have referred to the 'definitions' to visually identify and correctly name a symptom and associate it with a certain condition by both reading the text and by consulting the images, in order to recognize the way symptoms cluster and the body parts on which they typically occur. If Willan's text describes *Scrophulus confertus* as 'An eruption of numerous Papulæ, varying in their size, appears on different parts of the body in infants, during dentition, and has thence been denominated the Tooth Rash',[24] the image is as generic as this verbal account and does not pretend to refer to a specific case. It is not an individual baby observed at a particular moment, and the hand directed towards the mouth rather didactically points to the cause of the symptoms, the dentition.

Willan and Alibert and their respective draughtsmen thus have distinct approaches to the visualization of skin diseases. Alibert's atlases present themselves as collections of diseases observed at the Hôpital Saint-Louis. The portrait-style illustrations[25] suggest that they derive from looking at individual patients, even though they tend to conflate several cases, idealize physical features and emphasize certain elements of the pathological condition in order to render it more 'characteristic'. Despite the differences, however, Alibert's and Willan's dermatologies share their dependency on images and the associated challenge of matching the visual and the verbal, as well as the challenge of managing the transition between observation, delineation and verbal account.

Be that as it may, by the time Carswell came to study skin diseases in Paris, the distinction between the two schools had become less clear-cut. Swiss-born Laurent-Théodore Biett, a student of Alibert who later became leading physician of the St Louis, had become acquainted with the classification scheme of Willan and his successor Thomas Bateman during a trip to London in 1816, and introduced it thereafter in France.[26] The 1828 *Abrégé pratique des maladies de la peau* lauds it, despite some shortcomings, as the best existing system and takes up Willan's distinction between eight types of skin lesions.[27] In 1826–7 Pierre-François Rayer, a physician then working at the Hôpital Saint-Antoine in Paris, had already published a tract on skin diseases in which he adopted not only the nomenclature and associated classification system of the British dermatologists, but also the image concept of the isolated symptom on flat surface.[28] The distinctive feature of this publication is that it renounced portrait-like representations entirely, and referred to the human body, if at all, only in the form of segments: noses, eyes or nails indicating the typical location of the lesion. The largely even-sized compartments come in assemblages of four to ten units, with the charts as a whole having a highly decorative appeal despite their topic, turning the symptoms into a pattern on the skin. Equally attractive as the large-sized atlases, they were compiled as a small-sized book that was not only more affordable but also easy to transport, especially when the section with images was bound separately.[29] Such a book could have assisted the observation and description of an individual case with a symptom chart and matching nomenclature for reference.

Carswell's delineations of cutaneous diseases combine elements of both pictorial strategies. At times Carswell drew the full clinical picture in portrait-style images that share many characteristics with the illustrations for Alibert's atlases. In other watercolours, he employed small compartments to isolate individual symptoms. In one case, several drawings are assembled like a stripe on a single sheet of paper, forming a list of individual, yet segregated, symptoms (see Figure 10.2). Inscriptions in pencil name them as 'pimples, pustules, scales, macula' and so forth. Unlike Carswell's drawn case studies, this sheet is not dated, but it makes sense to assume that Carswell produced it at the outset of his visual concern with skin diseases, taking previous symptom charts as his model, in order to fabricate his own reference system. Such a reference made it easier to be consistent in the use of certain hues of watercolour for the rendering of specific symptoms, and to match a visual account of a distinctive morbid phenomenon with its name.

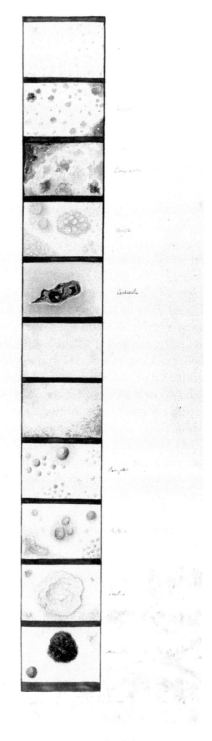

Figure 10.2: R. Carswell, 'Skin. Various eruptions' ([n.d.]). University College London
Collections, Fd 830; image reproduced by kind permission of
UCL Library Special Collections.

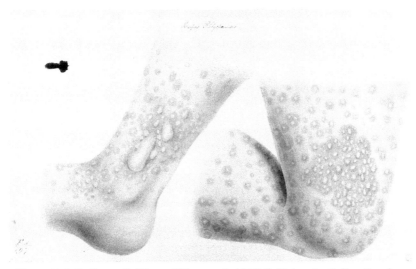

**Figure 10.3: R. Carswell, 'Herpes Phlyctanodes' (1826). University College London
Collections, Fd 197; image reproduced by kind permission of
UCL Library Special Collections.**

In another of Carswell's watercolours, drawn at the Hôtel-Dieu in April 1826
and representing a case of *Herpes phlyctanodes*, the focus is equally on the appearance and distribution of one particular symptom. Rather than elaborating on
any details of a sick person's dress and/or their situation in a sickbed, as in the
drawing of the 'variola and psoriasis' case discussed at the outset of this chapter,
this image concentrates on a lower leg and heel on the left side of one rectangular
sheet, and a knee with parts of a thigh and shank on the right (see Figure 10.3).
The depicted body parts are discontinued without the use of draperies or other
pictorial devices that conceal cuts in many medical illustrations, but drain off
at their margins into the foggy white ground of the image. Without evoking an
actual encounter with a sick person by means of anecdotal detail, this drawing
suggests that it was a product of an acute observation made in sight of a live phenomenon. It focuses on certain affected limbs while fading out (without visual
comment) anything outside the medial attention at the moment of observation.
In contrast, the related log book entry, one of Carswell's most elaborate case
notes, reports some details about this patient's life conditions prior to his entry
into the hospital and gives a sense of temporality as it recounts the development
and cure of the disease. The latter also indicates that Carswell followed this man's
case over a period of time, and that the report must have been finished later than
the initial 'at present' when the man's condition was at its peak and image made:

> James Peter, aged 30, married shoemaker, of middle stature, stout black complexion,
> entered Hotel Dieu the 30th April 1826 – Lives exterior to the City during summer,
> and at home in winter – manner of living very irregular, subject to privations – some-
> times eating little, at other times much – not given to drinking – says he has often
> had little pimples around the knee – [?] is at present (2nd May) 15 days since he fell

unwell previous to which, his health was good – He has then [?] very severe – Ophthalmia – coughed and expectorated a great deal for the first time – this began on 13th
April. Got acquainted with a woman at the 23 – with whom he passed the night [?]
On the following Wednesday and Thursday, thirst, violent itching, and on making
water slight pain in the extremity of the urethra. Scratched himself a great deal – on
the morning following says he observed a great many pimples of a red colour, which
he says [?] became larger – On Friday & Saturday fever – on the day of entry gonorrhoea torments him much – Entry – Pulse regular – tongue swollen as well as the lips,
which are covered with a thick black crust – this however is only on the mucous part
– thirst mouth pain [?] as well as the throat – cough – sound of chest good – mucous
rale – expectoration [?] vicious resembling the white of an egg – says he had had
since yesterday morning nausea – violent ophthalmia, particularly of the left eye, and
which began previous to the gonorrhoea, abundant [?] – the palphebral and ocular
conjunction is highly inflamed – red as scarlet and thickened – burning pain –

The skin presents first on the face on the cheeks two or three red elevations, slightly
elevated above the skin – five or six on the front – they are round, the epidermis slightly
raised, the largest, has about the diameter of a fiver, red, of a dull hue – on the anterior
and lateral part of the neck, there are from 30 to 35 spots varying in extent, the largest
having the size of a sixpence, the smaller rather larger than the bites of a flea & similar
in colour – these patches are felt to be elevated above the surface of the skin. Some of
them are smooth whilst others, even the smallest, have a central elevation formed by the
epidermis – this elevation is not transparent, but the epidermis is whitish – very few
on the breast and belly, from 20 to 30 of each – some of them round, others irregularly
oval – the most of them present an evaluation at the centre, some of which contain a
yellowish serosity – the epidermis is entirely separated from the cutis in a few of them,
which elevation has evidently followed the redness – nearly a hundred of these patches
are seen on the back and the lumbar region – chiefly on the latter – these, as the others
disappear or prefuse – few of them are no larger as a sixpence

Left leg – almost covered with red patches, almost all of which are surmounted
by phlygtena or bullae of the size of a pea – The anterior and inferior part of the
thigh presents a red surface about the size of the palm of the hand studded as it were
with phlygtena of a size of a pea, placed near each other and resembling entirely herpes phlygtenodes, filled with a yellow fluid. On the leg they are numerous separated
presenting [?] on the [?] there is an extensive red surface, here covered with small
vessels – there a larger bullae filled with serosity occupied the one half of it – the
mal exter. presents also a red surface covered by phlyctaenae of different sizes, but
in general small – Right inferior extremity – thigh resembling much the other leg,
nearly the same also on the internal malleolus 3, 4 or 5 of large bullae, filled with
yellow serosity, irregular – …

Left the Hospital towards the end of the month quite well.[30]

The first and second parts of the case description – quoted here almost entirely –
are quite distinct. Carswell's initial paragraph takes a narrative approach which is
very similar to Alibert's case descriptions: it recounts James Peter's circumstances
and the development of his disease, obviously following – for the period before
his entry into the hospital – Peter's own specifications upon being questioned by
a medic. The details about the man's habits match with what Alibert singles out as

the prime causes for skin diseases in his 1806 *Description*: poor or unhealthy diet, irregular intake of food and an unsteady lifestyle associated with, among other things, working conditions.[31] Contagion comes only as number seven of potential causes, well after climate or lack of hygiene, and is, in Carswell's case note, rather alluded to by mention of Peter's sexual encounter with a woman, which precipitated the itching – an episode that is recounted in a neutral, non-moralizing tone. Moreover, Carswell's description of the patient's general condition, beginning with his complexion and stature, results from a close examination by sight and touch.

The second part, on the other hand, has a tone of its own and reflects the particular focus of the drawing pathologist. It minutely describes the appearance of the disease: the location, size, number and colour of the individual eruptions were obviously recorded after close inspection of the entire body. In the passage referring to the legs, the focus of the language is the same as that of the drawing: the large number of 'red patches ... surmounted by ... bullae of the size of a pea' are patiently recorded, and Carswell visibly took pains to suggest elevations and their different degree of transparency via the use of light shading. Furthermore, he attempted to render both the individual blisters and the red patch roughly the size of a palm visible on the thigh precisely to scale. At this point of concentration, the visual and verbal recording of the observed symptoms seamlessly blend into the diagnosis: 'The anterior and inferior part of the thigh presents a red surface about the size of the palm of the hand studded as it were with phlygtena of a size of a pea, placed near each other and resembling entirely herpes phlygtenodes'. Visual and verbal descriptions coalesce and fall into place when they match with a disease already known. This interplay confirms the inextricable relationship between 'seeing and knowing', between the 'visible and the legible' characteristic, according to Foucault, of the nineteenth-century clinic. This observation certainly applies to dermatology. With its dependency on surface scrutiny and the concern with nomination and classification, the discipline relied on the coordination of observation and enunciation. As much as the table (*tableau*) that Foucault talks about in this context, the dermatological atlas integrates 'into a structure that is at the same time visible and legible, spatial and verbal, that which is perceived on the surface of the body by the clinician's eye and that is heard by the clinician in the essential language of the disease'.[32] Carswell opens up a similar space of words and images, when delineating the disease and making notes, and later on by using the watercolours for teaching, showing and speaking simultaneously. He initially notices the same thing in writing as in drawing, due to the trust in the immediacy of the visual observation and recording, as well as the belief in the possibility of a 'faithful description'.[33]

The focused point of view taken up particularly in Carswell's drawing of a case of *Herpes phlyctanodes* disregards the sick person in favour of a fragment of the body almost flattened into a surface, turning the disease into a pattern on the surface of the body and of the sheet of paper. This disregard for the sick subject, however, does not mean that the doctors did not regard them. It might be worth in this respect to return to the French term 'regard' originally used by Foucault, a term that can designate both an attentive look and a concern.[34] As Jacyna has argued for Alibert, if there was a medical gaze in the nineteenth century, it was certainly not clinical in the sense of being cool or detached. Alibert, for example, shows himself as terrified by the manifestations of diseases he had to face. In a remarkable passage from his 1806 atlas, he argues for the use of images not only because of their potential to produce evidence, but also for their emotional impact:

> In order to imprint a seal of authenticity upon what I have written, to augment the energy and power of my discourses, to perpetuate and animate, as it were, all my descriptions (tableaux), I have felt it necessary to have recourse to the ingenious contrivances of the paintbrush and of the engraver's needle. I have wished to reinforce the impression by the physical image of the objects that I want to offer to the contemplation of the pathologist; finally, I desired, by means of the terrifying colours [couleurs effrayantes] of the painter, to instruct, so to speak vision by vision ... to strike the senses of my readers, and to reproduce vividly before them the various phenomena that have surprised my eyes.[35]

Alibert declares himself affected by the affections he saw both in the sick subjects themselves and on the images, for it is not always clear whether he talks about persons or images – the sight of both seems to provoke the same emotional response. Particularly striking is his expression 'the terrifying colours of the painter', which seems like a displacement of the terrifying diseases stressing at the same time the fact that colours are significant in order to convincingly render pathological symptoms.

It is well known that one of the most feared conditions was smallpox, a killer disease that was widespread at the time. Alibert, who was among those promoting vaccination as a form of prevention, deemed it dreadful not only because of the physical suffering it caused, but also due to the potential disfigurement of the face, something explored in detail in Matthew Newsom Kerr's contribution to this volume. A person with a face entirely covered by the signs of smallpox was drawn by Carswell in the watercolour discussed at the outset, and a very similar looking (or possibly even the same) case was published in Alibert's 1833 *Clinique de l'hôpital Saint-Louis*.[36] Alibert explicitly discusses the disfiguring effects in his description of 'Variole Confluente' (Conflating Variola):

> But when the eruption is at its apogee, the eyes and the lids are horribly swollen, the face reaches this extraordinary puffiness that effaces all the traits of the physiognomy; it is no more than a masque the colour of which is white like mother of pearl.[37]

In the eyes of Alibert, such an extreme stage of smallpox led the physiognomy of a person to disappear. It thus takes away the legibility of the face, the potential for expressing emotions as well as the link between appearance and character that was at the heart of eighteenth- and early nineteenth-century physiognomy. Considering that the rendering of the characteristic traits of a person was widely regarded as the aim of portraiture at the time, one might argue that the disease dismantled the idea of physiognomic portraiture as much as it distorted the face. What comes to the fore instead is what Alibert, appropriating the language of physiognomy and portraiture for pathology, calls the characteristic traits of the disease.

At the same time, there is in Alibert's description of variola, a remarkable conflation of terror and beauty, transported likewise in the print presenting the shape that once was a face, framed by a headscarf and some curls, resting peacefully and expressionless on a pillow. The pustules, which Alibert associates with pearls, lay on the surface covering the face as if unable to harm the flesh underneath. There is both in the language and in the pictorial strategies of the image an attempt to ease the condition. Some images, among both Carswell's watercolours and the illustrations for Alibert's atlas, engage (wittingly or not) with the horrible sight and seem not fully disciplined by the regime of focused medical observation. Especially those images showing the head and bust of a sick person often include details of clothing and bedding, and frequently render the pattern of a fabric with particular care. 'Syphilide Pustuleuse en Grappe', from Alibert's description, is one example.[38] The pustules are distributed in clusters over the otherwise smooth skin, and attention is drawn away by the diverse chequered patterns of the blue and white scarf wrapped around the woman's head. In Carswell's 'Variola and Psoriasis' and in a watercolour representing a case of lupus (see Figure 10.4), morbid symptoms are balanced with the pattern of a fabric. The woman with lupus is represented both in profile and frontally, with a body part – an open mouth – placed between the two views, lending the image as a whole, to some extent, a diagrammatic character. The frontal view pushes the face to the foreground, flattening it as much as the disease has bereaved the face of its relief by aggressing the nose, an effect of lupus that seems to be the main purpose for unusually including a second view in profile. What pulls both the body and the image into the surface is simultaneously what points most clearly to the fact that this condition is not at all a surface phenomenon. This is even more apparent with the fragment of the open mouth, an orifice opening an abyss in the picture plane and granting an uneasy view into an undefined depth of the body where the disease has intruded the flesh. The chequered scarf around the neck of the woman takes up this fickle relationship between flatness and depth, abstraction and embodiment: a pattern *per se* is a flat pictorial element, but folded, as the patterned fabric is in this case, it has a three-dimensionality and hides some parts from plain view. It is thus tied to the skin condition, an element also enhanced by the use of the same colours for the rendering of the lesion and the chequered scarf. This choice of the same colours also gives the watercolour an aesthetic balance that certainly exceeds the mere task of documenting a pathological phenomenon.

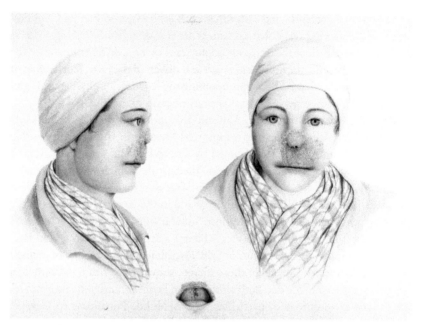

Figure 10.4: R. Carswell, 'Lupus' (1829). University College London Collections, Fd 358; image reproduced by kind permission of UCL Library Special Collections.

It is a moment when the medical eye goes astray and becomes attentive to a pattern other than that of a rash, spending as much time with the rendering of a striped scarf as with the signs of lupus. In those cases, the eye-catching pattern diverts attention from the disease while keeping it within the image. It serves as a formal balancing device that eases the pain of looking at the image (while simultaneously attesting to it) by making the symptoms themselves look like a pattern. These apparently random accessories are not so much a reference to the genre of the portrait, but rather a different kind of symptom, indicating that even the likes of Robert Carswell were sometimes affected by what they saw and sought pictorial strategies to avoid getting sick of delineating morbid phenomena.

11 ATAVISTIC MARKS AND RISKY PRACTICES: THE TATTOO IN MEDICO-LEGAL DEBATE, 1850–1950

Gemma Angel

The history of the tattoo in Western civilization has received sporadic and incomplete scholarly attention going back as far as the first century AD, according to some sources. Writing in 1869, the French naval surgeon Ernest Berchon cites a number of early works on methods of tattoo removal, of which Archigenes (AD 97) appears the earliest.[1] Indeed, if it were not for the researches of medical professionals and criminologists from the mid-nineteenth century onwards, the history of tattooing in Europe and North America during this period would be considerably more opaque.[2] The sudden effusion of publications in medical, military and criminological journals from c. 1850 into the early twentieth century reveals the emergence of strong scholarly interest in tattooing. These studies focused predominantly upon typically segregated social milieux – the hospital, barracks and prison – contexts that provided ample opportunity for research to be carried out amongst isolated populations. Occasionally, they also analysed tattoos of colonized peoples. But they mainly concerned tattoos of soldiers or sailors, or else of social 'deviants' – prostitutes, criminals or those whose reckless behaviour led them to a clinic for treatment.

Whilst there was often overlap between disciplinary fields, particularly within the developing disciplines of criminology or forensic science and the medical sciences, it is important to note the distinctions between discourses emerging from different geographical locations. For instance, historian Jane Caplan has pointed out that whilst there was a great deal of interest in the tattoo in continental European criminological debate, this preoccupation did not extend across the channel to Britain. She writes that 'not only was British criminology relatively dissociated from the continental schools, but tattooing was sufficiently normalized that it attracted virtually no official or scholarly attention.'[3] It is not surprising, then, that the first professional tattooists to establish successful trades and international reputations in the later nineteenth century were British and American. Whether their success was enabled by the lack of a socially pathologizing discourse in the UK and USA, or their sheer visibility within popular culture precluded the development of such discourses, is difficult to establish. However, a survey of the contemporary British and American medical literature reveals that there was some concern for the public health risks associated with tattooing – particularly in the transmission of infectious diseases such as syphilis and tuberculosis.

Although they follow different intellectual trajectories in differing national contexts, interesting analogies between criminological and medical studies of tattooing provide useful narrative linkages to trace the history of the European and American tattoo. In particular, an analysis of the visual material gathered by criminologists and doctors suggests an intriguing congruence in conceptual formulations centring around the visual nature of their objects of study – tattooed skin and skin disease, respectively. In what follows, I will explore some of the similarities in the pictorial strategies employed by criminologists and medical researchers alike in their pursuit of standardized knowledge objects – the criminal and the disease, respectively. I will then move on to consider the complex relationship between medical and folk knowledge of tattooing as health benefit or health risk, and the surprising ways in which these opposing epistemological formulations interacted and were variously taken up by tattooists and medical professionals alike.

Criminological Perspectives on Tattoos: Atavism and Degeneration

With the emergence of the 'new' criminology in continental Europe during the 1880s, tattoos developed a particular significance for researchers concerned with identifying reliable signs of criminality within their populations. The antecedent 'classical school' of criminology, or penology, came under criticism from the new 'positive' school, which challenged the prior emphasis on the nexus of legal code, criminal act and penalty.[4] The classical school's formulation proposed a 'typology of crimes', which Italian lawyer and sociologist Enrico Ferri termed a 'juridical anatomy' of deeds. This was rejected by the positive school in favour of a typology of criminals, which sought epistemological grounding in the scientific measurement of 'dangerous bodies' and the construction of an 'anatomy of deviance'.[5] According to this new discourse, 'Crime [became] a "risk" that human scientists proposed to manage through knowledge of statistical laws and a new attention to the bodies of the criminal'.[6] Citing Cesare Lombroso, the most famous criminologist of the positive school in his day, historical anthropologist David Horn puts his finger on two central aspects of the new discipline's approach: 'Numbers had shown crime to be "an unfortunate natural production, a form of disease, which demanded treatment and isolation rather than penalty and vendetta"'.[7]

The analogy drawn here between criminality and disease is intriguing: according to Lombroso and his contemporaries, criminality was a pathology located *within* the criminal body, revealed only by the forensic specialist who employed the appropriate statistical tools to access the truth within. Moreover, the signs of latent criminality lay on the body's surface, in much the same way that the morphology of cutaneous skin infections revealed evidence of underlying disease. Various physical features, from skull measurements to peculiarities of the ear and anomalies of the palm, were scrutinized by criminologists when constructing taxonomies of deviance. However, of all of the supposed outward signifiers of atavism, tattoos seemed to hold a particular fascination. Tattooing was at this time frequently associated with the 'primitive' body and art of the 'savage' Other,[8] familiar through both colonial experience and public displays of natives in fairs and anthropological exhibits.[9] The apparent popularity of tattooing amongst certain groups within European society was viewed by some as a dangerous regression or sign of degeneration.[10] In his essay 'The Savage Origin of Tattooing', which appeared in *Popular Science Monthly* in April 1869, Lombroso condemned the 'fashion' amongst 'prominent society ladies' of London in no uncertain terms:

> Tattooing is the true writing of savages, their first registry of civil condition ... Nothing is more natural than to see a usage so widespread among savages and prehistoric peoples reappear in classes which, as the deep-sea bottoms retain the same temperature, have preserved the customs and superstitions ... of the primitive peoples, and who have, like them, violent passions, a blunted sensibility, a puerile vanity, long-standing habits of inaction, and very often nudity. There, indeed among savages are the principal models of this curious custom.[11]

Thus Lombroso translates the 'savage' character of the foreign tattooed 'Other' into the criminal nature of the tattooed European. This view is representative of the Italian school of criminology in particular, which proclaimed the 'inborn' nature of criminality and emphasized the atavistic. However, *fin de siècle* scholars throughout Europe advanced similar ideas on tattooing and criminality. Much of the continental debate revolved around the relative popularity of the concepts of atavism and degeneration in the explication of theories of criminality. The French school, championed by physician and forensic scientist Alexandre Lacassagne, advanced the theory of *dégénérescence*, which highlighted the social etiology of crime. For Lacassagne and his followers, it was the *milieu social* which was the determining factor in criminal behaviour: 'The social milieu is the breeding ground of criminality; the germ is the criminal, an element which has no importance until the day where it finds the broth which makes it ferment'.[12]

The criminological preoccupation with tattoos may be elucidated through a consideration of two factors pertaining to the peculiar nature of the tattoo itself: firstly, the tattoo mark occupies a peculiar boundary, both physiologically and socio-culturally. It appears at the body surface, but is suspended indelibly *within* the flesh; as Julie Fleming writes, 'lodged on the border between inside and outside, the tattoo occupies the no-place of abjection'.[13] Thus embodying an internal-external dichotomy paralleled in the new criminological formulation of atavistic character and stigmatized body, the tattoo may be viewed as the ultimate symbol of abjection in the context of nineteenth-century criminological discourse – a self-imposed stigmata which scholars themselves found both abhorrent and irresistible. Moreover, as a socially *acquired* yet permanent physical mark, the tattoo seems to articulate something about the relationship between social atavism and corporeal 'degeneration', which, we will see, influenced discussions linking tattooing and skin disease.

The criminological study of tattoos produced an effusion of drawings taken directly from the skin of prison inmates, as well as soldiers and sailors in barracks – all conveniently isolated populations accessible to researchers. Tattoos were categorized according to their symbolism, and motivations read in turn from the symbols; they could signify desire for vengeance, group allegiance, whether regimental or criminal organization, vanity, imitation or idleness. Moreover, their crude 'hieroglyphic' style read as evidence of the primitive writing of the criminal. As Lombroso succinctly put it, the study of tattoos 'serve a psychological purpose, in enabling us to discern the obscurer sides of the criminal's soul'.[14] They also provided reliable, self-selecting evidence of social pathology. Thus the second aspect of the new disciplinary approach is revealed in a shift away from 'penalty and vendetta', which focused punishment upon the body, and towards 'treatment and isolation', which sought to manage the 'criminal soul'.[15] The newly developing technologies of power-knowledge, which read, interpreted and categorized the surface signs of the body, isolated these characteristics in their data in a process parallel to the isolation of criminals themselves, in prisons and asylums.

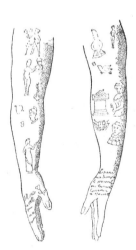

Figure 11.1: Ink drawing, 'Arms of a Criminal whose Whole Body was More or Less Tattooed', in H. H. Ellis, *The Criminal* (London: Walter Scott Ltd, 1895), p. 102. Image reproduced courtesy of the Wellcome Library, London.

Figure 11.1 is exemplary of the kind of visual data gathered by criminologists. Reproduced in the second edition of Henry Havelock Ellis's *The Criminal* (1895), a drawing of two disembodied arms float on a flat, featureless ground, with numerous tattooed figures decorating each limb. The primary purpose of the image is to illustrate the distribution and relative coverage of tattoos over the arms of an anonymous criminal. In this case, the tattoos are not as significant in isolation as in their cumulative effect, and indeed the claim was made that the extent of a criminal's tattoos often marked him out from his non-criminal tattooed contemporaries, such as sailors and ordinary working-class men.[16] Havelock Ellis followed the pictorial conventions evident in Lombroso's *L'uomo delinquente*; the isolation of the arms in the pictorial space, their abruptly ending delineation and the almost complete two-dimensionality of the image has the effect of conceptually abstracting the tattoo from the three-dimensionality of the body. This abstraction made it possible to devise a visual taxonomy, which in turn facilitated the shift away from the 'anatomy of crime' and towards the 'anatomy of the criminal' that the positive school advocated.

Interestingly, this pictorial strategy paralleled dermatological imagery of the nineteenth century. Figure 10.3 in Fend's chapter shows an 1826 watercolour and pencil drawing of two isolated segments of a leg afflicted with an outbreak of *Herpes phlyctanodes*. The artist, Robert Carswell, took care to paint only the afflicted body part, the legs appearing like neatly dissected specimens, fading at the margins, while the patient becomes generic and the disease is afforded greater specificity. As Fend demonstrates, this visual strategy facilitated the development of dermatology as an independent discipline in the nineteenth century. The creation of 'characteristic morphologies', which could be used for comparison and diagnosis – much like those explored in Stark's chapter – allowed physicians to perceive diseases as discrete entities, whilst implementing a degree of standardization. This was particularly important in the case of the 'Great Imitators' such as syphilis and tuberculosis, whose visual symptoms and effects could easily be misread and misdiagnosed prior to the development of microbial testing.

Whilst the tattoo was mobilized as a kind of socio-pathological signifier within the context of continental European criminology, medical professionals across the channel and the Atlantic turned their attention to the question of tattooing as a factor in disease transmission. In one context, the tattoo was re-coded as social disorder; in another, it appeared as corporeal malaise.

Medical Reports on Tattoos: Risk and the Inoculation of Disease

One of the earliest sources to link disease transmission and tattooing is M. F. Hutin's 'Recherches sur les Tatouages', published in 1853. He relates the case of a tattooed soldier, allegedly a virgin, who had been admitted to the Hôpital du Val de Grâce with syphilis. His tattooist was apparently to blame; as the tattoo ink dried, he re-moistened it using his saliva. With needle thus loaded with ink and *Spirochaetaceae*, the unfortunate soldier was simultaneously tattooed and inoculated with syphilis. The resulting infection was so severe, Hutin relates, that the arm almost required amputation.[17] Hutin shows that French doctors took an interest in the possibilities of disease transmission through tattooing, as did their German counterparts. Nevertheless, criminologists continue to dominate continental discourses on tattooing through the later nineteenth century. The relative absence of criminological debates in Britain and America, in contrast, invites further investigation of medical reports on inoculation via tattooing, allowing a picture, though partial, of an otherwise historically obscured tattooing practice to emerge.

After Hutin, and until the end of the century, only five cases of primary syphilis caused by tattooing appear in the major British and American medical journals. There is only one reported incident of tattooing-inoculated tuberculosis during this period. Reports from 1900 onwards discuss cutaneous lesions of secondary syphilis that were affected by tattoos, but there is no mention of tattooing as potentially causing disease, which may indicate a shift in the professional practices and standards of tattooists.[18] Of the nineteenth-century cases dealing specifically with skin disease inoculated by tattooing, two stand out, both of which are illustrated. The first report, 'Notes of Cases on an Outbreak of Syphilis Following on Tattooing' by British army surgeon F. R. Barker, appeared in the *British Medical Journal* in 1889. The images are of particular interest. They are highly unusual amongst the medical literature concerning tattooing and disease, because they clearly illustrate the tattoo itself as the site of infection. Barker's report describes an outbreak of syphilis at the Portsea army barracks in Hampshire in 1888, in which twelve soldiers were infected with the disease by a single tattooist, who is referred to simply as 'S.'. Barker located the tattooist, who was said to be a discharged soldier of the regiment and a 'hawker in the barracks'.[19] After interviewing him about his health and working methods, Barker established that he was indeed infected with syphilis. The article goes on to describe the tattooing method that Barker argued undoubtedly led to the transmission of infection – the tattooist had used his saliva variously throughout the process, either using it to mix his inks, moistening his needles in his mouth, or rubbing saliva directly onto the skin before, during and after tattooing. In all, twenty-three men where tattooed by S. over a three-month period, although only twelve showed signs of infection. The first four cases presented were photographed, and these images appear in Barker's article, one of which is reproduced here (see Figure 11.2).

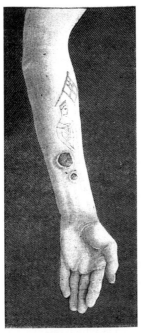

Figure 11.2: Illustration in F. R. Barker, 'Notes of Cases on an Outbreak of Syphilis Following on Tattooing', *British Medical Journal*, 1:1479 (1889), pp. 985–9, on p. 985. Image reproduced courtesy of the Wellcome Library, London.

The first two images in Barker's text show the flexor and extensor surfaces of the forearm, with ulcerated sores emerging from the margins of the tattooed lines themselves. Figure 11.2 reproduces the first of these, identified as 'Case I', and depicts the flexor surface of a left forearm tattooed with a flag and a female figure, the lower portion of the tattooed figure corroded by two large syphilitic ulcers. This image bears the typical features of cropping and isolating the affected limb in space common to contemporaneous medical illustrations of skin diseases, and in this respect it shares formal similarities with Carwell's watercolour in Fend's chapter (Figure 10.3). In contrast with the forearms depicted in Figure 11.1, however, there is a distinct voluminous three-dimensionality to the limb in this image, which has been reproduced from a photograph. The third image plate in Barker's article (not shown) presents a much more abstracted image of the infected tattoo, which fills the pictorial space. The syphilitic eruptions have a greater specific character, appearing to 'bloom' out of tattooed images of flowers in a pot. It is interesting to note Barker's subtle aesthetic judgements of these particular syphilitic manifestations: 'The rupiæ were very perfect, like limpet-shells. The ulcers were situated over the site of a flower and a flower pot tattooed by S. on the flexor surface of his left forearm'.[20] Barker's description of the rupial sores as a perfect representation of a morphological type suggests an important linkage between production of medical imagery and diagnostic standardization, particularly in the case of syphilis, whose surface manifestations are varied and may be confused with other conditions. This third image incorporates a different visual style, essentially presenting an isolated symptom on a flat surface; the skin only becomes legible as such through the surface sign of the disease, and in this case by the inclusion of the submerged tattoo. Similarly, in the work of criminologists of the same period, the surface sign of the tattoo is flattened out and 'removed' from the context of the body in the collections of drawings that accompany numerous criminological texts on tattooing.[21] It may be argued that these acts of visual abstraction and isolation contributed to the construction of visual taxonomies within the disciplines of medicine and criminology alike.

Tattoo, body and medical historian James Bradley comments upon Barker's report of the outbreak with reference to anthropologist Alfred Gell's metaphor of the 'epidemiology of tattooing': 'we see the quasi-dermatological illness of the tattoo spreading plague-like through a segment of the regiment, followed swiftly by the real disease of syphilis, which asserted its ascendancy by transposing its own mark upon the crudely etched tattoo patterns'.[22] Gell's formulation, which Bradley adopts, is based upon his observation that tattooing has an observable 'pattern of occurrence, which resembles the uneven, but at the same time predictable, incident of an illness'.[23] Though seeming to suggest that this pattern is metaphorical, he nevertheless refers to the empirically and theoretically tenuous work of Lombroso, who had identified 'imitation' and 'idleness' to be two of the primary motivating factors amongst criminals who acquired tattoos. Furthermore, he suggests that in this historical case there may be some veracity in his ideas. This metaphor, which proposes a mechanism of 'social contagion' for the spread of physical stigmata (the tattoo), reproduces many of Lombroso's questionable assumptions. Yet it is also intriguing, in light of these assumptions, to consider the ways in which nineteenth-century medicolegal professionals represented tattooing as a risk factor in the transmission of disease *associated with* disreputable behaviours.

A second case from the British medical literature concerning the tattoo as the site of skin disease – on this occasion tuberculosis – presents a particularly interesting example in light of the above. This extremely short report is accompanied by two images, which share stylistic similarities to those in Barker's report, although they are engravings rather than photographs. The transmission agent in this case, as in that involving the Portsea tattooist, was also saliva, although the artist on this occasion was a fifteen-year-old boy who had died of phthisis[24] shortly after tattooing his younger brothers, aged ten and thirteen. He is said to have used Indian ink 'rubbed up with his saliva in the palm of his hand'. In the first image accompanying the case notes, the tuberculosis infection has destroyed the lower portion of the tattoo, which is described to resemble a rose, heavily scarred and covered with a mass of pustules.

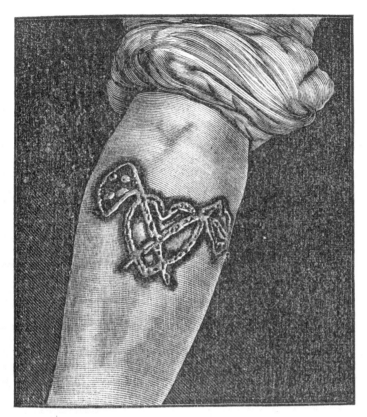

Figure 11.3: Illustration in D. W. Collings and W. Murray, 'Three Cases of Inoculation of Tuberculosis from Tattooing', *British Medical Journal*, 1:1796 (1895), pp. 1200–1, on p. 1201. Image reproduced courtesy of the Wellcome Library, London.

The second image depicts the flexor surface of the forearm, which is tattooed with a heart crossed by two flags, and described in the report as 'leaving in lines of the pattern deep ulcers with hard, round, smooth edges and granulating bases. The whole design was raised and surrounded with an erythematous border' (see Figure 11.3).[25] The infection has completely engulfed the tattoo such that the disease itself has taken on the pattern of the design. Thus, according to Bradley and Gell's formula, we are able to visualize the tattooed sign and symptom of infection merging into one single stigmata of social and physical disorder. It is possible to imagine the tattoo during the late nineteenth and early twentieth centuries as a kind of doubly pathological signifier, inflected with the spectre of social disreputability or even criminality in one social context, and stigmatized disease in another. There may even be overlap between the two: conspicuous diseases such as syphilis were implicated in the spread of social degeneration through the transmission of infectious diseases. Thus in response to outbreaks such as those described, some medical and military professionals were led to conclude that tattooing might pose a risk significant enough to be banned outright, as suggested by the American physicians F. F. Maury and C. W. Dulles in 1878.

> Tattooing, we think, might well be forbidden in the army and navy, as a useless and
> perhaps pernicious practice, one which may injure the men and prove an expense to
> the government, by bringing into hospital and on the pension lists some who might
> otherwise be in active service.[26]

Comments such as these may be considered within the broader development
of bacteriology and public health as disciplines. In the United States, bacteriology was introduced in the 1880s, and though American scientists initially made
limited contributions to the field, historian George Rosen notes that 'they were
more alert than their European confreres to its practical implications'.[27] The
development of the American public health laboratory service in the late 1880s
paralleled the emergence of bacteriology, demonstrating the medical community's willingness to employ new scientific techniques for the 'greater good' of
public health. According to Rosen, the USA was ahead of the trend in this regard,
with the earliest bacteriological laboratory established by Joseph J. Kinyoun in
1887, as part of the Marine Hospital on Staten Island, New York. Despite the
health warnings of medical professionals such as Maury and Dulles, the tattooing profession encountered few legal challenges based on associated health
risks, and then not until the mid-twentieth century.[28] Tattooing largely escaped
official regulation altogether, until 1988, when three states banned tattooing
outright and sixteen introduced some form of regulation. That said, thirty-one
states chose not to regulate tattooing.[29] Throughout the profession's early days,
it was largely left up to the tattoo practitioners themselves to adopt some form
of antisepsis in their working methods. Whilst some tattooists observed basic
hygiene, others relied on lay understandings of the practice propagated through
oral tradition, which often owed more to folk belief than modern medicine. In
practice, a far more complex cultural exchange involving different understandings of the body and medicine was transforming the tattooist's craft, as well as
that of the medical practitioner, as we will see.

Medical versus Folk Knowledge of Tattooing:
Tattooing as a Healing Art

From the late nineteenth century onwards, anthropologists, colonial officials and
amateur observers had begun to show an interest in the tattooing practices of the
native cultures they encountered. Reports from all corners of the globe recounted
the high regard in which tattooing was held within these societies, often as a powerful magical and therapeutic treatment for a variety of ailments and illnesses.
Some of these stories were based on careful research, others wild conjecture; many
were undoubtedly invented by the new breed of American and European tattooists themselves.[30] These new professionals were, by all accounts, a contradictory
and somewhat evasive lot. By the early twentieth century, many leading tattooists

where careful to advertise their practice and studios as 'sanitary', and were rightfully wary of suggestions that tattooing could spread disease.[31] However, many retained – and even cultivated – a mythology surrounding their practice, which owed more to sailors' stories and the half-digested foreign reports of the magical properties of tattooing than to the discoveries of medical science. That many had been sailors themselves is telling – sailors' tattoos being amongst the most talismanic of Western designs. One way or another, by the mid-twentieth century stories of the protective and healing powers of tattooing had filtered into popular culture and entered into the mythology of Western tattooists.[32]

An academic source which mentions the healing function of tattoos appeared in the *Journal of the Anthropological Institute of Great Britain and Ireland* in 1903. In his study, conducted amongst the lower-ranking soldiers of the Egyptian army, Dr Charles S. Myers aimed to determine 'by descriptive, metric and photographic methods' what differences may exist between the inhabitants of different regions of Egypt, although it seems his data was insufficient in this regard.[33] What emerges instead is a summary comparison of the tattooing practices of different groups in North Africa. As well as reproducing tattoo marks themselves, Myers also presented numerous anthropometric measurements and the specific ethnicity of the 1,006 participants in his study. Throughout his report, he regularly refers to the perceived protective health benefits of tattooing. For instance, in his discussion of Arab and Kabyle tattooing, he observes that 'the operation is performed by the mother on her child, often for mere decoration's sake, at other times to ward off or to cure disease'.[34] The study also sought to establish similarities between modern and ancient Egyptian peoples. To this end, he explores the origins of contemporary tattooing, citing the following reference:

> It is true that Fouquet, when unwrapping the mummy of a Theban priestess (the Lady Ament) who lived in the eleventh dynasty, observed many white and blue *ante mortem* linear 'cicatrices' on the abdomen and elsewhere; whence he concludes that the priestess had been treated for chronic pelvic peritonitis in a manner still practiced among the fellahin of the present day.[35]

Myers concludes that this apparently medicinal use of 'linear scars and tattoo marks' is a very ancient Egyptian practice. He subsequently reports that Egyptian mothers take their babies to be tattooed 'according to some for the sake of ornamentation, according to others in order to ward off the evil eye and disease', and then claims that 'even the Copts tatu the cross, in many cases, at least, on account of sickness'.[36]

A later, more considered anthropological study conducted by Winifred Blackman into the culture of the fellahin of Upper Egypt, also mentions the healing properties of tattoo marks in Africa: 'according to one of my informants, the dot tattooed at the side of the nostril is sometimes done as a cure for toothache'.[37] She also describes the use of tattooing to cure other specific ailments, such as headache, 'weak eye' and possession. To her contemporary readers, it may not have come as a surprise that long-standing or ancient cultural practices of tattooing were bound up with magic and healing ritual. However, what is perhaps more unexpected is the occurrence of similar beliefs within the twentieth-century American and European tattoo community.

Writing in 1933, Albert Parry notes that 'many Americans and immigrants see medicinal qualities in the very act of tattooing'.[38] He relates the example of John Solinsky, who apparently visited his tattooist, 'Professor Ted', every time he felt unwell, and asked to be tattooed on the skin nearest the discomfort. Parry goes on to quote two more New York tattooists, Billy Donnelly and the famous Charlie Wagner (1875–1953), both of whom confessed to having clients who requested this kind of 'therapeutic' tattooing. This would sometimes be done without the use of inks, and usually involved tattooing the area around their clients' rheumatic joints, in order to ease pain and discomfort. Most surprising of all is the San Francisco tattooist Louis Morgan's statement that 'It is well known that a good-sized tattoo is as good an innoculation [*sic*] as any vaccination, and people who have considerable tattoo work on their bodies are generally more healthy than those who have none'.[39] Moreover, it would seem that some of the imported folklore surrounding the healing properties of tattooing were conflated by some American tattooists with contemporary medical reports about the health risks associated with the practice, as this quote from Samuel M. Steward's memoirs of working as a tattooist in 1950s Chicago reveals:

> Old Randy in the arcade shop insisted that a tattoo cured syphilis. Possibly in his dim way he had heard of an article in the Journal of the American Medical Association stating that a syphilitic ulcer on a man's arm, originating on his wrist and travelling upwards, was stopped dead when it reached the red pigment of a tattoo. No wonder: the red pigment was a spirocheticide – mercuric sulphide, one of the old specifics against syphilis before the days of penicillin. The presence of mercury in the skin was enough to arrest the progress of a shallow skin ulcer; after that, the bugs went undercover.[40]

Somewhat ironically, the influences of folk belief and medical discourse conspire to produce an unfortunate amalgam, resulting in the assertion that a tattoo can, in fact, cure syphilis – apparently encouraged by the unexpected therapeutic side effects of the cinnabar-based[41] red tattoo pigments in early usage. There are a number of articles in British and American medical journals spanning from 1878 to around 1957 dealing with both the adverse and therapeutic effects of mercury-based tattoo pigments.[42] However, the article Steward referenced is most likely University of Michigan dermatologist George H. Belote's 'Tattoo and Syphilis', which appeared in the *Archives of Dermatology and Syphilology* in 1928. Belote examined tattooed patients with secondary syphilitic eruptions and observed:

On both forearms there were tattoo designs done in dark blue, green and vermilion (mercuric sulphide). In all the designs papules were present in the green and blue, but apparently not in the red. This was made more apparent by the fact that here and there papules occurred in the blue outlining the red, but appeared to stop sharply when the red portion was reached. Since this eruption was extremely profuse, it is assumed to have been more than a mere coincidence that all the red was spared.[43]

Another commentator in the medical periodicals, Lieutenant Commander Frederick Novy of the United States Naval Reserve, took a particularly dim view of the 'so-called artists' who practiced tattooing with 'no concept of antisepsis', and thought even less of their premises and methods, which he generally regarded as 'filthy'. However, he conceded that 'a theoretic explanation of low incidence of infection may be found in the fact that one of the red dyes contains cinnabar, which is mercuric sulphide. This chemical may act as an antiseptic as the needles are constantly dipped into the dye'.[44]

Not all medical writers regarded the practice of tattooing with such disdain, however. Intriguingly, some dermatologists explored the use of tattooing for therapeutic and cosmetic purposes from as early as the 1890s. A number of interesting accounts appear in the historical literature describing how doctors adopted tattooists' techniques and tools for medicinal purposes. These accounts reveal little of the moralizing frequently encountered in the continental criminological literature on tattooing during the period; rather, it seems that some medical professionals had a genuine interest in the new technology of tattooing. The electric tattoo machine in particular, which was invented in 1891 by the American tattooist Samuel O'Reilly, presented a novel method for the introduction of substances other than ink into the skin in a relatively controlled manner. For example, Leeds physician C. Butler Savory tattooed a solution of carbolic acid into the skin of patients with various dermatological ailments. In 1899 he published a report on this 'original method', which he termed 'hypodermic medication'.[45] He writes:

> For localised patches of ringworm, etc., this method of treatment proves eminently successful. I have not as yet tried the treatment for skin diseases depending upon constitutional conditions, but I see no reason why the result of tattooing some of the chronic localised rashes of syphilis liq. hydrarg. perchlor. should not prove successful.[46]

In this example, we see the argument coming full circle: whilst to some medical professionals tattooing represented a dangerous threat to public health as a vector in the transmission of highly stigmatized diseases, not least syphilis, to others the tools and process of tattooing could be appropriated in the treatment of the very same conditions. Tattooing as a method of introducing therapeutic compounds (often mercury sulphide) into areas infected with skin disease was also suggested as a treatment for *pruritus ani* in numerous sources throughout the 1930s and 1940s.[47]

Moreover, the potential artistic or cosmetic merits of the practice were also gradually appreciated by medical professionals. In 1930, New York physician Ludwig Filips advocated in the *Archives of Dermatology and Syphilology* for the cosmetic uses of tattooing for numerous skin defects, including scars and pigment disorders, to apply colour to grafted skin or to treat skin damaged by such diseases as lupus or epithelioma. He went on to discuss colour theory, the appropriate methods and formulas for mixing pigments, and application techniques utilizing a modern electric tattoo machine.[48] One might speculate about the apparent appeal of tattooing to physicians such as Filips; the process of tattooing itself suggests certain affinities with medical practices such as inoculation and vaccination. This was clearly not always to beneficial effect – but perhaps the source of medical interest in tattooing was the tattooists' very possession of a tool so like that of any doctor's trade. Medical historian Stanley Reiser writes that 'in general, technologies are created by the existence of possibilities that the prevailing ideas, culture, and social climate of an era suggest to an innovator could be useful, interesting, or profitable.'[49] This was certainly the case for the tattooists who benefited from Samuel O'Reilly's electric tattoo machine – it improved accuracy, was far less painful for the client and increased both the refinement of tattoo designs and the speed with which the tattooist could operate. In the twentieth century, new and innovative therapeutic treatments for diseases developed rapidly;[50] it is no wonder that the tattoo machine was seized upon by some medical professionals as a novel therapeutic tool. The development of many medical specialisms were in fact dependent upon technological innovations; similarly, it may be argued that the success of late nineteenth- and early twentieth-century tattoo artists such as O'Reilly, Burchett and Wagner was enabled by the invention of the electric tattoo machine.

Conclusions

In the context of late nineteenth-century criminal anthropology and forensic science, the tattoo was mobilized as a symbol for the transfer of meanings that sought to render the criminal and the 'savage' body analogous to one another. Paralleling the processes of segregation and isolation of the patient and disease within the hospital, a similar shift took place within criminology, in which criminals and their outward signs of criminality became the new focus of researchers, who conducted much of their work on the conveniently segregated and isolated populations in military barracks and prisons.

But whilst the influence of criminological anthropometrics gradually waned through the early twentieth century, and the idea of identifying the criminal character through tattoos with it, the medical concerns with the decorative practice remained. The associated risk factors shifted from syphilis and tuberculosis in the late nineteenth and early twentieth centuries to hepatitis from around the 1950s right up until 1980,[51] and HIV in the 1980s and 90s.[52] The association of tattooing with the disreputable and criminal element in society persisted within American and European popular culture well into the twentieth century, long after the tattoo ceased to be a source of serious criminological debate. As tattooing became more professionalized and hygiene practices improved, the stories of associated health risk also waned. As a parting remark in his autobiographical account of tattooing in 1950s Chicago and Oakland, Samuel Steward takes a pessimistic view of the future of tattooing: 'I am personally glad that I ended my tattooing career in 1970; I would not for anything in the world be tattooing in this day of AIDS. The time of gravest danger lies ahead for both the customer and the tattooist, who needs whatever advice and help a doctor can give him in setting up the system of antisepsis for his shop.'[53] Despite his concerns, and frequent mention of tattooing as a HIV risk factor in the medical literature from 1980 until the present day, to date there have been no documented cases of HIV infection caused by tattooing. The regulation of tattooing by public health authorities has undoubtedly made some difference to the conditions and working practices of contemporary tattooists. In the USA these regulations operate at state level, and may take a number of forms, including: requiring the licensing of the tattoo studio, or the tattoo artist; allowing only licensed medical or dental practitioners to carry out tattooing; setting down hygiene standards for studios; or prohibiting tattooing of minors.[54] In the UK, as in some American states, regulation is a relatively recent development. The Tattooing of Minors Act (1969) made it illegal to tattoo a child under the age of 18. It was not until the passing of the Local Government (Miscellaneous Provisions) Act (1982) that both tattooists and their premises required registration with local health authorities. This licensing may well have given the tattooists' clients greater confidence – an official health authority registration certificate on the wall provides an air of respectability to the tattoo studio – and it is certainly interesting to note that this period coincided with the 'tattoo renaissance' within popular culture and a general decline in the number and frequency of medical reports of tattooing-inoculated infection.

Thus the status of the tattoo as a signifier of disreputability – whether considered as a sign of atavism or criminality, or stigmata of infectious skin disease – gradually declined in scholarly discourse over the course of the twentieth century. Though it has not disappeared from discussions of public health risk entirely, improvements in the hygiene practices of tattooists and government regulation of the profession have enabled a shift in cultural perception such that tattooing is no longer considered to be the risky practice it once was.

12 'KISSED BY THE SUN': TANNING THE SKIN OF THE SICK WITH LIGHT THERAPEUTICS, *c.* 1890–1930

Tania Woloshyn

Introduction

Among civilized people, the skin is universally anemic [*sic*] and enfeebled by the universal practice of over-clothing. In view of the important functions of the skin, there should be a widespread campaign to introduce sun-bathing and the construction of sunny open-air gymnasiums. The tanned skin is able to defend itself against cold and to protect the body against disease much more efficiently than the pale, anemic [*sic*] skin which has not been 'kissed by the sun'.[1]

To tan skin is to brown it, dye it, transform its properties. Whether one refers to the process of turning raw hide to treated leather (the verb's etymological origins), or that of pigmenting human skin from pallid whiteness to a bronzed, luxurious surface, the concept of tanning remains the same. In contributing to this edited volume on skin and its medical histories, this chapter focuses on an under-explored topic in early twentieth-century medicine: bodily exposure of tubercular patients to light, or, perhaps better put, a therapeutics of tanning. From the early 1890s onwards, physicians internationally became increasingly fascinated by the natural healing powers of light. The primary, though not sole, target of both heliotherapy (natural sun therapy) and phototherapy (artificial light therapy) was to treat tuberculosis in its various manifestations. This included pulmonary tuberculosis, Pott's disease, scrofula, bone and joint ('surgical') tuberculosis, and *lupus vulgaris* (tuberculosis of the skin). Heliotherapists and phototherapists sought to rid the body of tubercle bacilli, heal the disfiguring and suppurating wounds caused by them, and prevent further recurrences by building up the patient's physiological defences. For these physicians, light had the miraculous, natural ability to conquer the ravages of disease. Directed onto the patient's skin, natural sunlight and artificial light were perceived to stimulate the body's mechanisms, the tissues, organs and blood, and those internal processes were signalled by external signs occurring on the surface, most notably through the ongoing pigmentation of the skin.

This is a history of tanning skin that must be understood as distinct from – although it is contextually related to – popular sun-tanning as we know it today. The narrative of the latter typically gives vague historical roots in medical practices to account for its mass appeal from the 1920s onwards, especially through the fashionable practices of rich holidaymakers on the French Riviera.[2] That history needs to be complicated and enriched, not least because it takes little to no account of the role of physicians and patients, who actively contributed to naturalizing tanned skin – both in their visual and textual production – as healthy and beautiful, and well before the 1920s.

In this chapter I wish to contextualize the practice of tanning through the primary literature and visual culture of light therapeutics, of phototherapy and heliotherapy. While the history of light therapeutics has been discussed in scholarly and popular literature, for example by Ina Zweiniger-Bargielowska, Simon Carter, Robert Mighall and Richard Hobday (Britain), by Pascal Ory, Bernard Andrieu, Arouna Ouédraogo and Arnaud Baubérot (France), and by Michael Hau and Maren Möhring (Germany), in such works it is situated within larger life reform movements and naturist practices.[3] As an adjunct of naturism and life reform programmes, bodily exposure to the sun (heliotherapy) was clearly a prime focus for its international practitioners with both aesthetic and sociopolitical, even eugenic, ends.[4] But rarely does secondary literature take account of the history of light therapeutics in and of itself, in which phototherapy and its technological processes remain a vital part, or of its dissemination through its visual and material production.

For this reason I specifically concentrate here on medical perceptions and aesthetic representations of tanning the skin of the tubercular patient with artificial and natural light, *c.* 1890–1940. I contend that during this period, the path to health for the tubercular patient undergoing light therapy was aesthetically driven by the eyes and hands of the physician. Photographs of patients before and after light treatments were employed to document that process, yet the aesthetic language utilized within them, such as their lighting and background choices, reveal a complex relationship between the aesthetics and the therapeutics of bronzed skin. This is also evident in popular culture of the period, particularly the literary production of the French writer André Gide (1859–1951), a tubercular patient who experienced and represented in his writings sun-tanning as a sensuous, erotic process. The aim of this chapter is to explore this relationship through medical texts and images as well as Gide's evocative literature, in order to investigate the medical desirability of being, in the words of John Harvey Kellogg, 'kissed by the sun'.

The Process of Pigmentation

The historical development of light therapeutics is attributed to the pioneering work of Danish physician Niels Ryberg Finsen, the inventor of phototherapy or artificial light therapy.[5] Importantly, for this discovery he won the Nobel Prize in 1903, the third winner in medicine to do so. Only one year later he died from Pick's disease, a rare neurodegenerative condition. In 1896 he had founded the Medical Light Institute in Copenhagen, which was later renamed the Finsen Institute. The Institute welcomed physicians from across the globe to observe its work, and it was funded by the state, indicating that its medical advancements were widely accepted and encouraged.[6]

Finsen began experimenting with natural and, soon afterwards, artificial light from the early 1890s, in order to treat variola (smallpox) and *lupus vulgaris* (tuberculosis of the skin). His research was initiated by an observation of light's negative influence on smallpox, discovering that ultraviolet (UV) light catalyzed its symptoms. To counter this he placed the patient in a darkened room within the first stages of smallpox, known as the stage of vesiculation or blistering of the skin; if this measure was taken quickly enough, the disease did not develop into the stage of suppuration, in which pus would discharge from the small blisters. By doing so the patient could heal with little or no scarring. To do this Finsen created a room where all the windows were covered with thick, red cloth or a dense, red glass, to filter out all but red rays. In other words he created a darkroom, ensuring its suitability by hanging photographic plates in the middle of the room to test for any invading light exposure.[7] For Finsen, 'the skin during small-pox is as susceptible to daylight as a photographic plate, and must be kept from the chemical rays in the same way and almost as carefully'.[8] Aware of these photographic practices, he explained that red light is the weakest of visible and invisible light rays on the spectrum in terms of concentrated chemical action. Red light is furthest on the spectrum from UV and violet light, which are highest in chemical or 'actinic' as well as bactericidal action. Finsen then began experimenting with the UV end of the spectrum to treat lupus, using them, in the words of Charles W. Allen, as a kind of 'a cauterant of mild character or a reducing agent'.[9] UV rays were therefore employed by Finsen for their destructive action.

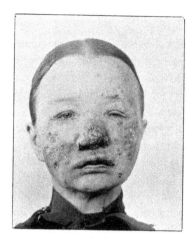 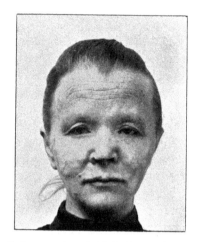

Figure 12.1: Before-and-after photographs of a lupus patient, in N. R. Finsen, *Die Bekämpfung des Lupus vulgaris: Vortrag bei der Herbstkonferenz im 'Internationalen Central-Bureau zur Bekämpfung der Tuberkulose', Berlin 1902* (Jena: Fischer, 1903), unpaginated plate. Author's collection.

He published his findings throughout the 1890s in Danish, and as early as 1901 these were gathered and translated into English in a book simply titled *Photo-therapy*; the French version appeared in 1899, though journal articles and reports of his had already been published in French, English and German by the mid-1890s. Before-and-after photographs of lupus patients were included in these publications. The photographs were employed for their documentary function, to record the progress of the treatment and of healing, as evidence of the efficacy of light therapy. In a pair of before-and-after photographs in Finsen's 1903 *Die Bekämpfung des Lupus vulgaris*, we are presented with two faces that seem incomparable (see Figure 12.1). In the former, a woman's face is shown ravaged by the disfiguring and painful-looking effects of *lupus vulgaris*. Inflammation has made it difficult for her to open her eyes fully, and her nose is almost totally engulfed by the disease. In the latter, she is shown again, equally expressionless, and yet miraculously healed. Subtle differences in her hairstyle and clothing add to the sense that she is a changed woman, healed and whole. Traces of the lesions may be detected by the slight uneven texture of her skin, particularly on her cheeks, but otherwise she appears to be entirely recovered. Phototherapists were clear to establish early on that the major advantages of the treatment were that it caused no pain and no scarring, producing new skin that was 'smooth, and supple, quite unlike ordinary cicatricial tissue' and thus, unlike scraping or cutting, a far more aesthetically appealing outcome for the patient.[10] In the photographs the therapeutic process is absent, merely implied in the spaces between them, and it must have been difficult for readers to believe that such dramatic results had been achieved simply through exposure to light.

In his writings, Finsen explained that he began with natural sunlight modified through lenses made of glass, then quartz (which allows UV rays to pass through them, whereas ordinary glass does not). Shortly afterwards, he employed electric light devices in an interior setting, as his patients required UV light in strong, consistent doses on a daily basis, beyond the restrictions of weather and season. He had various devices and instruments to facilitate the penetration of artificial light into lesions, including not only round lenses but also skin compressors, which wedged the skin and tissues around the lesion, removing blood from the area. He had discovered draining blood from around the sore greatly facilitated the penetration of light beyond the surface.[11] The skin, however, was the point of activation. As Hugo Bach explained,

> The *stratum basale sive germinativum*, the vital and active layer of the epidermis, is the organ which regulates the relation of the human body to light. It is a light-organ; the organ of bio-chemical relationship of man, and is the point of attack for that light which we have in mind when we speak of the effects of light on the living human body. It is, however, not only an organ for the reception of light, but also for the transformation of radiant energy of light; an organ of light-assimilation. It is an organ of secretory character, an organ which we must class on the same plane as the internal secretory glands.[12]

As a 'light-organ' and 'organ of light-assimilation', the skin's receptivity to light was judged through its ability to pigment. Though the belief was sometimes contested, the majority of light therapists agreed that patients who pigmented well were those who recovered quickly.[13] As the well-known promoter of 'helio-hygiene' and smoke abatement laws in England, Dr Caleb W. Saleeby, noted in his 1923 book *Sunlight and Health*:

> we must remember that pigmentation of the skin is a marked feature of the sun-cure, and that patients who do not pigment well do not progress well[;] no one who has seen and touched the typical pigmented skin of a heliotherapeutic patient can doubt that very active chemical processes are there occurring.[14]

Much earlier, in 1907 Dr François Chiaïs, based in Menton, posed the tanning process in starker terms: 'If pigmentation does not develop, the prognosis is most dire'.[15] For Professor Louis Landouzy, dean of the Paris medical school, 'pigmentation is the barometer of the sun-cure', a tool to make heliotherapy a legitimate and progressive science beyond mere empiricism.[16]

Kellogg wrote that 'the skin may play an important part in defending the body against infection by raising the immunizing power of the blood under the influence of light rays'.[17] He noted specific histological changes to the skin when exposed to light, including swelling of the collagen, increasing numbers of active tissue cells and notable dilating of blood vessels.[18] This was also stated by the most famous of heliotherapists, Dr Auguste Rollier, who added that sunlight catalyzed tissue repair, the elimination of pus and necrotic bone and the production of hae-moglobin and phosphorus in the blood.[19] According to the Nice-based naturist physician Dr Albert Monteuuis, 'the accentuation of pigmented colour is a sign of the increase of nutritive activity and as a result of vigour'.[20] As such, the skin's physiological reaction to the sun's rays initiated the body's natural defences to withstand disease, suggesting that the tan signalled deeper, interior processes at work. In other words, in addition to it denoting the therapeutic process successfully underway, the tan was a marker of prophylaxis. Not only itself a protective measure for further surface exposure to light rays, it was also a visual sign of ready preventive measures within the body. As Möhring has noted, in relation to German nudist practices, the tan 'became a signifier for stored solar energy'.[21]

Absorbed through the skin, light rays were perceived to activate the body's vital forces, initiating a reaction that would spread throughout it entirely. And in keeping with the latest laboratory experiments in bacteriology, they described its effects using the emerging vocabulary of germ theory to promote sunlight as naturally antiseptic and bactericidal.[22] Heliotherapists and phototherapists frequently cited the work of Arthur Downes, Thomas Blunt and Robert Koch, who had published studies on the antibacterial properties of light. The experiments of the destructive action of light on bacteria by Downes and Blunt in 1877 were considered irrefutable proof of the efficacy of sunlight in combating tuberculosis,[23] while Koch had demonstrated that UV rays destroy bacteria, most importantly the tubercle bacillus. If sunlight could kill bacteria spread onto a microscope's glass slide, it could kill bacteria living in the blood and tissues of the tubercular patient. With this scientific evidence behind it, light was understood as a natural regenerative agent, whether naturally obtained or artificially produced, with unforeseen potential within modern, progressive medicine. And as Zweiniger-Bargielowka, Hau and Baubérot have discussed in relation to life reform practices in England, Germany and France, respectively, a diverse range of practitioners within both orthodox and 'alternative' medicine believed in light's natural powers of transformation.[24] For these physicians, describing and visualizing the pigmented skin of the healing patient was paramount to ascertaining light's therapeutic efficacy.

Visualizing Pigmentation

Known as the 'High Priest of modern Sun-worshippers',[25] Rollier created several outdoor sanatoria in Leysin, an alpine resort in Switzerland for tubercular adults and children, from 1903 onwards. Rollier advocated a total body treatment to natural sunlight, not simply for specific lesions on the surface but for a holistic, immune-boosting regeneration of the entire body. While Finsen reported successful treatments of tuberculosis by directing concentrated natural or artificial light solely onto the visible lesion on the skin's surface, Rollier professed having obtained the same excellent results with general exposure of the whole body to alpine sunshine. In Figures 12.2 and 12.3, Rollier employed the same visualizing tactics as Finsen, before-and-after photographs with neutral nondescript backgrounds and tight cropping around patients' bodies; but here differences of skin tones are made far more legible. These are photographs of the same child, once riddled with tuberculosis of the bones and joints and, following heliotherapy, totally healed. The 'before' photograph features the tubercular child seated atop a dark cushion and before a uniform, black background, reminiscent of a photographer's studio. By contrast, the 'after' photograph has been shot with a white background, created by a hanging white cloth and a table covered in white sheets, set up outdoors within bright, natural daylight. Such simple props and choices aid enormously in marking out changes to the patient's skin tone. Posed with a toy in his hands and facing the camera, the boy in the 'after' photograph proudly displays his body, sitting purposefully upright, confidently staring at the viewer, his body plump and bronzed. Unlike the more frontal lighting of the 'before' image, the natural lighting in the 'after' image is discernibly directed from the left, casting shadows all over the boy's deeply tanned body. With photographs like this in mind, it is unsurprising that heliotherapists like Dr Monteuuis would declare, 'The regenerating action of the sun is so profound that it produces ... actual resurrections'.[26] The 'after' photograph serves to mark out changes that are physical (his healed, tanned skin), psychological (his smile) and moral (his respectable appearance, emphasized further in subsequent photos of the boy, older and healthy, at work in the fields[27]). As Rollier stated, the sunshine's *'joie de vivre'* produced 'a desire for activity' and a strong work ethic that was morally driven, substantiating his philanthropic initiatives to educate his young patients and have them perform light work at his facilities.[28]

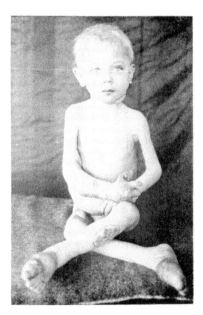 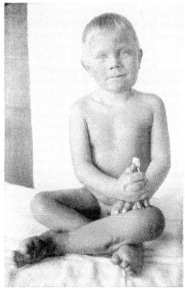

Figure 12.2 (left): 'Sick child aged 4.5 years old, with 34 foci of osteitis, periostitis and adenitis, numerous fistulae, advanced tuberculosis of the two feet, of the right hand and the left lung, peritonitis, cachexia', *c.* 1908.

Figure 12.3 (right): 'The same sick child, one year later. Cicatrization of fistulae, reconstitution of the musculature and the general state', *c.* 1910. Both figures in A. Rollier, *La Cure de soleil* (Paris: Baillière et fils; Lausanne: Constant Tarin, 1914), figures a and b of plate XL, unpaginated plate. Permission kindly granted by Suzanne Chapuis-Rollier and Martine Gagnebin.

I do not believe these strategies of visualization were unique to light therapeutics; neither do I believe it was exceptional to perceive physical health as the path to moral improvement: '*mens sans in corpore sano*'. I am, however, fascinated by the attempts to make explicit the success of the cure, including the changes beyond simple pigmentation of the skin or, rather, that as a surface marker pigmentation became naturally associated with such changes: that the 'whole, healed, happy flesh'[29] of the respectable citizen *was* tanned.

The Hardening Process

For physicians, the tan was regarded as a necessary trace and indicator of the cure's efficacy; it traced the progress of the cure on the invalid's body. The tan was also perceived to transform the body to withstand further exposure and, as such, little different from a callous: a physiological reaction to protect the skin from overexposure. The protection the tan afforded was perceived by physicians eventually to 'harden' the body. Möhring has discussed that German nudists even privileged sunburn to produce this hardening and the subsequent new skin, in addition to rubbing, oiling and polishing the skin to 'train' it.[30] In Rollier's 1923 English publication *Heliotherapy*, his surgeon Dr E. Amstad explained the process:

> By means of frequent and regular cold baths or douches and by continual exposure to fresh air, the patient should harden himself until he is no longer painfully susceptible to cold and draughts. Such hardening is also obtained by sun-treatment. Anyone who has seen the balconies of the Leysin clinics during a spell of cold weather will have observed the tolerance of cold shown by the majority of naked and sunburnt patients when the sun is temporarily hidden by clouds – goose-flesh is quite unknown to them. The pigmented (*i.e.* physiological) skin forms a protecting apparatus against chills ...[31]

Amstad implied that as the invalid absorbed the sunlight (tanning in the process), his or her body became closed, hard and protected. The hardening of the body was synonymous with its healing, the closure of wounds and lesions and the tanning of skin equated with the return to health. Kellogg specified that other physicians had reported patients' skin becoming denser and literally harder under the influence of light, the 'protoplasm [in the skin's cells] being reduced to keratin'.[32] Others spoke of the process in more abstract terms, conceptualizing the hardening process as akin to the skin being 'weathered' by exposure to the elements. But the closed, healed skin of patients in 'after' images would suggest much more than metaphor at work here, the light rays being perceived as having the natural potential to seal the open, suppurating wounds, to regenerate the surface and to protect the body from future attack. 'Weathering' is therefore a particularly apt notion, especially when we consider that invalids were regarded as rendered weak by their physical state and easily susceptible to the elements. As Thomas More Madden, an obstetrician and authority on European health reports, stated in 1864:

If such be the influence of climate on entire races of man, modifying not only their external form, and the relative importance of the functions of many of their internal organs ... how great then must be its influence on individual men, more especially when these are in a weak and delicate state of health, and therefore infinitely more susceptible of all the good effects of a suitable change of climate ...[33]

Madden made clear that the invalid's body was more receptive to and more quickly affected by the influence of a new climate than the healthy body. This was doubtless a fundamental principle underlying the widespread international use throughout the nineteenth century of climatotherapy, a natural therapy from which light therapy emerged.[34]

Patient experiences of the tanning process are absent in heliotherapeutic and phototherapeutic literature. They are, however, provocatively described by the French writer and Nobel Prize winner André Gide. In his novels and autobiography, Gide offers insight into invalid experiences of light therapeutics, experiences that can enrich our understanding of its history and visual culture. Much like the visual material, Gide's writings are aesthetic products and agents actively contributing to the popular dissemination of these therapies.

During the 1890s, at the same time that Finsen was experimenting with light in Denmark, Gide spent time in French-colonized Algeria convalescing from pulmonary tuberculosis. His choice of undergoing a climate-cure in Algeria was not unique; doctors had been recommending Algeria's dry, warm climate for tuberculosis from the 1870s and 1880s. In fact, one source from 1883 noted that tuberculosis was the main disease among invalids choosing Algeria to convalesce.[35] Gide and his biographers described his recovery as a miraculous rebirth, a new life initiated by life-threatening illness.[36] We find fascinating descriptions in his quasi-autobiographical novel of 1902, *The Immoralist*, which is set in Algeria as well as in the Italian towns of Sorrento and Ravello on the Amalfi coast. In the novel, Gide's protagonist, the tubercular Michel, travels south and begins a self-healing process by forcing himself to walk in the open air of Algeria and expose his enfeebled body to the Italian sun. In one memorable scene set in the hilltop recesses of Ravello, Michel is inspired to try sun-bathing as a way to regenerate his weak body:

The sight of the beautiful, brown, sun-burned skins which some of the carelessly clad peasants at work in the fields showed beneath their open shirts, made me long to be like them. One morning, after I had stripped, I looked at myself; my thin arms, my stooping shoulders ... but above all the whiteness of my skin, or rather its entire want of colour, shamed me to tears. I dressed quickly and ... turned my steps towards some mossy, grass-grown rocks, in a place far from any habitation ... where I knew no one could see me. When I got there, I undressed slowly. The air was almost sharp, but the sun was burning. I exposed my whole body to its flame. I sat down, lay down, turned myself about. I felt the ground hard beneath me; the waving grass brushed me. Though I was sheltered from the wind, I shivered and thrilled at every breath. Soon a delicious burning enveloped me; my whole being surged up into my skin.[37]

As Gide makes clear, Michel's desire to tan stems from his admiration of the bronzed skins of Italian peasants labouring in the fields. His intimate descriptions and escapades throughout the novel make it clear to the reader that Michel, in fact, lusts after labourers like these, especially young men and boys, their dark skin deeply attractive to him.[38] Michel repeats the act of sun-tanning every day for two weeks, describing it as a 'cure' that arrests his continuous sweating and chills and allows him to walk in the open air with less need for clothing. Both poetically rendered and medically significant, Gide's seemingly self-regimented, spontaneous act of exposing his skin to the sunshine correlates to the methods of direct sun-bathing as advocated in heliotherapy manuals.[39] Gide's prior knowledge of the practice of heliotherapy eludes the reader, since he makes it appear in every way a natural act of instinct. However, in his 1920 autobiography *Si le grain ne meurt...*, Gide reveals not only a familiarity with heliotherapy, but also the fact that his own personal experience did not take place on the Amalfi coast, but in the hinterlands of Italy and Switzerland. In 1894 Gide spent time at the mountainous spa resorts of Lecco and Champel, following his trip to Algeria.[40] Not fully recovered, he consulted a Dr Bourget, and it was this physician who introduced him to heliotherapeutic practice. His autobiography recalls his memories of the sun-bath:

> My body, shot through with rays, seemed to enjoy some chemical benefaction; with
> my garments I laid aside anxieties, constraints, solicitudes, and as my will evaporated,
> I felt myself becoming porous as a beehive, and let my sensations secretly distil the
> honey that flowed into the pages of my *Nourritures* [*Les Nourritures terrestres*, pub-
> lished in 1897].[41]

Interestingly, Gide's claim to feeling porous in a state of illness implies that the invalid's body was regarded as open, soft, weak and easily receptive to the sun's beneficial rays. He described the sensation of sun-bathing as penetrative, transformative and inspirational. Like the passage from his novel *The Immoralist*, it is also intriguingly saturated with sexual innuendo.

Kissed by the Sun

Gide dramatized Michel's act of heliotherapy, and indeed his own, as one of physical, sensuous contact with the sun, through which he became intensely aware of his own skin. The desired result of his repeated bodily exposure to the sunlight was, of course, a tan. Claudia Benthien, in her cultural history of skin, has remarked that 'sensual and emotive touches are understood as nondiscursive, invisible traces that, nevertheless, inscribe themselves on the skin.'[42] But what if that process of inscription did leave a visible trace on the body? Is the tan not a visual marker of the body's contact with sunlight?

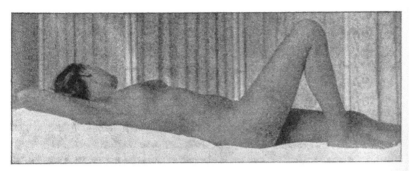

Fig. 5.—A 19-year-old girl, with multiple tuberculous lymptomata, who came for treatment in an emaciated and wretched condition. Cured by ten months' heliotherapy. Note her fine physique with the smooth, superb bronzed skin.

Figure 12.4: Photograph, *c.* 1917, in O. Bernhard, *Light Treatment in Surgery*, trans. R. King Brown (London: Edward Arnold & Co., 1926), p. 66. Author's collection.

In Figure 12.4, a photograph from Oskar Bernhard's 1926 edition of *Light Treatment in Surgery*, the composition of the image is as intriguing as its accompanying caption. A nineteen-year-old girl is seductively laid atop a soft white cloth, her faced turned away from the camera and her body arranged to allow total visual access to the length of her body. Her arm is raised so that her right breast is fully exposed and her right leg artfully posed to hide her genitals, tantalizing the viewer more. She is a veritable *Venus pudica*, arranged like a model for a traditional oil painting or marble sculpture. From the limited medical information, claiming she suffered from 'multiple tuberculosis lymptomata', it is impossible to distinguish within the photograph the specific portions of her newly healed skin from the rest of her body. In other words, what are we looking at? What is the purpose of this image? It is clearly a kind of 'after' image, and yet without a 'before' image to precede it, its purpose becomes obscure. From the caption, we are advised by Dr Bernhard to '[n]ote her fine physique with the smooth, superb bronzed skin'. Here is an example of aesthetic considerations that complement therapeutic preoccupations of the attendant physician, where perceptions of beauty and health converge on to the tanned body, employing a vocabulary laced with desire.

After visiting Rollier's clinic in Leysin, Saleeby recorded his observations of the patients' bronzed, healed skin:

> Properly aired and lighted, the skin becomes a velvety, supple, copper-coloured tissue, absolutely immune from anything of the nature of pimples or acne, incapable of being vaccinated, and its little hairs usually show considerable development. When the visitor touches such a skin, in the cool air, he is surprised to find it quite warm.[43]

The aesthetic effect of the tan was also considered by Kellogg, who wrote in 1927 that:

> The change which takes place during the process of pigmentation, is most remarkable. Instead of becoming thicker and harder, as might be expected from exposure in the so-called hardening process, the very opposite change occurs. The pigmented skin becomes thinner, softer, more elastic and altogether finer and more delicate ... Under the process of tanning in the open air, the skin not only becomes delicate and elastic, but loses its wrinkles, acquires an under-padding of fat, and is thus 'beautified' in a manner which no cosmetic can equal.[44]

Bernhard similarly described the tanning process as beautifying the skin.[45] The emphasis in these texts, quite aside from the images within them, evokes strong sensory engagement of the physician with his patient, and of the patient with the light. Saleeby mentioned physically touching the patient to feel the texture and heat of the skin as a way to convince himself of the efficacy of the treatment. Gide's fictional and autobiographical writings further conflate the tanning process as overtly sensory, even a kind of sexual contact with the invisible, penetrating rays of the sun. Bernhard's photograph and accompanying caption (Figure 12.4) equally draw the sexual desirability of tanned skin to the fore.

Möhring has stated that 'Regulating one's body according to a physiological and aesthetic ideal had a strong normalizing impact', and that German nudists paid particular attention to skin care as a practice both hygienic and aesthetic requiring strict self-monitoring and self-control. She continued: 'Within the nudist procedures of hygienic and aesthetic self-normalization, however, there were still sensual moments not completely controllable'.[46] Möhring implies that the enjoyable sensual experience of nudist practices, including sun-bathing, was regarded as a latent, guilty pleasure other to, or dichotomous with, their hygienic aims ('however', 'still'). Primary texts and images suggest that physicians and patients of light therapy, in fact, encouraged and sought after this sensuality, conflating the experience of tanning as sensory (its look and feel) and sensuous (pleasurable and desirable).

The quote by Kellogg at the outset of this chapter affirmed healthy skin as having been 'kissed by the sun', declaring that pale city workers of the 'civilized' races (that is, white Europeans and Americans) remained unhealthy because they did not have access to its transformative rays.[47] For Kellogg, it was the liberated, progressive, nature-loving being who gave himself or herself to the light, accepting and embodying the sunshine as an act towards physical health. The visual trace or mark of the sun, its 'kiss', tanned or 'weathered' the skin, making it desirable and beautiful. Gide portrayed Michel's sun-bath as sex with the sun, while Kellogg viewed the tan as 'sun-kissed' and others noted even the scar (cicatricial) tissue of a unique kind both soft and smooth (quoted above). Such language, driven by aesthetically explained visual and tactile attention, makes obvious how tanned skin came to be associated with sexual liberation and the pleasure of bodily exposure as practised through naturism.[48] So too does that sensuous language, along with the visual culture of light therapeutics, account for how tanning could become naturalized so seamlessly within popular culture as desirable.

Conclusion

That tanned skin became aesthetically desirable – that is, a visual marker of beauty – at the same moment that it became perceived as signifying health is not, to my mind, happenstance. Proponents, practitioners and patients of light therapeutics gauged the cure's efficacy through changed sensuous qualities to the skin: its look (pigmentation) and feel (composition). Heliotherapists and phototherapists placed considerable visual focus on the pigmentation of the skin of the tubercular patient. Indeed, what I have tried to emphasize throughout this chapter is that the very 'look' of the tan was integral to the therapeutic process, a visual indicator of the patient's state of healing. As a visual marker it denoted a sensuous process at work, what Kellogg called the sun's 'kiss', and the skin's receptivity to that kiss – with all its evocative, erotic undertones – was explained by its photosensitivity through knowledge of light physics and photography.

This is clear both in light therapeutics' visual culture and its literature. The photographs I have shown, and the literature by Gide, are aesthetic representations of light therapy's effects on the tubercular patient, and the transformations they describe are remarkable: from open, suppurating wounds, disfiguring and unsightly manifestations of tuberculosis, or painful-looking bone malformations to bronzed, closed skin, bodies whole, upright and healed, and smiling faces. Such representations mediate between evoking light therapy as simultaneously scientifically advanced *and* magically healing, and this seeming contradiction is embedded within the medical literature itself:

> Under the magic influence of these miracle-working rays, the elements found in earth, air and water are organized into molecular groups, some comprising thousands of atoms, the breaking up of which, as the result of vital activity, liberates the light energy employed in holding together these organic unities, permitting the energy thus set free to manifest itself in muscular and mental effort, and various other forms of vital work.[49]

This passage, by Kellogg in his 1910 edition of *Light Therapeutics*, is as evocative and prose-like as any of Gide's sensuous descriptions. Note not only his use of the words 'magic' and 'miracle-working', but also the metaphor of power and liberation to describe the process of light upon life, all the while employing a scientifically informed vocabulary and conception of the elements. The desire to tan the skin of the tubercular patient during the early twentieth century was, in this context, as much an aesthetic issue as a therapeutic one. Or rather, what emerges from the visual and textual material is that when it came to tanning skin by light therapy, they were, in fact, one and the same.

13 'CLASSIC, CHARACTERISTIC OR TYPICAL': THE SKIN AND THE VISUAL PROPERTIES OF EXTERNAL ANTHRAX LESIONS

James F. Stark

The appearances [of external anthrax] are in the highest degree characteristic.[1]

Cutaneous anthrax is associated with a characteristic skin lesion.[2]

An examination of almost all recently published texts on pathology, industrial medicine and bacterial diseases reveals a common underlying assumption that the appearance of external anthrax is somehow distinctive and easily recognizable.[3] In addition, this is not a new phenomenon, as the gap of 145 years between the two quotations above demonstrates; the idea of a 'characteristic' appearance for anthrax lesions on the skin was established long before a cause for the disease itself was identified. The pustules that indicate the presence of an anthrax infection in the skin are said to be large and almost exclusively black in colour. Nor is this a phenomenon restricted to contemporary descriptions of the disease: the French word for the disease, *charbon*, means 'coal', 'charcoal' or 'carbon', reflecting the colour of the external lesions.[4] The association between anthrax pustules and their colour and general appearance is therefore one which earned the disease, and its supposedly characteristic pustules, its name. This view is deeply embedded within the visual culture of anthrax; as far back as the late fourteenth century, English texts referred to the 'coal-fire' appearance of the disease on human skin.[5] Historians of medicine have likewise taken the nature of the pustules of external anthrax for granted. Studies addressing the visual properties of anthrax have largely focused on the causative organism – *Bacillus anthracis* – and the manner in which representations of this bacillus were exchanged between centres of research.[6] The seeming visual ubiquity of anthrax pustules was established long before the bacillus had even been observed, however, and the idea of the characteristic anthrax pustule remained almost completely intact despite the emergence of the germ-theoretic cause of anthrax lesions during the second half of the nineteenth century. The appearance of these lesions in accounts of the history of the disease is agreed on by scholars to be somehow 'classic, characteristic or typical'.[7] Whilst histories of anthrax neglect critically to examine this view, the disease is similarly marginalized within the literature on the history of dermatology; anthrax, after all, was and is a disease not specific to the skin.[8] Claudia Benthien has noted that the skin represents the major medium through which bodies can encounter one another.[9] These encounters also apply to practitioner-patient relationships and diagnostic practices, however, and the 'anthrax-encounter' has been and remains one based around the visual properties of lesions on the skin.

This chapter interrogates the widespread (indeed, almost universal) understanding amongst clinicians, historical actors and historians of medicine that anthrax pustules are somehow 'classic, characteristic or typical'.[10] The focus here will be on the efforts of one British medical practitioner and leading authority on anthrax during the early twentieth century – Frederick William Eurich – to show that the pustules could present in a variety of different fashions. Eurich was based in Bradford, West Yorkshire, a locality that became intimately connected with the incidence of anthrax during the late nineteenth century.[11] After extensive first-hand encounters with the disease, Eurich went on to state of anthrax: '[i]ts most common form, the "malignant pustule", is often said to be a characteristic structure when fully developed. This is an error'.[12] The chapter will, accordingly, outline the origins of the 'classic' anthrax pustule, as well as the emergence of anthrax in nineteenth-century Bradford, before addressing his work in more detail. Eurich encouraged practitioners and workers to abandon the notion of a characteristic pustule; his approach shows how one of the foremost British anthrax researchers made an attempt to dispel what he saw as an erroneous and misleading diagnostic marker.

Recent scholarship on the history of the skin and its relationship with disease has made such an analysis possible, and the complex connections between symptoms on the skin and diagnoses of particular diseases are further illuminated by the case of external anthrax. The conjunction and significance of skin disease and colour has been remarked upon most notably by Steven Connor, who observes that 'so many diseases are identified by the chromatic changes they induce in the skin or bodily products'.[13] However, whilst Connor cites the etymology of anthrax as a case in point, he further argues that contemporary understandings of the skin have somehow dissociated colour from specific diseases as part of 'the colourless, galvano-mechanic body of modern conception'.[14] This chapter examines in detail the manner in which the appearance of anthrax pustules, especially their colour, on human skin has become deeply embedded as a sign and symptom of that particular disease, and questions how such views have continued to persist despite resistance to the notion of an 'idealized' anthrax pustule.

Anthraxes Ancient and Modern: The Origins of the 'Classic' Pustule

The earliest frequently cited examples of outbreaks liable to have been caused by the anthrax bacillus are the fifth and sixth plagues of the Old Testament, where cattle were given 'over to the pestilence; blotches and blains broke forth on man and beast'.[15] Another appearance of an anthrax-like disease in ancient texts comes from Virgil's *Georgics*, where the author describes in detail a condition that ravages grazing animals and those handling them with a burning fire and leads to rapid death.[16] Early descriptions of the disease in English continued to classify a condition as anthrax according to its external appearance. Anthrax thus became synonymous with the 'burning coal', and the lesions were described in both medical and nonmedical literature as dark purple or, more commonly, black, and surrounded by an area of redness and swelling. This became the 'classic' pustule of anthrax, an example of which can be seen in Figure 13.1. Classifying diseases according to external appearance and sets of symptoms was the predominant mode of thought until the late eighteenth century. The presence of a black carbuncle was thus the principal diagnostic marker in confirming a case of anthrax. It was not until the work of French physicians and veterinarians such as Philibert Chabert and Jean Fournier, in the 1770s and 1790s respectively, that anthrax was re-cast as a disease that had both an internal (respiratory and intestinal) and external (cutaneous) form.

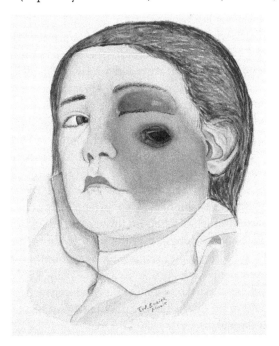

Figure 13.1: Anthrax pustule, painting (*c.* 1910) by Frederick William Eurich. CHSTM Anthrax Papers, uncatalogued, University of Manchester.

Chabert, Fournier and others moved beyond a symptomatic understanding of anthrax and attempted to demonstrate that there was a common underlying *cause* for these apparently disparate conditions.[17] Understanding diseases in a causal fashion is more generally associated with the work of nineteenth-century medical scientists, however, and it was not until the work of Robert Koch, Louis Pasteur and others in the 1870s and 1880s that micro-organisms themselves were linked in a formal manner to the occurrence of specific illnesses.[18] Whilst anthrax was for Pasteur, Koch and their continental colleagues primarily a disease of animals and therefore treated as an economic problem facing rural areas, the disease in Britain was bound up with the wool trade and occurred principally in the manufacturing centres of West Yorkshire.

The dramatic increase in the importation of fleeces from areas where anthrax was endemic – East India, Persia and Peru – brought a rise in the number cases observed amongst those working in the wool trade. In this period, Bradford was widely regarded as the wool capital of the world: 'worstedopolis'.[19] The industry had grown throughout the nineteenth century, and by 1889 there were some 338 mills in the Bradford borough. Even as late as 1910, when the Bradford economy had become far more diverse, 17 per cent of adult males and 50.2 per cent of adult women were directly employed in the textile industry.[20] Alongside this dependence on a single industry and its tightly knit group of workers came the birth of the Independent Labour Party in the 1890s; Bradford was at the heart of this reconfiguration of left-wing politics following the dominance of Gladstonian liberalism characteristic of the 1870s and 1880s.[21] Spurred on by the resulting highly organized labour force, as well as an active and vocal duo of local newspapers – the *Bradford Observer* and *Bradford Daily Telegraph* – practitioners studied the nature of anthrax and possible preventive methods from the late 1870s.[22]

Particularly prominent amongst local investigators based in Bradford was John Henry Bell. He kept meticulous records of cases that he encountered from 1876 onwards.[23] He gave a paper to the Bradford Medico-Chirurgical Society on 3 February 1880, at which meeting his support for the causative role of *Bacillus anthracis* was poorly received by fellow members. In light of this lack of consensus, the Society established a Commission on Woolsorters' Diseases, composed of fourteen of its members, to investigate the underlying nature of the disease(s) affecting those engaged in the wool industry. The Commission reported in 1882, and although it recommended a number of preventive measures, such as improving factory ventilation and the daily washing of floors, it remained deeply divided as to the nature of the condition in question.[24]

Whilst the cause of the disease (at least in Britain) remained a point of significant contention through the early 1880s, the idea of a typical external anthrax lesion, following its ancient roots, was becoming still more firmly engrained within medical literature. For example, in 1882 J. N. C. Davies-Colley, a surgeon and lecturer on anatomy at Guy's Hospital, published detailed case histories of two instances of malignant pustule (cutaneous anthrax) that had come under his care. He described at length 'the characteristic vesicular eschar', making particular reference to 'the blackened part in the centre'.[25] Accompanying his description of the pustules was a colour plate showing the characteristic lesion that presented in the second of his cases. As with Figure 13.1, the central black area was clearly visible, and even though there was only a very small area of redness and minimal swelling in Davies-Colley's case, he readily identified this as the typical appearance of external anthrax.

Significantly for the purposes of this chapter, Davies-Colley also asserted:

> As a rule diagnosis is easy. The raised indurated [hardened] area with its central blackish depression surrounded by small vesicles can hardly be mistaken for any other affection ... and the occupation of the patient will give some clue to the recognition of the disease.[26]

Medical practitioners throughout the 1880s therefore subscribed to the idea of a 'classic' or 'characteristic' pustule associated with external anthrax, often explicitly citing the observations of Davies-Colley on this matter. In 1884, for example, J. H. Hemming read a paper before the South Midland Branch of the British Medical Association where he acknowledged that consensus which had emerged surrounding the appearance of anthrax lesions. Hemming noted that 'you [the readers] will all readily follow my description. In each case there was a black shrunken eschar, from an inch to an inch and a half in diameter, round, surrounded by a raised zone of blebs or vesicles'.[27] Further, in 1886 Arthur Barker, Professor of Surgery at University College Hospital, remarked on the 'eschar so characteristic of the disease'.[28]

John Henry Bell, who had encountered a great number of cases of suspected anthrax first-hand, was also of the opinion that blackness was an important diagnostic indicator in this condition. By the turn of the twentieth century Bell was a national authority on the subject, and he described in a series of cases published in 1901 'an ulcer 1 inch in diameter, somewhat circular in shape, and with a base composed of dark-brown or black sloughing tissue'.[29] These detailed descriptions of pustules by Bell, Davies-Colley and others reinforced the idea of a 'classic' anthrax pustule. The lesions described in the medical literature were remarkably consistent and served as a key component of the patient-practitioner encounter. The observation of the location, size and colour of the pustule on the skin provided the practitioner with a very swift opportunity to rule in or out the possibility that he was dealing with a case of anthrax without further laborious tests.

The other option available to practitioners was to take a sample of fluid from the small vesicles surrounding the central eschar and attempt to culture *Bacillus anthracis*, the presence of which would confirm the diagnosis of anthrax. This was a lengthier process, however, and the rapid progression of anthrax – with death observed as few as six hours after hospital admission – necessitated early intervention. Culturing *Bacillus anthracis* was certainly not regarded as being essential prior to carrying out treatment. In one suspected case where the pustule 'was perhaps not markedly characteristic', Bell nevertheless advised the 'speedy removal of the infected area' before results of culturing were obtained.[30] Establishing a common understanding of the 'classic' anthrax lesion thus ensured a swift diagnosis was possible, based on cutaneous appearance and patient history. This meant that the practitioner was able to excise the pustule – the most common treatment in this period – at an earlier stage.[31] Intriguingly, the anthrax bacilli themselves were also well established as being of a distinctive size and shape and displayed 'characteristic feather-like growth' when cultured in gelatin.[32]

By the turn of the twentieth century, therefore, the typicality of the external anthrax pustule was a matter of universal agreement amongst medical practitioners who had encountered cases (or even simply read about them). The following section will examine how this assumption was challenged by a Bradford-based anthrax investigator – Frederick William Eurich – whose institutional affiliation ensured that he observed many cases of suspected anthrax at different stages of development.

Formalizing the 'Anthrax Encounter': The Anthrax Investigation Board

The beginning of the twentieth century saw an increase in the number of anthrax cases experienced by workers in Bradford's wool industry. This was in spite of local and national preventive regulations of the 1880s and 1890s, and their failure led in part to increasing political and social pressure on organizations representing both capital and labour to institute a major investigation, involving local wool industry representatives.[33] The Bradford Chamber of Commerce (BCC) and Bradford Trades and Labour Council (BTLC), bodies of employers and workers respectively, accordingly established the Bradford and District Anthrax Investigation Board (AIB) in 1905 for the principal purpose of devising a method through which the raw fleeces might be made safe. The Board was composed of fifteen individuals from both the BCC and BTLC, and they recognized at their first meeting on 17 July 1905 that 'the services of a bacteriological expert' were necessary in order to meet their goal.[34] Just three days later the Board reconvened for an 'informal meeting', having invited the local medical practitioner and bacteriologist to the City Council, Frederick William Eurich, to join them. At this meeting Eurich was charged with establishing what resources might be necessary to carry out investigations into protecting workers, neutralizing dangerous fleeces and observing suspected cases across the region of the Board's operations – effectively the entire reach of the West Riding wool industry. In October of that same year, the Board 'resolved "[t]hat Dr Eurich be appointed bacteriologist"', and his work in that regard began in earnest.[35]

Eurich at once sought the assistance of local medical practitioners by sending a circular requesting that they bring any suspected case of anthrax to his attention immediately. Medical men were also issued with capillary tubes for collecting samples, and a set of instructions to standardize the process. The reasoning behind recruiting practitioners in this way was to identify not only the distribution of the disease across local employers, but also to determine with more certainty which types of wool posed the greatest risk to operatives.[36] Previously, the individual practitioner was required (occasionally in consultation with colleagues) to judge qualitatively the nature of the pustule shortly after a cursory inspection of what might in all probability be his first encounter with this relatively rare disease. Now, however, Eurich was able to record details of a large proportion of the cases that occurred within the West Riding. The death of John Henry Bell in 1906, the year after the formation of the AIB, left Eurich as the local anthrax expert, and he observed over twenty cases in the first year of his work for the AIB.[37]

Eurich's activities with the Anthrax Investigation Board brought him face-to-face with more cases of anthrax than any other British-based practitioner in this period. He was, therefore, in a privileged position with respect to devising therapeutic and preventive measures. More than this, however, his call to local practitioners to notify him at the earliest available opportunity of any cases which arose meant that he observed cases at a variety of different stages of development. The increasing awareness amongst those engaged in the trade that expert medical advice should be sought at the earliest possible opportunity also meant that Eurich was able to examine suspected cases first-hand, in some cases just a few hours after the appearance of a possible anthrax pustule.[38]

Despite this increased contact with patients, Eurich still lamented the high mortality rate of cases of external anthrax a full ten years after the AIB's formation. In 1915 he noted that the previous decade's mortality for cases had been 14.9 per cent in the Bradford area. This, he attributed to two related factors:

> (1) Advice may be sought too late, the innocent-beginnings of the pustule having deceived the patient. Careless disregard of symptoms is also responsible ... (2) The nature of the disease may be recognized too late by the doctor in attendance – either from want of experience ... or, more frequently, because the pustule does not show the characteristic appearances.[39]

Eurich saw the 'characteristic' anthrax pustule as a misleading and dangerous concept. In addition to the perhaps expected failure on the part of the patient to recognize an early-stage pustule, he also felt that medical practitioners were so fixated on the 'classic' anthrax lesion that cases which did not adhere to this visual configuration were not being recognized until treatment was too late.

The bacteriologist also noted that internal cases of anthrax – more difficult to recognize and to treat – were likewise liable to be overlooked by practitioners: 'only in one out of the twenty-two cases [recorded in Bradford that year] was the diagnosis made reasonably early; in the remainder either no medical advice was sought, or suspicion was not aroused till the patient was dying or actually dead'.[40] It was Eurich's claim that cases of anthrax were being diagnosed too late to allow for therapeutic intervention that prompted the Home Office – which contributed the sum of £100 annually to subsidize the work of the AIB – to explore the possibility of distributing posters to factories where workers were handling materials potentially laden with anthrax spores.[41] An earlier poster produced by the Factory Inspectorate and based on images of external anthrax painted by John Henry Bell had been issued around 1905, but had little effect in prompting workers to seek swift treatment.[42] The following section will explore in more detail the second poster issued by His Majesty's Stationary Office (HMSO) in 1916, the contribution made by Eurich to this notice, and the poster's life in factories in West Yorkshire and further afield. Skin lesions in cases of anthrax formed a key part of this notice, and served as an important vehicle by which the conception of the 'classic' anthrax pustule was challenged.

'Different Appearances of Anthrax on the Skin': A Cautionary Notice and Attempts to Establish Lesion Plurality

Members of the Anthrax Investigation Board had initially forecast that their work would take around three years. By the time that this had stretched to five, interested locals, including Fred Jowett, the Labour MP for Bradford West, began to make their anxieties about the lack of progress known.[43] The AIB's failure to establish an economically and practically viable system of disinfection of fleeces meant that calls from local employers and workers for a Home Office Departmental Committee of Inquiry (DCI) to investigate the problem could no longer be ignored. Such a Committee was duly established by the newly elected Conservative-Unionist government in 1913.[44] In that same year, Eurich had noted that 'with the lengthening interval between the first appearance of symptoms and the date of medical attendance the number of moderately severe and of the severe cases increases'.[45] It was to this delay in seeking medical advice that he attributed the unnecessarily high mortality amongst patients suffering from cutaneous anthrax. As a member of the DCI, Eurich was able to use his knowledge of the condition in industrial Bradford to persuade the medical inspector of factories, the renowned Thomas Morison Legge, to introduce a cautionary notice through the auspices of the Home Office. This poster would prove to have a long life in factories across Britain.

Eurich himself provided the images of anthrax cases that were to be used on the poster. An enthusiastic amateur artist, he photographed many unusual medical conditions that he encountered. In addition to keeping the photographic records of external anthrax cases, however, he also used these as the basis for a series of paintings, some of which he completed with the help of his daughter Margaret.[46] In choosing to record the appearance of anthrax pustules through paint rather than black-and-white photography (colour photography was available, but still an expensive and unwieldy technique unsuited to hospital-based use at short notice), Eurich was able to capture additional visual information, particularly in relation to the colour of the lesions (see Figure 13.1). In painting, he was able to record the extent of the redness and swelling in addition to the colour of the central pustule on the skin.

These images were made not simply for Eurich's own records, however. The Anthrax Investigation Board and the Home Office collaborated to produce a cautionary notice which carried warnings about the dangers of handling material potentially contaminated with anthrax spores, and also showed nine anthrax pustules at various stages of development, all of which were taken from paintings completed by Eurich (see Figure 13.2). This poster was issued to local firms in 1916 with instructions that it should be displayed in factories prominently.[47]

The hope of both the AIB and the Home Office was that 'every case of suspected Anthrax be immediately brought to the notice of the [Anthrax Investigation] Board's Bacteriologist [Eurich] in order that advantage may be taken of the various laboratory methods of diagnosis'.[48] Indeed, Eurich asserted that 'the diagnosis of cutaneous anthrax is primarily a bacteriological one'; a judgement on the part of either the worker or consulting practitioner as to the nature of the disease based purely on the appearance of the pustule was untrustworthy.[49] In this respect Eurich differed markedly from his predecessor, Bradford's previous anthrax authority, John Henry Bell. Although their work on the disease overlapped only briefly during 1905–6, a particular incident demonstrates their different views concerning the relative merits of bacteriological and visual diagnosis. Bell was of the opinion that a case of suspected anthrax in a 48-year-old blacksmith from Cleckheaton 'was [external] anthrax in spite of negative [microscopical and cultural] results'. This observation was recorded in the first annual report of the AIB alongside Eurich's assertion that bacteriological tests were the only reliable way of establishing the diagnosis of anthrax.[50]

The importance of maintaining the visual attributes of the cautionary notice is revealed by the instructions at the bottom of the poster: '[i]n order to preserve this Form and prevent fading of colours, it should be mounted on cardboard and varnished on both sides and should not be exposed to direct sunlight.'[51] Those responsible for the creation of the poster, including Eurich, thus recognized that keeping the colour and appearance of the images was integral to the

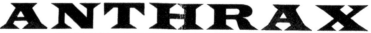
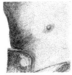

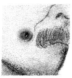
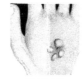

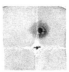
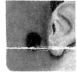

Figure 13.2: Anthrax poster issued by His Majesty's Stationary Office (1927). Papers of Dr Donald Hunter (1898–1977), Wellcome Library, CMAC PP/HUN/B/17; image reproduced courtesy of the Wellcome Library, London.

poster's continued use.[52] This was in marked contrast to cautionary notices for other industrial conditions of this period, which were almost universally printed in black and white, had detailed prevention instructions and offered guidance rather than warnings.[53]

Although it might be assumed that the motivation of both Eurich and the Home Office Factory Department in issuing the poster was to better educate at-risk workers of the appearance of anthrax pustules, his comments on the abuse of the cautionary notice reveal a rather different attitude. In 1926, the year before the poster was re-printed in order to widen its coverage to different industries, Eurich noted that the poster:

> is meant only to arouse suspicion and to keep vividly before the worker the risk which he is running, not to be an aid to diagnosis. The diagnosis is the doctor's duty, which should not be arrogated to himself by the foreman or manager, as I have known done, with disastrous results.[54]

Eurich therefore encouraged workers in trades liable to anthrax not to compare suspected pustules with those displayed on the cautionary notice, but rather to seek medical advice when any abnormality on the skin arose. Whilst this was a criticism of potential patients, he also attacked practitioners' assumptions that anthrax pustules presented universally with a 'characteristic' appearance, noting that:

> [t]ext-books often tell us that the appearance of the pustule is characteristic. This is not so ... It cannot be urged too strongly that it is a grievous error to allow the picture of the fully developed pustule to dominate the mind.[55]

This was a concerted attempt on the part of Eurich to dispel what he regarded as a misleading mythology about anthrax's presentation on the skin. By the time the poster was re-printed in 1927 (with the same images as the original 1916 notice), the AIB had been wound up and the Anthrax Prevention Act (1919) passed. This piece of legislation stipulated mandatory disinfection of certain classes of fleece through a system devised by members of the Departmental Committee of Inquiry.[56] The re-issuing of the poster clearly demonstrates that notwithstanding the gradual drop in the number of recorded anthrax cases, concern over the disease persisted amongst workers, researchers, such as Eurich, and Home Office officials.[57]

The cautionary notice itself had a lengthy life in the factory environment and moved far beyond the confines of the traditional industries associated with anthrax – the wool, hide and tanning trades – and into abattoirs, docks and elsewhere across Britain.[58] A Royal Mail film – *Men in Danger* – about the health risks posed by specific occupations showed the poster behind a woolsorter going about his work, whilst the celebrated occupational health expert Donald Hunter noted in 1950 that regulations required that 'cautionary placards be displayed in certain factories… show coloured pictures of the skin lesion in anthrax at various stages'.[59] By this stage, Hunter noted, workers in occupations associated with an increased risk of anthrax infection carried a card, issued by the Factory Department of the Ministry of Labour, to 'suggest tactfully' to medical practitioners that anthrax might be suspected.[60]

The occurrence of industrial, cutaneous anthrax was not limited to Britain; the cautionary notice also had a role to play elsewhere. In 1952 a representative of the Hides, Tanning and Allied Industries Bureau in Nairobi – T. M. Loudon – contacted the Colonial Products Advisory Bureau in London. Loudon had heard that 'a series of posters relating to anthrax and anthrax prevention' were in use in Britain, and he asked for a set to be sent to Kenya.[61] The addressee – R. W. Pearman – duly obliged, indicating that there were in fact three such posters in use, one of which was Form 410, the anthrax poster bearing Eurich's images.[62]

Loudon received the posters in early November 1952 and wrote to thank Pearman for sending them so promptly. However, he also revealed that the representations of cutaneous anthrax pustules created by Eurich were less useful than he had hoped, writing: '[u]nfortunately as far as the illustrations are concerned the colour of the African skin makes it very difficult to produce a poster to illustrate the symptoms of this unpleasant disease.'[63] Similar difficulties attended diagnosis of vitiligo (skin depigmentation) during the nineteenth and early twentieth centuries, particularly in the context of European colonies. This visually striking ailment presented in very different fashions on dark and white skins and caused some consternation as to how practitioners who were unfamiliar with patients of a certain skin tone might recognize the condition.[64]

For the case of anthrax, Loudon's observation serves to further reinforce the point made by Eurich: that the appearance of anthrax lesions on the skin was anything but 'characteristic'. The visual configuration depended not just on the stage of development of the pustule, but also the colour of the patient's skin. The firmly established idea of the classic anthrax pustule was thus dependent on the properties of the skin itself, in addition to the colour of the lesion and its natural progression. Eurich clearly believed that keeping the variety of appearances of anthrax pustules in view meant that workers and practitioners would be more alert to the possibility that this was the disease with which they were dealing. Nevertheless, despite concerted Home Office-backed attempts to instil this view, the prevailing perception remained that anthrax displayed a 'classic, characteristic or typical' lesion on the skin.

Conclusion

In a striking similarity with other (albeit less fatal) conditions that present on the skin, such as meningitis, modern-day textbooks continue to refer to anthrax pustules as displaying a near identical appearance in all cases. As Eurich noted, bacteriological analysis should be used in all suspected instances of anthrax in order to arrive at a more certain diagnosis; the visual aspects of the pustule became marginalized in the diagnostic process. This view fits neatly with Steven Connor's characterization of 'the colourless, galvano-mechanic body of modern conception'.[65] Nevertheless, the mere fact that 'blackness' continues to be used as an important signifier of anthrax demonstrates that the association between colour and specific diseases remains deeply embedded in medical (and wider) culture. The cultural significance of different skin types has likewise been the focus of recent scholarship in the history of the skin, and the failure of the anthrax cautionary notice to operate outside of the social and cultural boundaries within which it was conceived serves to further highlight the erroneous notion of a 'classic' anthrax pustule.[66]

Eurich argued that incorrect diagnoses were made as a result, and even when anthrax was identified correctly, the patient often delayed seeing a practitioner to such an extent that chances of successful treatment were greatly reduced. Modern textbooks on dermatology regularly assert the importance of visual observation in diagnosis. One such widely used text notes that 'the dermatologist can often make a rapid and correct diagnosis simply by looking at the patient'.[67] With such emphasis placed on determining the nature of disease simply by visual observation of a symptom on the skin, Eurich's warning from 1926 that 'it is a grievous error to allow the picture of the fully developed pustule to dominate the mind' seems to carry added significance for modern dermatology.[68] So too does the use of white skin predominantly in illustrations remain an issue in this field.

What remains unclear is why the view of the 'classic' anthrax pustule persisted despite the efforts of Eurich and others. One possible explanation is that the greatly reduced incidence of the disease across the twentieth century simply meant that general practitioners (and indeed workers) almost invariably did not encounter anthrax, and therefore had little reason to question the received view. Alternatively, a general shift in anthrax diagnostic practices from simple visual observation towards laboratory-based culturing of bacilli may have caused the reduced emphasis placed on the appearance of pustules in suspected cases.

The skin itself was the first site of encounters between patients, practitioners and pustules. The absence of pain in most cases of external anthrax meant that the appearance would be the primary indicator of abnormality to the patient, whilst the practitioner was informed of the likely diagnosis in the same way. Culturing *Bacillus anthracis* was a technique widely available from the turn of the twentieth century, but this was not able to provide the rapid diagnosis afforded by observing the pustule itself. Indeed, whilst the characteristic appearance of the pustule was contested by Eurich, a different facet of anthrax was also considered characteristic: the causative organism. *Bacillus anthracis* presented under the microscope, on agar and in capillary tubes in a typical fashion. Establishing agreements about the visual nature of these growths proved to be far more fruitful than regarding the pustules as similarly classical in appearances. However, the skin lesions were viewed as characteristic prior to the implication of *Bacillus anthracis*; these observations of the skin at the macro-pathological level offered a parallel diagnostic pathway for the practitioner. Furthermore, whilst the word 'anthrax' referred to any kind of malignant carbuncle prior to major research into the disease in the mid-nineteenth century, its usage was confined to lesions caused by *Bacillus anthracis* thereafter. Despite this, the visual signs that indicated anthrax remained identical after these links were established.

As Canguilhem has argued, historians might usefully challenge other notions of typicality in disease.[69] Conditions that present primarily on the skin are excellent candidates for such analysis, as little or no technological mediation is required for both practitioners and patients to observe such signs. Consensuses surrounding such appearances reveal much about the cultural and classificatory heritage of specific diseases, and provide important insight into the relationship between medico-cultural practices and human skin.

AFTERWORD: READING THE SKIN, DISCERNING THE LANDSCAPE: A GEO-HISTORICAL PERSPECTIVE OF OUR HUMAN SURFACE

Philip K. Wilson

Contributors to this volume frequently alluded to ways of perceiving the skin beyond that of a mere bodily part or a platform for disease. Many of these perceptions bear a striking similarity to geo-history.[1] Geo-history depicts the accurate, orderly and rational description and interpretation of variable characteristics at the earth's surface – and that of its underlying strata – over the course of time.[2] Additionally, the term encompasses explanations of the life forms whose existence depends upon interaction with surface substances or with subterranean strata.

As this volume has shown, the skin is a surface that, like the earth, is subject to bouts of disruptive erosion and disordering decay. Those who study the skin, like those who study the earth, are keenly interested in morphology, distribution patterns and classificatory schemes. By reflecting upon key points drawn from this volume's collective focus, some interesting similarities arise from comparing contemporaneous periods of thought about the terrestrial landscape with those marking the human landscape – the skin.

Reading the Skin as Space and Place

Since at least the Enlightenment, humans have viewed their skin as a single entity, as an enveloping environment, and as a connecting point to the world around them.[3] Reading the skin as a bidirectional conduit connecting the inner self with the outer world is central to a number of works in this volume, particularly those of Lie, Moran and Minard. A perception of our skin represents a spatial view in that discreet areas are connected – or disconnected – from that which lies either beneath or beyond. Thus the study of skin and its diseases is, on one important level, a study of space and place.[4] As the authors in this volume have demonstrated, skin diseases have often been linked to, and even identified according to, particular places. Pellagra was called 'Italic scurvy', endemic syphilis came to be named after Quebec's 'St Paul's Bay', anthrax was termed '*la maladie de Bradford*' and scabies became known as the 'Scotch itch'. But the medical and surgical world also envisioned deeper links between skin and geo-history. This overview expands upon these links in offering a slightly nuanced spatial analysis of the skin and diseases incident to the skin over representative periods of Western history.

To convey precise meanings about space and place, a common language and an ability to pinpoint specific areas are necessary. Early modern explorers and geographers envisioned the introduction of maps as a new visual language that clearly and precisely delineated certain areas. Those who developed a special study of the skin also found – though much later in history – that mapping common skin conditions into a comparative collection of images, i.e. the derma-tologic atlas, gave them a special, new visual language through which they were able to convey more precise visions of the geo-history of skin. In doing so, such renderings gave the skin a new conceptual meaning.

The map has been an increasingly common and useful metaphor for the body as well as for the skin. The body in its skin has often been referred to as a terrain to be mapped. As a form of visualizing meaning, maps artfully produce images that spatially portray patterns of connectedness. They provide orientation and direction; they concisely depict phenomena in relationship to each other; they convey meaning through the power of synopsis; and they are perspectival in that their features depend upon the aims, needs, interests, biases and mindsets of the cartographers. Maps 'provide a way of noting differences as well as establish[ing] a sense of self among space, time and other elements. Maps mark location as well as act as a means to monitor sites of transgression.'[5] As such, maps of our bodily covering convey the landscape of the skin, or 'skinscape'.[6]

Skin has also frequently been metaphorically referred to as a text – a 'surface upon which something can be written'. Skin and its inscriptions 'can be read like any other text'. Combining metaphors, we can envision skin as a map of text with 'characteristics of both surface and depth' that provides 'a particular type of terrain'.[7] More precisely, skin is a palimpsest – a structure upon which some-thing can be written, scraped off, and later, different messages can be written. This structural metaphor is particularly useful as it implies the additional need for deciphering something that, though faintly apparent, may lose particular meanings to later generations. Kerr's work on smallpox highlights such a repre-sentation where, following the advent of vaccination, the skin was 're-imagined as a new type of text upon which were written entirely new messages about vis-ibility, exhibition, beauty and safety'.

Admittedly, geo-history and skin history have distinct methodologies, and they have developed along their respective professional lines of inquiry. How-ever, they share many perspectives. For example, both are based on correlative viewpoints.[8] The spatial thinking and techniques that geographers employed for visual representation played vital roles in developing a 'science' of skin, a finding corroborated by Benthien's suggestion that early medicine is best perceived in terms of 'anatomical cartography',[9] and by Connor's analysis of the early Salpêtrière neurological pathologist Jean-Martin Charcot's attempt to 'map' the 'strange double topology' of hysteria.[10] Borrowing further insight from that most ancient field of investigation – geo-history – may well provide a more solid, unified and relational approach towards better understanding the seemingly myriad classificatory groupings, etiologies and even approaches to treating the diseases incident to the skin.

Geo-historical Groundwork

To more fully appreciate these shared views, let us turn to some specifics of geo-history and landscape. Geography has frequently been characterized as one of the 'oldest fields of intellectual inquiry'.[11] According to the earliest accounts, the ancients distinguished two different areas of geographical investigation: topography, the study of places as discreet units, and chorography, the study of interconnecting systems of space and place. Yet as the ancient Greek historian Herodotus's *Geographica* noted, both of these areas were organized around a regional focus. This regionalism remained the predominant geo-historical outlook until the Renaissance. Then, as influential works like that of the German physician and geographer Bernhardus Varenius's *Geographia Generalis* (1650) demonstrate, a general, systematic approach was posited whereby whole earth processes and operations complemented the long-entrenched, specific regional geo-historical investigations. The Enlightenment which followed presented both geography and history as descriptive synthetic bodies of knowledge that focused upon 'totalities' – or, in a sense, bringing it all together.

Early Romantic-era thought pointed to difficulties that arose when attempting to distinguish boundaries. These difficulties were evident not only in the materials of the world being studied but also in attempts to define distinct fields or specialties of investigation. According to the prolific and influential French historian Jules Michelet, history was 'at first entirely geography', but gradually, 'society overcomes nature', and 'history efface[d] geography'. One of Michelet's most enduring figurative and literal images was that of geography as a tableau upon which the drama of history was unfolded.[12]

The nineteenth century was also marked by the re-emergence of regional thinking about geo-history in ways that philosophically captured concepts of both landscape and lifestyle in each of the regions (or *pays*) described. This interconnectedness reflected a refined focus at that time upon the environment and its associated life forms. The *pays* approach also became apparent in the growing

discourse of national personalities, as prominently conveyed through the influential nationalist-based history writings of University of Berlin professor and
Royal Historiographer Leopold von Ranke.[13]

Skin and its Diseases over the Ages

Following this geo-history timeline, we encounter a number of parallels when
we focus upon the skin and its diseases. If we accept anthropologist Nina Jablonski's claim, then for 'thousands of years before the birth of modern medicine',
skin 'alone testified to the state of a person's health, displaying most of the
known signs and symptoms of disease'.[14] Indeed, 'no other organ in the body
can boast so many diverse and important roles'.[15] Primary sources frequently
convey similar ideas. Noted seventeenth-century English physician Sir Thomas
Browne claimed that the 'consideration of the skinne takes up ... the cosmeticall
and exornatorie part of physic for which men have sett downe more recepts than
for any ... [other] part of the body'.[16] Yet, ironically, it is difficult to envision the
skin as holding such extraordinary importance, when throughout so much of
its history it remained merely the invisible backdrop to medicine. Physicians of
old 'paid little heed' to the skin.[17] And like the depiction of geo-history as being
'what's left after someone has found a use for everything else',[18] the skin has long
had to grapple for visibility.

When it was discussed in antiquity, Greek physicians advocated the Hippo-
cratic vision of the skin in both local and constitutional frameworks. The Greeks
read changes in skin colouration – both locally and systemically – as a 'reliable
manner' of diagnosing 'bodily well being'.[19] The prolific Roman physician-phi-
losopher Galen described the skin more in regional terms, distinguishing those
visibly apparent skin diseases that occurred on the scalp from those that presented elsewhere on the surface of the body. This regional landscaping shaped
the framework of dermatological discourse for centuries to come.

During the medieval period, the physical body commonly and literally became
viewed as the cosmos in miniature. To study the human was to know the cosmos,
and to know the cosmos was to know oneself. Medieval zodiac man depicted specific heavenly geographic signs as holding special powers over correlative human
bodily regions. By the 1600s, macrocosm/microcosm analogies were routinely
used to explain human body function in both medical and popular writings. To
aid such thought, the outer layer of the body – the skin – became the physical site
for mapping earth and sky. Such maps were more than mere analogy, though, for
the diagnosis and treatment of disease were routinely based upon wisdom derived
from reading specific geo-historical patterns upon the skin.

University of Padua Chair of Medical Practice Geronimo Mercurialis's *De
Morbis Cutaneis* (1572) is routinely viewed as a milestone in skin thought.[20]

Though it retained the common Galenic divide, Mercurialis also prompted a further parcelling of the body in terms of skin surfaces. His work also conformed to a new breed of anatomical thinking in which humanists of the period turned their gaze away from medieval scholastic commentaries upon Galen and towards the natural world itself. Nature's secrets, they exclaimed, were revealed by peeling away its structure layer by layer. Such new findings in medicine were also thought to be uncoverable by the natural philosophical flaying the body of its skin. Indeed, analogies between skin and tree bark became increasingly common in contemporary writings.

Throughout the Renaissance, the skin, much like Edgar Allan Poe's purloined letter of a later period, remained 'Hidden in Plain View'.[21] As Javier Moscoso noted in the guide accompanying the 2010 Wellcome Collection Skin Exhibition in London, 'skin has historically enjoyed an independent life'. At the time when Renaissance artists focused considerable attention upon their canvas, the skin – that human canvas – remained relatively invisible. When anatomists, revelling after the long-banned opportunity to practice human dissection, chose to depict the skin, it typically appeared as a superfluous, expendable covering, cast off like a coat 'in order to reveal the body's "inner" truth'.[22] Though admittedly humanistic-centred in their thinking and privileged with inner views of the body unlike those before them, these anatomists did not regard the cadaver, flayed of its skin, as having been stripped of its 'dynamic personhood'.[23]

Some Renaissance medical authorities extended the long-held view of skin protecting the more valued inner, hidebound body from physical harm to beliefs that the skin also shielded against disease-causing agents in the external environment. Girolamo Fracastoro, University of Padua medical professor and physician of the Council of Trent, specified this role of the skin in the three types of contagion he famously discussed: direct contact with disease, contact with belongings of the diseased and bad air. In another work, Fracastoro created a geo-historical connectedness of the skin to syphilis. Quite distinct from our common notion of syphilis as a single disease entity, it has historically represented, as Siena reminds us, a broader range of diseases, some of which spread venereally. Syphilis has also typically carried the connotation of both moral and environmental uncleanliness, each of which contributed to its prolific propagation.

Blame for syphilis's origin and spread quickly became construed xenophobically in terms of regional, geographical medical nomenclature. Fracastoro, an Italian, proclaimed syphilis to be the French disease, as did those in Germany and Poland. The French claimed it as the Italian disease; the Russians, the Polish disease; the Dutch, the Spanish disease; the Turks, the Christian disease; and in later centuries, the Tahitians referred to it as the British disease.[24] Nationalism and transgression of space loomed large in the nomenclature of other skin-level diseases. Norway's radesyge and Quebec's St Paul's Bay disease signified, as we have seen, threats to national strength. French colonialists inflicted repulsive stigma upon their Algerian subordinates through their use of the truly geo-historical labels 'Kabyle leprosy' and 'Arab syphilis'. Further cultural studies of the geographical nomenclature relevant to skin disease (as well as disease in general) would expand the current scope of our history of both global health, as well as medical geography.

As Siena and Reinarz, Lie, Moran, Minard and Angel have discussed, syphilis redirected considerable medical thinking and practice to the skin. In short, the skin as a medical map marking the pathogenic spread of syphilis became more pronounced. Information gathered from reading the skin made individuals at the frontier of syphilology more surefooted as they entered new terrain.[25] One such syphilological frontiersman was the English surgeon-turned-physician and pioneering dermatologist of the English language, Daniel Turner, an individual frequently mentioned in the historical annals of skin disease whom we have already encountered in Siena's chapter.[26]

In his 1714 *De Morbis Cutaneis: A Treatise of Diseases Incident to the Skin*, Turner guides us even further into a new frontier in terms of the skin. Though the text is most commonly cited today as his entrée into the battleground over skin markings resulting from maternal impressions, Turner more broadly used this work to help his readers rethink the external/internal nature of this bodily covering.[27] Though certainly not the first to describe the skin microscopically (that was William Cowper),[28] Turner was the first to argue forcibly skin's peculiar role in the armamentarium against disease.[29] By more closely examining the strata of skin itself – and its geographical positioning – he concluded that skin served as more than the liminal separation of outer and inner bodies.[30] While acknowledging the skin's protective function for the inner body, he advocated that the skin's impressive and variegated structure allowed it to serve as both a mountainous blockade as well as a morphological passage through which a bidirectional flow could be properly controlled.

In geo-historical terms, Turner retained a regional focus along a planar surface, but he also directed further attention to how the skin's function was mediated by a third dimension through the threshold of its pores. Pores, as Payne has shown, became functional tools for surgeons who used them to relieve the inward build-up of inflammation and to relay externally applied medicines inwardly. It was porous skin, as Lie argues, that was deemed responsible for drawing in the radesyge and, when blocked, actually created this disease from within. Turner, as well as Payne and Lie, came to see the skin, to borrow a phrase, as 'a permeable map with characteristics of both surface and depth'.[31] Such a view corroborates the contemporaneous move towards considering the skin in its totality.

Later, during the eighteenth century, similar to the geographer's changing view of the global landscape, medical and surgical practitioners began to focus on the skin *en masse*. For example, at times the skin was found completely to change its anatomical and physiological characteristics in reaction to diseases. Some diseases affecting the skin remained local, causing little if any constitutional derangement.[32] Alternatively, some skin signs suggested significant systematic spread. Thus a looming concern about the skinscape remained: When does a cutaneous eruption indicate that the skin itself is diseased, and when is it a sign of systemic disease spreading cutaneously?[33] Leprosy, as Gentilcore notes, 'actually resides in the skin', in contrast to pellagra in which the skin is 'only affected periodically'. Payne's surgeons read changes in the skinscape in distinct ways. At times the ripple of a granulation or the valley of an abscess indicated the need for a locally applied treatment to allow the wound to heal itself from below. At other times the skin showed the systematic spread of inflammation, thereby indicating something particular about the nature of the disease lurking within.

Classifications and Atlases of Skin Diseases

To better ascertain which diseases affected the skin in a particular manner, physicians looked to natural philosophers' models of grouping together similar structures that they had found on the landscape. In efforts to order diseases of the skin, the late eighteenth century witnessed a flurry of creative classification schemes or nosologies. One striking difference between nosological camps of the period was the extent to which they viewed their schematic ordering of diseases as either natural or artificial. According to contemporary accounts, an artificial arrangement implied 'one in which the points of resemblance or difference between the objects brought into close approximation in the several orders or classes, have relation to obscure or trivial characters', whereas a natural arrangement is one that 'brings together objects' that were seen to 'correspond in their most obvious and important relations, phenomena, or characters'.[34]

Viennese physician Joseph Jacob Plenck's 1776 classification scheme depicted an artificial grouping of skin diseases based upon the 'ocular appearance' of 'certain salient [external] features or properties which the individuals comprising each of the general classes [of disease] had in common'.[35] Importantly, this systematic approach was based upon the type of lesion, thereby following the work of the renowned Paduan anatomist Giovanni Battisti Morgagni's *The Seats and Causes of Disease* (1761) rather than drawing on Galen's concept of regionalization. Such a view typified the descriptive morphology common to Enlightenment geography.

In the early nineteenth century we find an increasing number of examples that, though not strictly organized into Linnaean artificial classes, were grouped according to what were touted as natural similarities of morphological form. Premiere among this type of natural cutaneous eruption is London physician

Robert Willan's *Description and Treatment of Cutaneous Diseases*.[36] Willan, whose topographical work was discussed by Lie and Fend, strove to clearly differentiate diseases incident to the skin in terms of their essential pathognomonic lesions. Such an approach would, it was argued, make this work 'more practicable' than that of Plenck or Alibert; the latter, as Fend notes, sought to capture the image of disease only in its full bloom.[37]

A new format for representing skin disease soon followed in the form of atlases. Atlases, which had come to dominate geo-historical works of the period, were, in regard to skin diseases, textualizations of the flesh and iconographies of skinscape. Similar to the ways that geo-historical atlases focused upon *pays* in the landscape, skin atlases offered facsimiles of the pathognomonic signs of disease.[38] Hereafter, verbal descriptions, like those Payne identified in the work of James Moore regarding the geo-historical stages of inflammation and healing within the layers of the skin, became more universally visualized. Following Willan, a spate of skin atlases appeared, each attempting to out-naturalize its predecessor, meticulously improving upon the realistic lithography and colouration of skin lesions and then, starting with surgeon Alexander Balmanno Squire's 1864 atlas, rendering even more realistic representations through photography.[39] Fend's exposé adds a new dimension on how the colouration of atlas illustrations and, equally important, the 'inscription' of skin disorders on living individuals in the manner popularized by Robert Carswell helped humanize both the perception of and suffering associated with these truly visible diseases. Minard deftly envisions photographers' ability to capture skin disease as 'moving [away] from maps' and toward 'portraits of the sick'.

One aberration in this general move towards realism in depictions of skin disease was that of Hôpital Saint-Louis and later royal physician Jean-Louis-Marc Alibert's arboreal representation of disease. Alibert's work, noted by Minard and discussed in greater depth by Fend, which was acclaimed as the 'first systematic attempt to classify cutaneous diseases according to their inherent natural qualities',[40] presented dermatoses as sharing a common root, originating in some 'morbid action to which the skin was subject[ed]' and then branching out, in tree fashion, divergently from one another according to genera, species and varieties.[41] This pedigree, represented as growing singularly in front of a looming alpine mountainous backdrop, offered a literal geo-historical landscape of skin disease. Though his particular view of distinct divisions was later modified, Alibert successfully introduced the lasting concept of natural families of disease that affect the outer bark of humanity – the skin.

Living Skin

Building upon earlier views of the skin as merely a static enclosure, Anne Charles de Lorry's 1777 description of the skin as a living organism was concurrent with geo-historical worldviews.[42] This organicist view pervaded the popular and academic writings of contemporary luminaries, including Immanuel Kant, Johann Gottlieb Fichte, Friedrich Schelling, Friedrich Schiller, Johann Wolfgang von Goethe and, later, Friedrich Schleiermacher. Among geo-historians, Alexander von Humboldt and Carl Ritter were the most prominent proponents.[43]

As these geo-historians argued, if the earth appeared to be a static organism, it was only because the naturally counterpoised forces had reached some temporary state of resolution or equilibrium. All nature, they surmised, experienced an ongoing conflict between progress and regress over time. Humboldt envisioned the great importance of living beings in terms of *Zusammenhang* – or a literal 'hanging togetherness' of all things. In organicist terms, the earth was viewed as a whole, dynamic, developing organism, comprising nature, man and moral and intellectual life all interconnected or 'hanging together'. This interconnectedness implied a 'grand harmony' that unified many diverse and natural geographical parts. Ritter added that the dynamic, living organic earth contained regions of text like a book within which the history of all life forms could be found and upon which the history of mankind's progress could be read.

Von Humboldt's immodestly titled five-volume *Cosmos: A Sketch of a Physical Description of the Universe* further popularized these ideas of hanging together.[44] Yet in assembling this grand purview, Von Humboldt also drew particular attention to the regional differentiation that he had uncovered within this harmonious totality. Such regional focus is evident in the pictorial graphs derived from data he collected during perilous and painstaking travels across, upon and into the earth. By bringing together the physical descriptions of various regional locations, he – like many others in his era – sought to uncover the specific laws of nature responsible for the apparent harmony of a dynamic, living world.

By mid-century, a similar search for natural laws became evident in dermatopathological quests for specific anatomical seats of disease. These concepts, introduced by London surgeon Sir Erasmus Wilson and Viennese physician Julius Rosenbaum in the early 1840s, were furthered by Berlin Charité director of skin disease and syphilis Karl Gustav Theodor Simon, and became even more pronounced with Vienna School of Dermatology founder Ferdinand von Hebra's new objective outlooks and reclassificatory patterns of the skin and its diseases. Von Hebra microscopically searched the skin's anatomy for indications of local pathological processes.[45] This focus, particularly upon tissue pathology, prompted him to rewrite the known natural history of diseases that, at least in part, became associated with the skin. Many lesions appeared to derive from local, regional processes, whereas others reflected what he termed the 'consecutives' – local disease that spread geographically and developed, successively, into more widespread systemic disease.

Reading the skin increasingly became part of physical diagnosis.[46] Such a view, particularly in nineteenth-century thought, is substantiated by many chapters in this volume. Continuing the tradition of Edinburgh's educational prowess cited herein, nineteenth-century physicians like Joe Bell taught medical students in the Scottish capital to rely upon their ability to read the landscape of the skin in order to uncover clues about pertinent conditions regarding the human under that skin. Even if Bell's name escapes many historical accounts, his method of diagnosis was immortalized through his student, Arthur Conan Doyle, who used Professor Bell as the model of his masterful detective – Sherlock Holmes.[47]

Indeed, Conan Doyle designed the plot of his 1926 Holmes tale 'The Adventure of the Blanched Soldier' around skin disease. In it, James M. Dodd sought Holmes's assistance to locate his former Boer War army comrade, Godfrey Emsworth. After having once again caught a glimpse of Emsworth, Dodd exclaimed, 'never have I seen a man so white'. Holmes, following his own advice that 'when you have eliminated all which is impossible then whatever remains, however improbable, must be the truth', deduced that Emsworth, after being wounded, made his way to the nearest hospital – a leprosarium. Later, the 'bleaching of [Emsworth's] skin' was initially diagnosed as leprosy. A second opinion, which Holmes secured from Sir James Saunders, provided the less threatening and, in this case, correct diagnosis of 'pseudo-leprosy ... a scale-like affliction of the skin' which, although 'unsightly' and 'obstinate', was most likely 'curable, and certainly non-infective'. Conan Doyle then asserted a bit of Sherlockian elimination of the impossible in establishing a psychosomatic origin of Emsworth's skin disease as he provoked his readers to consider, 'Are we assured that the apprehension, from which this young man has no doubt suffered dearly since his exposure to its contagion, may not provide a physical effect which simulates that which it fears?' An interesting geographical mental and bodily transit underlying this skin disease, to say the least.[48]

Diagnosis, Design and Dwelling Places

Joe Bell's diagnostic method relied upon reading visible signs. In more recent decades, the once less visible skin has not only caught our ocular attention, but it is being read in myriad ways, too. This is apparent in photography and film, in the 'cosmeceutical' industry, in fashion design, in fiction and in plastic surgery, as well as in the increasingly accessible acts of bodily adornment, fetishism and sadomasochism.[49] Discourse and meaning regarding tattoos, as Angel has shown, vary widely over geographical regions. At times, Angel discovered, tattooing was even performed as a therapeutic healing art at the skin level, treating diseases lying beneath. Payne hinted that the desired aesthetics of wound appearance tempered rivalries between eighteenth-century proponents of particular healing methods all endeavouring to downplay any disruption of the terrain. Counter to earlier concerns about wound healing, more recently, skin mutilation has become, for some, a desired way to produce changes in body iconography whereby new expressions of one's identity can be mapped onto the flesh. In classificatory terms, such intentional changes upon the skinscape represent 'artificial' landmarks, whereas topographical changes resulting from disease are considered to be 'natural'.

Within the medical realm, the skin is no longer viewed as a mere screen or Michelet tableau upon which the drama of disease plays its part, nor as a mechanical membrane separating internal (proximate) function from external (remote) influences. As Connor has cogently argued, the skin has become an entire milieu –the grand geo-historical physical environment in which something happens.

Recent research has also come to show that not all skin is equal. For centuries, various skin pigmentation has denoted geo-historical meaning regarding particular regional, ethnic and class roots.[50] Now, even upon the same body, skin has distinct regional differentiation. In 1950, Montreal Neurological Institute neurosurgeons Wilder Penfield and Theodore Rasmussen famously correlatively linked specific sensory and motor areas of the body – in particular, areas of bodily skin – to precise regions of the brain.[51] Also dating back to the mid-twentieth century, skin surfaces called dermatomes became readable as specific organizational areas, each of which represents a geographical region of skin where sensory nerves all derive from a single spinal nerve root.[52] Additionally, though widely described throughout history, certain regions of the body's skin have recently been officially dubbed as erotogenic or erogenous zones. It is also notable that geo-historical rearrangements of skin via transplant grafts have drawn considerable attention in recent decades.

When we consider the skin in terms of created environments, its history becomes an environmental history. We begin to appreciate our skin in terms of ecosystems spread across a landscape. Skin study becomes a form of biogeography – a living landscape that is frequently invaded and ultimately inhabited by foreign beings, some of which establish new dwelling places that promote irreversible destruction of the terrain. Such a perspective is echoed throughout this volume.

A Medical History of Skin highlights a multitude of ways of thinking about, seeing and reading the skin in history. On one level, our skin helps to visualize meanings of identity, but it also visibly relays cultural and temporal messages about beauty, horror, age, stigma and race. Notably, skin, though at times acting as an opaque border of self, also allows for an extension beyond our selves. In its healthy state, the anatomical, multi-layered structure of our skin allows for a physiological connectedness with the world beyond us. But skin is also a platform for pathology; moreover, skin has a pathological basis in itself, too. It indicates pathology within the body as in the case of jaundice, or allows contagions to enter the body from the external world as with cutaneous anthrax, or in some as of yet fully known way, it assists the body's predilection for or resistance against disease as in the case of leprosy.

When viewed as text or palimpsest, skin becomes subjected to literary analysis. When seen as a canvas, a more visual cultural analysis is warranted. Here, we consider one further view, that of geo-historical comparisons that allow us more fully to comprehend all that our skin represents. Beyond mere historical representations, we must remember that our skin itself has a history, a story to be read and told. Indeed, skin is an historical artefact, and a primary source for historical interpretation. Our skin is marked with interpretable signs of experience. It is a place where identity and experience are 'both revealed and concealed'.[53] Like regions of the earth, regions of our skinscape have become 'heavily vested with symbolic importance'.[54] At times, the skin becomes an important site from which to interpret cultural power struggles and upon which to read, in philosopher Michel Foucault's terms, the inscribed surface of events.

As we become increasingly aware of the world around us, it is the skin that serves as our primary interface through which we, in the interior, learn more about our surrounds. Indeed, skin heightens our sensation of our environment. An intact sense of tactility, that geographical connectedness between skin and nerves, accentuates our feeling, both literally and figuratively, as well as physically and mentally.[55] We come to know more about who we are, where we are, and from whence we have come by looking at – and becoming in touch with – the terrain of the environment around us. We are regional beings. Through our skin and our mind, we detect what we have come to call the 'personal space' surrounding us. Part of the ability to look out and think beyond our skin offers us a better sense of self. Ultimately, it is this sense of self that helps us individually and collectively to envision what it means to be human. What we look like as humans, that is our appearance, whether in the geo-historical landscape we come to know in the mirror or from our shadows, is largely determined by our individual interface with reality through our skin.

NOTES

Siena and Reinarz, 'Scratching the Surface: An Introduction'

1. *The Proceedings of the Old Bailey*, Trial of Elizabeth Bradshaw, 5 December 1739, reference number t17391205-52, at http://www.oldbaileyonline.org [accessed 1 June 2011].
2. W. A. Pusey, *The History of Dermatology* (Springfield, IL: C. C. Thomas, 1933); P. E. Bechet and H. E. Michelson, *A History of the American Dermatological Association in Commemoration of its Seventy-Fifth Anniversary, 1876–1951* (New York: Froben Press, 1952); R. Friedman, *A History of Dermatology in Philadelphia* (New York: Froben Press, 1955); J. Crissey and L. Parish, *The Dermatology and Syphilology of the Nineteenth Century* (New York: Praeger Publishers, 1981); K. Holubar, *Zur Hundertjahr-feier der Österreichechen Gesellschaft für Dermotologie und Venerologie, 1890–1990* (Vienna: Institut für Geschichte der Medizin, 1990); R. R. Forsey, *Historical Vignettes of Canadian Dermatology* (Montreal: TRANS Canaderm Inc., 1990); W. B. Shelley and E. D. Shelley, *A Century of International Dermatological Congresses: An Illustrated History, 1889–1992* (Park Ridge, NJ: Parthenon Publishing Group, 1992); J. T. Crissey, L. C. Parish and K. Holubar, *Historical Atlas of Dermatology and Dermatologists* (New York: Parthenon Publishing Group, 2002); J. Reinarz, *Health Care in Birmingham: The Birmingham Teaching Hospitals, 1779–1939* (Woodbridge: Boydell & Brewer, 2009), especially chapter 6, 'The Importance of Good Teeth and Skin'. See also the 'Leaders in Dermatology' series published by Syntex Laboratories.
3. S. Ahmed and J. Stacey (eds), *Thinking Through the Skin* (London: Routledge, 2001); C. Benthien, *Skin: On the Cultural Border between Self and the World* (New York: Columbia University Press, 2002); S. Connor, *The Book of Skin* (London: Reaktion Books, 2004).
4. C. Taylor, *Sources of the Self: The Making of Modern Identity* (Cambridge: Cambridge University Press, 1989); D. Wahrman, *The Making of the Modern Self: Identity and Culture in Eighteenth-Century England* (New Haven, CT: Yale University Press, 2004).
5. D. Anzieu, *The Skin Ego* (New Haven, CT: Yale University Press, 1989).
6. M. Bakhtin, *Rabelais and his World* (Bloomington, IN: Indiana University Press, 1984).
7. B. Duden, *The Woman Beneath the Skin: A Doctor's Patients in Eighteenth-Century Germany* (Cambridge, MA: Harvard University Press, 1991).
8. M. Te Hennepe, 'Depicting Skin: Microscopy and the Visual Articulation of Skin Interior, 1820–1850', in R. van de Vall and R. Zwijnenberg (eds), *The Body Within: Art, Medicine and Visualization* (Leiden: Brill, 2009), pp. 51–65.
9. E. Grosz, *Volatile Bodies: Towards a Corporeal Feminism* (Bloomington, IN: Indiana University Press, 1994).

10. D. Outram, *The Body and the French Revolution: Sex, Class and Political Culture* (New Haven, CT: Yale University Press, 1989).

11. M. Flanagan and A. Booth (eds), *Re: Skin* (Cambridge, MA: MIT Press), pp. 1–2.

12. S. Gilman, *Making the Body Beautiful: A Cultural History of Aesthetic Surgery* (Princeton, NJ: Princeton University Press, 2000); E. Haiken, *Venus Envy: A History of Cosmetic Surgery* (Baltimore, MD: Johns Hopkins University Press, 1997); D. Sullivan, *Cosmetic Surgery: The Cutting Edge of Commercial Medicine in America* (New Brunswick, NJ: Rutgers University Press, 2001).

13. Benthien, *Skin*, pp. 37, 53–56, 102.

14. Wahrman, *The Making of the Modern Self*, pp. 260–4.

15. Early modern medical histories touching on skin include O. Weisser, 'Boils, Pushes and Wheals: Reading Bumps on the Body in Early Modern England', *Social History of Medicine*, 22:2 (2009), pp. 321–39; and D. Bhode, 'Skin and the Search for the Interior: The Representation of Flaying in the Art and Anatomy of the Cinquecento', in F. Egmond and R. Zwijnenberg (eds), *Bodily Extremities: Preoccupations with the Human Body in Early Modern European Culture* (Aldershot: Ashgate, 2003), pp. 10–47.

16. Connor, *The Book of Skin*, pp. 37–9, 59–60.

17. P. Di Folco, *Skin Art* (Paris: Fitway Publishing, 2004), p. 8; N. Jablonski, *Skin: A Natural History* (Berkeley, CA: University of California Press, 2006), p. 3.

18. S. Ahmed and J. Stacey, 'Introduction', in Ahmed and Stacey (eds), *Thinking Through the Skin*, p. 2.

19. Connor's reflections on skin's role as a filter are thoughtful in this regard; see Connor, *The Book of Skin*, pp. 65–7.

20. D. Howes, 'Skinscapes: Embodiment, Culture, and Environment', in C. Classen (ed.), *The Book of Touch* (Oxford: Berg, 2005), pp. 27–39.

21. Ahmed and Stacey, 'Introduction', in Ahmed and Stacey (eds), *Thinking Through the Skin*, p. 2.

22. Ibid.

23. D. Serlin (ed.), *Imagining Illness: Public Health and Visual Culture* (Minneapolis, MN: University of Minnesota Press, 2010); L. Cartwright, *Screening the Body: Tracing Medicine Visual Culture* (Minneapolis, MN: University of Minnesota Press, 1995).

24. K. Ott, 'Contagion, Public Health and the Visual Culture of Nineteenth-Century Skin', in D. Serlin (ed.), *Imagining Illness: Public Health and Visual Culture* (Minneapolis, MN: University of Minnesota Press, 2010), pp. 85–107, on p. 86.

25. B. Stafford, *Body Criticism: Imaging the Unseen in Enlightenment Art and Medicine* (Cambridge, MA: MIT Press, 1991), pp. xviii and 300–4.

26. M. Foucault, *The Birth of the Clinic*, trans. A. M. Sheridan Smith (London: Tavistock, 1973); E. Ackerknecht, *Medicine at the Paris Hospital* (Baltimore, MD: Johns Hopkins University Press, 1967); W. F. Bynum, *Science and the Practice of Medicine in the Nineteenth Century* (Cambridge: Cambridge University Press, 1994); R. C. Maulitz, *Morbid Appearances: The Anatomy of Pathology in the Early Nineteenth Century* (Cambridge: Cambridge University Press, 1987).

27. L. S. Jacyna, 'Pious Pathology: J. L. Alibert's Iconography of Disease', in C. Hannaway and A. La Berge (eds), *Constructing Paris Medicine* (Amsterdam: Rodopi, 1998), pp. 185–219, on p. 190.

28. M. Te Hennepe, *Depicting Skin: Visual Culture in Nineteenth-Century Medicine* (Wageningen: Ponsen & Looijen, 2007), p. 21.

29. Ibid.

30. Ibid., pp. 24, 28.
31. Ibid., pp. 36–7.
32. Foucault, *Birth of the Clinic*; M. Fissell, *Patients, Power, and the Poor in Eighteenth-Century Bristol* (Cambridge: Cambridge University Press, 1991).
33. Benthien, *Skin*, p. 57.
34. T. Schnalke, 'Casting Skin: Meanings for Doctors, Artists, and Patients', in S. de Chaderevian and N. Hopwood (eds), *Models: The Third Dimension of Science* (Stanford, CA: Stanford University Press, 2004), pp. 207–41, on p. 216.
35. Connor, *The Book of Skin*, p. 84.
36. Ibid.
37. R. Bivens, *Alternative Medicine? A History* (Oxford: Oxford University Press, 2007), p. 2.
38. J. D. Howell, *Technology in the Hospital: Transforming Patient Care in the Early Twentieth Century* (Baltimore, MD: Johns Hopkins University Press, 1995), p. 233; G. Weisz, *Divide and Conquer: A Comparative History of Medical Specialization* (Oxford: Oxford University Press, 2006), p. xxv. As Woloshyn demonstrates in this volume, new technologies had similarly elevated the status of dermatologists with the development of Finsen's lamp.
39. Te Hennepe, *Depicting Skin*, p. 125.
40. Schnalke, 'Casting Skin', p. 217. Given the importance of colour to early dermatological imagery, we must apologize for being unable to include colour images in the book.
41. L. U. Marks, *The Skin of the Film: Intercultural Cinema, Embodiment and the Senses* (Durham, NC: Duke University Press, 2000), p. 162.
42. Connor, *The Book of Skin*, pp. 53–59, 64.
43. See S. Romano, 'The Dark Side of the Sun: Skin Cancer, Sunscreen, and Risk in Twentieth-Century America' (unpublished PhD thesis, Yale University, 2006).
44. Connor, *The Book of Skin*, p. 119.
45. E. Goffman, *Stigma: Notes on the Management of Spoiled Identity* (Englewood Cliffs, NJ: Prentice Hall, 1963), pp. 8, 10, 12, 19, 47, 50–1, 118, 132.
46. Ibid., p. 127.
47. On pre-modern leprosy, see C. Rawcliffe, *Leprosy in Medieval England* (Woodbridge: Boydell Press, 2006); L. Demaitre, *Leprosy in Premodern Medicine: A Malady of the Whole Body* (Baltimore, MD: Johns Hopkins University Press, 2007); R. I. Moore, *The Formation of a Persecuting Society: Power and Deviance in Western Europe, 950–1250* (Oxford: Blackwell, 1987), pp. 45–59; and S. Brody, *The Disease of the Soul: Leprosy in Medieval Literature* (Ithaca, NY: Cornell University Press, 1974).
48. S. Gilman, *Disease and Representation: Images of Illness from Madness to Aids* (Ithaca, NY: Cornell University Press, 1988), pp. 246–56; see also J. G. Harris '(Po)X Marks the Spot: How to "Read" "Early Modern" "Syphilis" in *The Three Ladies of London*', in K. Siena (ed.), *Sins of the Flesh: Responding to Sexual Disease in Early Modern Europe* (Toronto: Centre for Reformation and Renaissance Studies, 2005), pp. 109–32.
49. On Hogarth's use of pockmarks, see F. Haslam, *From Hogarth to Rowlandson: Medicine in Art in Eighteenth-Century Britain* (Liverpool: Liverpool University Press, 1996), pp. 87–119; and R. Paulson, *Hogarth's Harlot: Sacred Parody in Enlightenment England* (Baltimore, MD: Johns Hopkins University Press, 2003), pp. 99–101.
50. J. Prosser, 'Skin Memories', in Ahmed and Stacey (eds), *Thinking Through the Skin*, pp. 52–68, on p. 55.
51. Connor, *The Book of Skin*, pp. 227–8.

52. On lepers, see the works cited in note 47; on the isolation of syphilitics, see J. Arriza-balga, J. Henderson and R. French, *The Great Pox: The French Disease in Renaissance Europe* (New Haven, CT: Yale University Press, 1994); K. Siena, *Venereal Disease, Hospitals and the Urban Poor: London's Foul Wards, 1600–1800* (Rochester, NY: University of Rochester Press, 2004); R. Jütte, 'Syphilis and Confinement in Early Modern Germany', in N. Finzsch and R. Jütte (eds), *Institutions of Confinement: Hospitals, Asylums, and Prisons in Western Europe and North America* (Cambridge: Cambridge University Press, 1996), pp. 97–116.

53. Connor, *The Book of Skin*, p. 96.

54. Thanks to Michael Stolberg and Claudia Stein for consulting on this point.

55. G. W. Rutherford, S. K. Schwarcz, G. F. Lemp, J. L. Barnhart, K. J. Rauch, W. L. Warner, T. H. Piland and D. Werdegar, 'The Epidemiology of AIDS-Related Kaposi's Sarcoma in San Francisco', *Journal of Infectious Diseases*, 159:3 (1989), pp. 569–72, on p. 569.

56. G. Bennett, *Bodies: Sex, Violence, Disease, and Death in Contemporary Legend* (Jackson, MS: University Press of Mississippi, 2009), p. 126.

57. R. Shilts, *And the Band Played On* (New York: St Martin's Press, 1987), p. 198.

58. D. Crimp, 'How to Have Promiscuity in an Epidemic', in B. Wallis, M. Weems and P. Yenawine (eds), *Art Matters: How the Culture Wars Changed America* (New York: New York University Press, 1999), pp. 237–71, p. 133.

59. F. Fanon, *Black Skin, White Masks*, trans. C. L. Markham (New York: Grove Press, 1967).

60. B. Rush, 'Observations Intended to Favour a Supposition that the Black Color (as it is Called) of the Negroes is Derived from the Leprosy', *Transactions of the American Philosophical Society*, 4 (1799), pp. 289–97.

61. D. Outram, *The Enlightenment* (Cambridge: Cambridge University Press, 2005), pp. 53–5.

62. R. Edmond, *Leprosy and Empire: A Medical and Social History* (Cambridge: Cambridge University Press, 2006), p. 112.

63. A. M. Kraut, *Goldberger's War: The Life and Work of a Public Health Crusader* (New York: Hill and Wang, 2003).

64. Benthien, *Skin*, pp. 54, 59; Te Hennepe, *Depicting Skin*, chapter 3.

65. P. Wilson, *Surgery, Skin and Syphilis: Daniel Turner's London (1667–1741)* (Amsterdam: Rodopi, 1999), pp. 60, 69–70.

66. Connor, *The Book of Skin*, pp. 11–18.

67. On searchers, see R. Munkhoff, 'Searchers of the Dead: Authority, Marginality, and the Interpretation of Plague in England, 1574–1665', *Gender and History*, 11:1 (1999), pp. 1–29; and K. Siena, 'Searchers of the Dead in Long Eighteenth-Century London', in K. Kippen and L. Woods (eds), *Worth and Repute: Valuing Gender in Late Medieval and Early Modern Europe* (Toronto: Centre for Reformation and Renaissance Studies, 2011), pp. 123–51.

68. J. Jacobs Brumberg, *The Body Project: An Intimate History of American Girls* (New York: Vintage, 1997), pp. 57–94.

69. K. Brown, *Foul Bodies: Cleanliness in Early America* (New Haven, CT: Yale University Press, 2009), pp. 42–57.

70. E. Scarrey, *The Body in Pain: The Making and Unmaking of the World* (Oxford: Oxford University Press, 1987); A. Synnott, *The Body Social: Symbolism, Self and Society* (London: Routledge, 1993); S. Gilman, 'Touch, Sexuality and Disease', in W. F. Bynum and R. Porter (eds), *Medicine and the Five Senses* (Cambridge: Cambridge University Press, 1993), pp. 198–224; R. Rey, *The History of Pain*, trans. L. E. Wallace, J. A. Cadden and S.

W. Cadden (Cambridge, MA: Harvard University Press, 1998); E. D. Harvey, *Sensible Flesh: On Touch in Early Modern Culture* (Philadelphia, PA: University of Pennsylvania Press, 2003); C. Classen (ed.), *The Book of Touch* (Oxford: Berg, 2005); E. Cockayne, *Hubbub: Filth, Noise & Stench in England* (New Haven, CT: Yale University Press, 2007); M. Smith, *Sensory History* (Oxford: Berg, 2007); Brown, *Foul Bodies*.

1 Payne, 'Drain, Blister, Bleed: Surgeons Open and Close the Skin in Georgian London'

1. W. Chamberlaine, *Tirocinium Medicina, or a Dissertation on the Duties of Youth Apprenticed to the Medical Professions* (London, 1812), p. 24.
2. 'A Letter from William Hallett, MD to Henry Pemberton, MD FRS & Chemistry Professor Gresham: Containing the Case of a Lad, Who was Shot through the Lungs: Drawn up by Mr. Nicholas Peters, Junior, Surgeon', *Philosophical Transactions*, 43 (1744–5), pp. 151–6.
3. Ibid., p. 151.
4. Ibid., p. 152.
5. Ibid., p. 154.
6. Ibid., p. 155.
7. Ibid.
8. Ibid., p. 156. Peters sent him to Hallett's hospital, the Devon and Exeter Hospital.
9. These figures are based on a survey of eighteenth-century surgical lecture notes made by medical men in London.
10. See M. Crumplin, *Men of Steel: Surgery in the Napoleonic Wars* (Shrewsbury: Quiller Press, 2007).
11. P. Clare, *An Essay on the Cure of Abscesses by Caustic and on the Treatment of Wounds and Ulcers* (London, 1779), preface, p. iv. Crumplin notes that the capital operations were amputation, trepanning, lithotomy, mastectomy, ligation of major arteries for aneurism, management of severe injury and treatment of irreducible strangulated hernia (*Men of Steel*, p. 157).
12. C. Benthien, *Skin: On the Cultural Border between Self and the World*, trans. T. Dunlap (New York: Columbia University Press, 2004), p. 40.
13. J. Elkins, *Pictures of the Body, Pain and Metamorphosis* (Stanford, CA: Stanford University Press, 1999), p. 51.
14. Details of Pott's life can be found in J. Earle, *The Chirurgical Works of Percivall Pott to which are Added a Short Account of the Life of the Author* (London: J. Johnson, 1790).
15. Crumplin, *Men of Steel*, p. 157. Also see S. Lawrence, *Charitable Knowledge: Hospital Pupils and Practitioners in Eighteenth-Century London* (Cambridge: Cambridge University Press, 1996).
16. Dressers worked on the wards and paid Pott approximately 50 guineas to do so, even when apprenticed to other surgeons, as for example Abernathy to Charles Blicke. Pupils, who only observed and did not dress patients, paid 25 guineas a year.
17. Crumplin notes that candles and lamps emitted perhaps a few hundred lux, while the modern operating theatre has a light intensity of 10,000–40,000 lux (*Men of Steel*, p. 220).
18. Clare, *An Essay on the Cure of Abscesses*, p. 14.
19. Ibid., p. 15.
20. Ibid.

21. Ibid., p. 26.
22. J. Moore, *A Dissertation on the Process of Nature in the Filling up of Cavities, Healing of Wounds, and Restoring the Parts which have been Destroyed in the Human Body, which Obtained the Prize Medal Given by the Lyceum Medicum Londiense in 1789, and was Ordered to be Published for the Use of the Society* (London, 1789), p. 52.
23. Ibid., pp. 52–3.
24. Wellcome Library, MS 5590, 'Lectures on the Practice of Surgery by Percival Pott – F.R.S. and Senior Surgeon to Bartholomew's Hospital. Notes on a Course of 64 Lectures, 1765 or Later', fol. 6v.
25. Clendening Library, MS 1020 D2/1, 'Transcript of a Course of Lectures on the Theory and Practice of Surgery as Delivered in the Theatre of St. Barthelomew's [*sic*] Hospital by J. Abernethy F.R.S., Lecturer on Anatomy & Surgery & Assist. Surgeon to that Institution Collated from Notes taken by Wm. Robarts Anno 1810', fol. 32v.
26. Clare, *An Essay on the Cure of Abscesses*, p. 1.
27. Moore, *A Dissertation*, p. 26.
28. Royal College of Surgeons of London, MS 0071, 'Mr. Pott's Surgical Lectures, Oct. 2nd 1767, in an Anonymous Hand', Box 1, fol. 3v.
29. Moore, *A Dissertation*, p. 26.
30. Wellcome Library, MS 3957, 'Lectures on Surgery by Percival [*sic*] Pott Esq. Given at the Theatre at Bartholomew's Hospital, *c*. 1770', fol. 17v.
31. Wellcome Library, MS 3957, 'Lecture on the Cessation of Menses', fol. 19v.
32. Moore, *A Dissertation*, p. 33.
33. Ibid., p. 46.
34. Royal College of Surgeons of London, MS 0071, 'Heaviside, John, Lectures on Surgery by Mr. Pott, Senior Surgeon to St. Bartholomew's Hospital begun Oct. 9th, 1769', Box 10, fol. 1v.
35. P. Pott, *Observations on the Nature and Consequences of those Injuries to which the Head is Liable from External Violence* (London, 1768), p. 200. This treatise includes description of an indolent tumour of the scalp now associated with intracranial abscesses and known as 'Pott's Puffy Tumour'.
36. Ibid., pp. 200–2.
37. Clendening Library, MS 1020 D2/1, fol. 75v.
38. Ibid., fol. 80v.
39. Ibid., fol. 35v. At St Bartholomew's Hospital, people applied for admission as patients on Thursday mornings.
40. Clendening Library, MS 1020 D2/1, fol. 60v.
41. Ibid.
42. Ibid., fols 141–9.
43. Clare, *An Essay on the Cure of Abscesses*, p. 3.
44. Clendening Library, MS 1020 D2/1, fol. 88.
45. Clare, *An Essay on the Cure of Abscesses*, pp. 7–9.
46. Wellcome Library, MS 3956, fol. 1v.
47. Ibid., fol. 14v.
48. Ibid.
49. Royal College of Surgeons of London, MS 0071, 'Mr. Potts Lectures taken in 1777, Lecture 18 Wounds of the Thorax/Milk Abscess in Female Breasts/ Schirrus & Cancer of the Breast', Box 10, fol. 5v.
50. Wellcome Library, MS 3957, fol. 36v.
51. Ibid., fol. 37r.

52. See W. E. Thomas, *Dr. Johann Hunczovsky, Surgeon 1752–1798, Life – Work – Times* (Pierpont, SD: Nemsi Books, 2006), pp. 53–6.

53. The Gordon Riots of 1780 were an anti-Catholic uprising against the Papists Act of 1778; they centred on areas close to the hospital.

54. Wellcome Library, MS 4337, 'Medical Notes taken at Barts 1778–81', fol. 62.

55. Wellcome Library, MS 3957, fol. 143r.

56. Royal College of Surgeons of London, MS 0071, Box 10, fol. 46v. The embarrassment of young surgeons could also have been related to handling the female breast.

57. Ibid., fol. 144v. Included in the Heaviside MS 0071 are twelve loose-leaf folios that describe how opium was distilled, and its limited use.

58. J. Hemlow (ed.), *Fanny Burney: Selected Letters and Journals* (Oxford: Clarendon Press, 1986), p. 140.

59. See Crumplin, *Men of Steel*, pp. 216–20, for a discussion of what little was available or used to provide pain relief.

60. Royal College of Surgeons of London, MS 0071, 'Mr. Pott's Lectures taken in the Courses of 80 & 81 by Heaviside, Lecture 24th on the Imperforate Anus', Box 10, fol. 120v.

61. Ibid., 1769, fol. 33v.

62. Wellcome Library, MS 3957, 'Lect. 15th, The Hare Lip', fol. 60v.

63. The best description of the types of sutures used in the later eighteenth century can be found in the multivolume *A System of Surgery* by Benjamin Bell (Edinburgh, 1787), pp. 18–26.

64. J. Abernethy, *Surgical Observations on Tumours and on Lumbar Abscesses* (London, 1816), p. 36.

65. Royal College of Surgeons of London, MS 129, Folder 3, fols 253–4. 'Mr. Wilson on Opening Dead Bodies, May 7th', pp. 252–4. This was Lecture 1 on a course of anatomy, 1798, at the Great Windmill Street Anatomy School.

66. Wellcome Library, MS 3957, fol. 9v.

67. A translation of *A Dissertation on the Inutility of the Amputation of Limbs* by Bilguer had been published in England in 1764, to which Pott had responded with *Remarks on the Necessity and Propriety of the Operation of Amputation* (1770). See P. Pott, *Chirurgical Works*, 3 vols (London, 1779), vol. 3, pp. 386–424.

68. T. Kirkland, *Observations upon Mr. Pott's General Remarks on FRACTURES, etc IN Three LETTERS to a young SURGEON Intending to Settle in the Country. With a Postscript, Concerning the Cure of the Compound Dislocations; in which the Usual Method of Treating WOUNDS of the TENDONS and LIGAMENTS is Briefly Considered* (London, 1770), pp. 14–15.

69. Ibid., pp. 19–21.

70. Ibid., pp. 42–3.

71. Ibid., p. 44.

72. Ibid., p. 45.

2 Lie, 'Abominable Ulcers, Open Pores and a New Tissue: Transforming the Skin in the Norwegian Countryside, 1750–1850'

1. The minister Rasmus Peter Langhorn, in a letter to the Radesyge Commission, 4 November 1778; The Norwegian National Archive, Cabinet No. 9 ('Radesykeskapet'), Package 165 A–C. All subsequent references to this package will be referred to as NA.

2. This story is narrated by Nicolaus Arbo in his treatise on radesyge, N. Arbo, *Afhandling om Radesygen eller Salt-Flod* (Kiøbenhavn: C. L. Buchs Forlag, 1792), pp. 87–93.

3. 'Chamber councillor' was an honorific title granted to successful officials in the state. It is not clear from the text what kind of formal position he held in the local community.

4. Collegium Medicum to the Chancellery, 17 September 1772, NA.

5. 'A disease which creates so many incapable, even harmful subjects, cannot be eradicated quickly enough, and every parsimony that postpones the general cure must be considered most harmful', was the message from the Collegium Medicum in Copenhagen: Letter from Collegium Medicum to the Lieutenant Scheel of the County of Stavanger, 29 September 1774, NA.

6. The district commander (*stiftsamtmann*) had military command over an area equal to a diocese. There were four dioceses in Norway at this time.

7. Hans Hagerup in a letter to King Christian VII, 12 January 1769, NA.

8. 'til Hospitals Lemmer reducerede', Ibid. The word 'patient' is not a very good translation; the Danish-Norwegian original *Lem* signified 'limb' or 'member'.

9. To that figure can be added about nine master and twenty-five journeymen surgeons, and five to six physicians in private practice. In any case, the country, which at that time had about 800,000 inhabitants, was very sparsely populated with medical personnel.

10. See, for instance, F. Holst, 'Sygehuse for venerisk Syge, Radesyge og andre ondartede Hudsygdomme i Norge i Decenniet fra 1822 til 1831', *Eyr*, 10:1 (1834), pp. 1–44. The actual number depends on whether the hospitals for venereal disease are included. For a more elaborate discussion of the rise of the radesyge hospitals, see O. G. Moseng, *Ansvaret for undersåttenes helse 1603–1850*, ed. A. Schiøtz, 2 vols (Oslo: Universitetsforlaget, 2003), vol. 1, Det offentlige helsevesen i Norge 1603–2003, pp. 189–210; and A. K. Lie, 'Treatment Politics. The Rise of the Norwegian Radesyge Hospitals', in K. Stene-Johansen and F. Tygstrup (eds), *Illness in Context* (Amsterdam: Rodopi, 2010), pp. 139–63.

11. J. Utheim, *Oversigt over det norske civile Lægevæsens historiske Udvikling og nuværende Ordning* (Oslo: Johannes Bjørnstads Bogtrykkeri, 1901), pp. 2, 4. The extent of the authorities' concern is exemplified by the donation of 20,000 riksdaler from the absolutist state in 1789 for measures to deal with the problem of radesyge. (For comparison, a physician would earn about 300 RD annually.)

12. Arbo, *Afhandling om Radesygen eller Salt-Flod*; H. Møller, *Forsøg i det som angaaer det Norske Folks Sundhed*, vol. 1:8, Nye Samling af det Kongelige Norske Videnskabers Selskabs Skrifter (Kiøbenhavn: Christian Gottlob Prost, 1784); J. C. Mülertz, *Bidrag til Oplysning om Radesygens Natur og bedste Lægemaade* (Kiøbenhavn: P. M. Liunge, 1799); C. E. Mangor, *Underretning om Radesygens Kiendetegn, Aarsager og Helbredelse* (Kiøbenhavn: Johan Frederik Schultz, 1793); J. Matthiessen, *Anviisning til at kiende og helbrede Radesygen* (Kiøbenhavn, 1796); H. Deegen, *Noget om Radesygen, observeret ved Sygehuuset i Flechefiord og udgivet til Nytte for Almuen* (Christiansand: Andreas Swane, 1788). For a later summary see, for instance, F. L. Hünefeld, *Die Radesyge, oder Das skandinavische Syphiloid: aus skandinavischen Quellen dargestellt* (Leipzig: L. Voss, 1828).

13. F. Holst, *Morbus quem radesyge vocant quinam sit quanamque ratione e Scandinavia tollendus?* (Christiania, 1817).

14. Surgeon Daniel Touschen to Governor Scheel, 6 March 1774, NA.

15. See, for example, J. Belart, 'De morbo quem Radesyge nominant. Dissertatio inauguralis pathologica' (Berlin: Humbold Universität, 1830); C. A. Gedike, 'Dissertatio inauguralis medica de morbo, quem Radesyge dicunt, in Norvegia endemico' (Berlin: Starck, 1819); J. J. Hjaltalin, 'Dissertatio inauguralis de Radesyge, Lepra et Elephantiasi

septentrionali quam ... in Academia Christiana – Albertina' (København: Københavns Universitet, 1839); G. Rullmann, 'De ulcere radesyge' (Würzburg: Universität Würzburg, 1844); W. G. Pfefferkorn, *Über die norwegische Radesyge und Spedalskhed, als eine Probeschrift zur Erlangung der Doctorwürde* (Altona: Hammerich, 1797); and B. Steidel, 'De natura radesyges' (Jena: Universität Jena, 1851).

16. E. Gabler, *Lateinisch-deutsches Wörterbuch für Medizin und Naturwissenschaften* (Berlin: Hermann Peters, 1857), p. 302.

17. R. Frankenau, *Det offentlige Sundhedspolitie under en oplyst Regiering: især med Hensyn paa de danske Stater og deres Hovedstad: en Haandbog for Øvrigheder og Borgere* (København: Poulsen, 1801), p. 78.

18. Andreas Faye to the Radesyge Commission, 10 October 1778, NA.

19. R. Porter, *The Greatest Benefit to Mankind: A Medical History of Humanity* (New York: W. W. Norton and Co., 1997), pp. 121–2.

20. For a discussion of the nosological determinations of radesyge in relation to the categories of cachexiae in de Sauvages and William Cullen, see A. K. Lie, 'Radesykens tilblivelse' (PhD dissertation, University of Oslo, 2008), pp. 96–102.

21. B. Duden, *The Woman Beneath the Skin: A Doctor's Patients in Eighteenth-Century Germany* (Cambridge, MA: Harvard University Press, 1991).

22. Møller, *Forsøg i det som angaaer det Norske Folks Sundhed*, p. 219.

23. Ibid., p. 220.

24. Holst, *Morbus quem radesyge vocant*, p. 71.

25. Ibid.

26. A. Corbin, *The Foul and the Fragrant: Odor and the French Social Imagination* (Cambridge, MA: Harvard University Press, 1986), p. 56.

27. N. Elias, *The Civilizing Process*, trans. E. Jephcott (1937; New York: Urizen Books, 1978).

28. Møller, *Forsøg i det som angaaer det Norske Folks Sundhed*, p. 219.

29. Mangor, *Underretning om Radesygens Kiendetegn, Aarsager og Helbredelse*, p. 22.

30. On the notion of the *vix medicatrix naturae*, see M. Neuburger, 'An Historical Survey of the Concept of Nature from a Medical Viewpoint', *Isis*, 35:1 (1944), pp. 16–28; and M. Neuburger, *Die Lehre von der Heilkraft der Natur im Wandel der Zeiten* (Stuttgart: Enke, 1926).

31. For a discussion of the healing powers of nature in Denmark–Norway at the time, see, among others, H. Callisen, *System der neuern Wundarzneykunst: zum öffentlichen und Privatgebrauche* (Kopenhagen: Christian Gottlob Proft, 1788), p. 18.

32. J. Møller, 'Schreiben des seeligen Doctors und Landphysikus Möller zu Porsgrund bey Scheen in Norwegen, vom 29. aug. 1787', *Medicinisch-Chirurgisches Journal*, 5:1 (1800), pp. 45–61; Arbo, *Afhandling om Radesygen eller Salt-Flod*, ch. 2.

33. J. Starobinski, *Montaigne in Motion* (1982; Chicago, IL: University of Chicago Press, 1985).

34. H. Munk, 'Om Bratsberg Amts Sygehus i de siste forløbne 12 Aar', *Eyr*, 6:1 (1831), pp. 1–16.

35. J. J. Hjort, 'Bidrag til Kundskab om de endemiske Hudsygdomme', *Norsk Magazin for Lægevidenskaben*, 1:1 (1840), pp. 1–25, on p. 10.

36. M. Foucault, *The Birth of the Clinic: An Archaeology of Medical Perception*, trans. A. Sheridan (1963; London: Tavistock, 1973), p. 136.

37. R. Willan, *On Cutaneous Diseases*, vol. I (London: Johnson, 1808). For the history of the development of dermatology and venereology in the nineteenth century, see J. T. Crissey

and L. C. Parish, *The Dermatology and Syphilology of the Nineteenth Century* (New York: Praeger, 1981).

38. G. Tilles and D. Wallach, 'Robert Willan and the French Willanists', *British Journal of Dermatology*, 140:6 (1999), pp. 1122–6, on p. 1123.

39. Hjort, 'Bidrag til Kundskab om de endemiske Hudsygdomme', p. 25.

40. C. W. Boeck, 'Klinik over Hudsygdommene og de syphilitiske Sygdomme', *Norsk Magazin for Lægevidenskaben*, 2nd series, 6 (1852), pp. 273–330, on p. 273.

41. Ibid.

42. For the history of syphilization, see A. Dracobly, 'Ethics and Experimentation on Human Subjects in Mid-Nineteenth-Century France: The Story of the 1859 Syphilis Experiments', *Bulletin of the History of Medicine*, 77:2 (2003), pp. 332–66. For syphilization in the Norwegian context, see C. W. Boeck, *Recherches cliniques sur la syphilisation* (Paris: Dupont, 1854); and C. W. Boeck, *Syphilisationen studeret ved Sygesengen* (Christiania: Brögger & Christie, 1854).

43. Boeck, *Traité De La Radesyge*, p. 53.

44. J. H. Warner, *The Therapeutic Perspective: Medical Practice, Knowledge, and Identity in America, 1820–1885* (Cambridge, MA: Harvard University Press, 1986).

45. Boeck, *Traité de la Radesyge (Syphilis Tertiaire)*, p. 42.

46. C. W. Boeck, *Samling af Iagttagelser om Hudens Sygdomme* (Christiania: C. Tönsberg, 1855–62).

47. E. Ehlers, *Folkesyphilis i Danmark* (København: H. Koppel, 1919); Hünefeld, *Die Radesyge, oder Das skandinavische Syphiloid: aus skandinavischen Quellen dargestellt*; E. A. L. Hübener, *Erkenntnis und Cur der sogenannten Dithmarsischen Krankheit* (Altona: Aue, 1935); P. Brandis, 'Om den ditmarsiske Syge', *Bibliothek for læger*, 2:1 (1810), pp. 1–26; L. A. Struve, *Ueber die aussatzartige Krankheit Holsteins, allgemein daselbst die Marschkrankheit genannt. Ein Beytrag zur Kenntnis der pseudosyphilitischen Uebel* (Altona: Joh. Friedr. Hammerich, 1820).

48. L. Fleck, 'Scientific Observation and Perception in General', in R. S. Cohen and T. Schnelle (eds), *Cognition and Fact: Materials on Ludwik Fleck* (1935; Dordrecht: D. Reidel Publishing Company, 1986) pp. 59–78.

49. Ibid., p. 60.

50. S. Connor, *The Book of Skin* (Ithaca, NY: Cornell University Press, 2004).

3 Moran, 'Protecting the Skin of the British Empire: St Paul's Bay Disease in Quebec'

1. I would like to thank former UPEI students Norah Pendergast, Ian Lane and Cassandra Armsworthy for their help with research connected to this project. Partial funding for this research was provided by the University of Prince Edward Island's SSHRC Institutional Grant Program. Many conversations with Lisa Chilton have helped greatly to hammer this chapter into shape.

2. See, for example, S. Leblond, 'Le mal de la Baie, Etait-ce La Syphilis?', *Journal of the Canadian Medical Association*, 4:116 (1977), pp. 1284–90; J. Heagerty, 'Mal De La Baie St-Paul', in J. Heagerty (ed.), *Four Centuries of Medical History in Canada* (Toronto: MacMillian Company of Canada, Ltd, 1928), pp. 131–60; S. Leblond, 'Philippe Louis Badelart: Le Mal de la Baie', in S. Leblond (ed.), *Médecine et Médecins D'autrefois: Practiques Traditionnelles et Portraits Québecois* (Quebec: Presses de l'Universite Laval, 1986),

p. 69; L. P. Audet, 'Le Maladie de la Baie Saint Paul', *Revue de L'Université Laval*, 6:5 (1952), pp. 412–14; L. Chartrand, 'L'Epidemie Honteuse de la Baie St Paul', *Quebec Science*, 17:9 (1979), pp. 52–3; E. Des Jardins, 'Le Mal de la Baie Saint-Paul', *Union Médicale du Canada*, 102:10 (1973), pp. 2148–52; and N. E. Dionne, 'Le Mal de la Baie Saint-Paul', *Bulletin des Recherches Historiques*, 25:12 (1919), pp. 377–9.

3.   C. Roland, 'Dr James Bowman vs. Canada: A Struggle to Obtain Payment for Government Services', *XXVe Congrès International D'histoire de la Médecine*, Québec, du 21 au 28 aout 1976. Second Programme Provisoire; E. Des Jardins, 'James Bowman', in *Dictionary of Canadian Biography*, 4 (1979), pp. 82–3.

4.   S. Connor, *The Book of Skin* (Ithaca, NY: Cornell University Press, 2004), p. 21.

5.   Ibid., p. 23.

6.   P. K. Wilson, *Surgery, Skin and Syphilis: Daniel Turner's London, 1667–1741* (Amsterdam: Rodopi, 1999), pp. 59–84.

7.   K. Siena, 'Pliable Bodies: The Moral Biology of Health and Disease in the Enlightenment', in C. Reeves (ed.), *Cultural History of the Human Body in the Enlightenment* (Oxford: Berg, 2010), pp. 33–52.

8.   See R. Lessard, *Le Mal de la Baie Saint-Paul* (Québec, Université Laval: Rapports et Mémoires de reserche du Célat, no. 15, 1989), p. 51.

9.   Ibid., p. 6.

10.   J. Bowman, *Direction pour la Guerison du Mal de la Baie St Paul* (Quebec, 1785), Bibliothèque nationale du Québec. My translation.

11.   J. Cassel, *The Secret Plague: Venereal Disease in Canada, 1838–1939* (Toronto: University of Toronto Press, 1987), pp. 52–3.

12.   James Bowman's mercury concoctions can be found in: Memorial of James Bowman to the Board of Accounts, 1 December 1785, Miscellaneous Records Relating to St Paul's Bay Disease – 1785–1791, RG4 B43, vol. 1 (hereafter Misc. Records RG4 B43), Library and Archives of Canada (hereafter LAC); F. Swediaur, *Practical Observations of Venereal Complaints to which are Added an Account of a New Venereal Disease which has Lately Appeared in Canada* (Edinburgh: W. Berry and T. Kay, 1787), p. 173. See also R. Jones, *Remarks on the Distemper Generally Known by the Name of the Molbay Disease, Including a Description of its Symptoms and Method of Cure* (Montreal: Fleury Mesplet, 1786), pp. 17–18; Bowman, *Direction pour la Guerison du Mal de la Baie St Paul*; and Cassel, *The Secret Plague*, p. 52.

13.   Information for the next three paragraphs is drawn from Lessard, *Le Mal de la Baie Saint-Paul*, pp. 51–65.

14.   Governor Hamilton's Order the Captains of Militia, 19 May 1785, Misc. Records, RG4 B43, LAC.

15.   See N. Séguin, *Atlas Historique du Québec: L'institution Médicale* (Sainte-Foy: Les Presses de L'université Laval, 1998), pp. 5, 15.

16.   Letter from J. Olivier Briand to parish priests, 9 February 1783, in *Mandements des Évêques de Québec*, ed. H. Têtu and C. O. Gagnon, 4 vols (Quebec: Imprimerie Générale, A. Coté et Co., 1888), vol. 1 (hereafter *Mandements*), pp. 303–4, my translation.

17.   Letter from Louis Philippe Mariaucheau d'Esglis to parish priests, 12 April 1785, in *Mandements*, p. 31, my translation.

18.   O. Hubert, 'Ritual Performance and Parish Sociability: French-Canadian Catholic Families at Mass from the Seventeenth to the Nineteenth Century', in N. Christie (ed.), *Households of Faith: Family, Gender, and Community in Canada, 1760–1969* (Kingston: McGill Queen's University Press, 2002), pp. 37–76, on p. 47. See also C. Hudon,

'Beaucoup de bruits pour rien? Rumeurs, plaints et scandales autour du clergé dans les paroisses gaspésiennes, 1766–1900', *Revu d'histoire de l'Amérique Française*, 55:2 (2001), pp. 217–40; and O. Hubert, *Sur la terre comme au ciel: La gestion des rites par l'Eglise catholique du Québec (fin XVII–mi–XIX siècle)* (Quebec: Presses de l'université Laval, 2000).

19. Letter from J. Olivier Briand to parish priests, 9 February 1783, in *Mandements*, p. 304, my translation.

20. Hubert, 'Ritual Performance', p. 46.

21. Charles- François Perrault to James Bowman, 6 August 1785, Misc. Records, RG4 B43, LAC.

22. Letter from Louis Philippe Mariaucheau d'Esglis to parish priests, 12 April 1785, in *Mandements*, p. 318, my translation. See also Jones, *Remarks*, pp. 18–19.

23. Charles- François Perrault to James Bowman, 6 August 1785, Misc. Records, RG4 B43, LAC.

24. Father Jean-Baptiste Noël Pouget to James Bowman, 31 October 1785, Misc. Records, RG4 B43, LAC; Father St Germain to James Bowman, 9 June 1785, Misc. Records, RG4 B43, LAC. See also Father le Noir to James Bowman, 23 September 1785, Misc. Records, RG4 B43, LAC.

25. Father Morin to James Bowman, 5 October 1785, Misc. Records, RG4 B43, LAC; Father Huot to James Bowman, 21 November 1785, Misc. Records, RG4 B43, LAC.

26. On population estimates for the day, see F. Ouellet, *Histoire économique et sociale du Québec, 1760–1850, Structures et Conjuncture* (Montréale: Fides, 1966) p. 143.

27. Father St Germain to Lieutenant Governor Henry Hamilton, 13 October 1785, Misc. Records, RG4 B43, LAC.

28. Instructions to Dr James Bowman, 18 April 1785, Misc. Records, RG4 B43, LAC.

29. U. Tröhler, 'Quantifying Experience and Beating Biases: A New Culture in Eighteenth-Century British Clinical Medicine', in G. Jorland, A. Opinel and G. Weisz (eds), *Body Counts: Medical Quantification in Historical and Sociological Perspectives* (Montreal: McGill Queen's University Press, 2005), pp. 19–50, on p. 25. A.-H. Maehle, *Drugs on Trial: Experimental Pharmacology and Therapeutic Innovation in the Eighteenth Century* (Amsterdam: Rodopi, 1999), p. 16.

30. Maehle, *Drugs on Trial*, p. 16.

31. B. Curtis, 'The Canada "Blue Books" and the Administrative Capacity of the Canadian State, 1822–67', *Canadian Historical Review*, 74:4 (1993), pp. 535–65.

32. See Lessard, *Le Mal de la Baie St Paul*, p. 11.

33. T. Savitt, 'Slave Health and Southern Distinctiveness', in T. Savitt and J. H. Young (eds), *Disease and Distinctiveness in the American South* (Knoxville, TN: University of Tennessee Press, 1988), pp. 120–53.

34. M. E. Kelm, 'Diagnosing the Discursive Indians: Medicine, Gender and the Dying Race', *Ethnohistory*, 52:2 (2005), pp. 371–406.

35. A. Ray, *Indians in the Fur Trade: Their Role as Trappers, Hunters, and Middlemen in the Lands Southwest of Hudson Bay, 1660–1860* (Toronto: University of Toronto Press, 1974), pp. 188–9; J. B. Waldram, D. A. Herring and T. Kue Young, *Aboriginal Health in Canada: Historical, Cultural and Epidemiological Perspectives*, 2nd edn (Toronto: University of Toronto Press, 2006), pp. 154–5; T. Savitt, *Race and Medicine in Nineteenth-and Early-Twentieth-Century America* (Kent, OH: Kent State University Press, 2007), chapter 7.

36. James Bowman to Lord Dorchester, 16 November 1786, Misc. Records, RG4 B43, LAC.

37. James Bowman to Lieutenant Governor Hope, 7 February 1787, Misc. Records, RG4 B43, LAC.
38. James Bowman to Governor-General Hamilton, 19 October 1785, Misc. Records, RG4 B43, LAC.
39. R. Jones, *Remarks on the Distemper Generally Known by the Name of the Molbay Disease* (Montreal: Fleury Mesplet, 1786), p. 19.

4 Gentilcore, '"Italic Scurvy", "Pellarina", "Pellagra": Medical Reactions to a New Disease in Italy, 1770–1815'

1. F. Fanzago, *Memoria sopra la pellagra del territorio padovano* (Padua: Gio. Antonio Conzatti, 1789), reprinted in F. Fanzago, *Sulla pellagra. Memorie* (Padua: Tipografia del Seminario, 1815), pp. 45–83, on pp. 48–9.
2. J. Gregory, *Observations on the Duties and Offices of a Physician; and on the Method of Prosecuting Enquiries in Philosophy* (London, 1770); *Lezioni sopra i doveri e le qualità di un medico*, with a translator's preface by Fanzago, dated 20 March 1789 (Florence, 1789; Pavia, 1795). Fanzago dedicated the translation to his mentor, Frank.
3. On Fanzago, see A. Porro's entry in the *Dizionario Biografico degli Italiani*, at http://www.treccani.it/biografie/ [accessed 12 May 2011]. This however gives the publication date of Fanzago's *Memoria* as 1790, instead of the previous year, and refers to it as the first study of pellagra in the Veneto, even though Fanzago himself republished Jacopo Odoardi's 1776 paper, *Una specie di scorbuto*, in his 1815 collection of works on the subject.
4. Fanzago, *Memoria*, p. 75.
5. Ibid., p. 67.
6. Ibid., p. 76.
7. For the latter phase, from Italian unification to World War I, see A. De Bernardi, 'Pellagra, stato e scienza medica: la curabilità impossibile', in F. Della Peruta (ed.), *Storia d'Italia. Annali 7. Malattia e medicina* (Turin: Einaudi, 1984), pp. 681–704. The same historian is also the author of a broader social history: A. De Bernardi, *Il mal della rosa. Denutrizione e pellagra nelle campagne italiane from '800 e '900* (Milan: Franco Angeli, 1984).
8. Fanzago, *Sulla pellagra*.
9. J. Odoardi, *D'una specie particolare di scorbuto, dissertazione [...] recitata nell'Accademia di [Belluno] li 18 luglio 1776* (Venice: Simone Occhi, 1776), and reprinted in F. Fanzago, *Sulla pellagra*, pp. 1–31, from which I cite.
10. Odoardi, *D'una specie*, pp. 8–9, 21–2.
11. Ibid., p. 24.
12. Ibid., p. 25. The notion of 'insensible transpiration', that the body invisibly excreted much of what it ingested (in addition to the visible process of evacuation), was first developed by the Paduan physician Santorio Santorio in 1614. It was an important element of Pujati's work on regimen, *Della preservazione della salute de' letterati e della gente applicata e sedentaria* (Venice: Antonio Zatta, 1762). The work was published posthumously by Pujati's son Anton-Gaetano, to whom Odoardi dedicates his pellagra treatise.
13. Odoardi, *D'una specie*, p. 25.
14. F. Fanzago, *Paralleli tra la pellagra ed alcune malattie che più le rassomigliano* (Padua: Conzatti, 1792), reprinted in Fanzago, *Sulla pellagra*, pp. 93–202.

15. Giovanni Videmar had published a paper entitled *De quadam impetiginis specie morbo apud nos rusticis nunc frequentiori vulgo pellagra nuncupata* (Milan: Luigi Valadini, 1790).
16. For a detailed exploration of pellagra as a 'nosological problem', see D. García Guerra and V. Álvarez Antuña, *Lepra Asturiensis: la contribución asturiana en la historia de la pelagra (siglos XVIII y XIX)* (Madrid: CSIC, 1993), pp. 167–82.
17. F. Frapolli, in his *Animadversiones in morbum vulgo pelagram* (Milan: Giuseppe Galeazzi, 1771); G. Strambio, *De pellagra observationis, quas in regio pellagrosorum nosocomio collegit* (Milan: Giovanni Battista Bianchi, 1787 and 1789).
18. Fanzago, *Paralleli*, p. 107.
19. Ibid., p. 112.
20. Ibid., p. 113.
21. Fanzago refers to the German physician Karl Strack, although there is no note.
22. Fanzago, *Paralleli*, p. 114.
23. Ibid., pp. 124–5.
24. Ibid., p. 141.
25. Ibid., p. 144.
26. Ibid., pp. 146–7.
27. Ibid., p. 151.
28. Ibid., p. 163.
29. Ibid.
30. Ibid., p. 160.
31. Ibid., p. 164.
32. Ibid., p. 167.
33. Ibid., p. 172.
34. Ibid., p. 177.
35. Ibid., notes on pp. 178–9.
36. Ibid., p. 180, citing Videmar, *Impetiginis specie*.
37. Fanzago, *Paralleli*, pp. 184, 188, 190.
38. Ibid., p. 197.
39. F. Fanzago, 'Sulle cause della pellagra: memoria', in his *Memorie della Accademia di scienze, lettere ed arti di Padova* (Padova: Zanon Bettoni, 1809), pp. 22–46; reprinted in Fanzago, *Sulla pellagra*, part II, pp. 3–40.
40. G. B. Marzari, *Confutazione del sistema di Brown arricchita di nuove ed interessanti riflessioni indirette ai progressi della teoria e della pratica della medicina* (Venice: Francesco Andreola, 1802; Naples: Saverio D'Onofrio and Raffaele Palma, 1803). Marzari would have known Brown's work through a Latin translation published in Italy, *Elementi medicinae* (Milan: Josephus Galeatius, 1792). See J. Overmier, 'John Brown's Elementi medicinae: An Introductory Bibliographical Essay', *Bulletin of the Medical Library Association*, 70 (1982), pp. 310–17.
41. J. Pellizzari, *Discorsi dei presidenti e relazioni accademiche dell'Ateneo di Treviso* (Treviso: Andreola, 1834), cited in A. Chiades, *Un giornale, una storia: Il Monitor di Treviso, 1807–1813* (Treviso: Bepi Crich, 1982), p. 134.
42. G. B. Marzari, *Saggio medico-politico sulla pellagra o scorbuto italico* (Venice: Giovanni Parolari, 1810); *Della pellagra e del modo di estirparla in Italia* (Venice: Giovanni Parolari, 1815); and *Memoria ... nella quale rispondendo ad alcune obbiezioni riconferma la sua dottrina sulla causa della pellagra* (Treviso: Francesco Andreola, 1817).
43. C. Sprengel, *Stato della medicina nel decennio 1805–1814* (Venice: Giuseppe Picotti, 1816), pp. 259–60. The translation from the German was by Renato Arrigoni, a physi-

cian in Treviso, who would fill in for Marzari as editor of the newspaper *Il Monitor di Treviso*.

44. Marzari, *Saggio medico-politico*, p. 106. The italics are Marzari's own.
45. Fanzago, 'Appendice alla memoria sulle cause della pellagra', p. 43.
46. Ibid., p. 45.
47. Marzari, *Saggio medico-politico*, p. 87.
48. Ibid., pp. 28–9.
49. Ibid., p. 31; Fanzago, 'Cause della pellagra', pp. 9–10.
50. Fanzago, 'Cause della pellagra', pp. 5–6. The word *salso*, from 'salty', was used to describe 'that itching to the skin, caused by a salty humour'. G. Boerio, *Dizionario del dialetto veneziano* (Venice: Andrea Santini, 1829), p. 522; Marzari, *Saggio medico-politico*, p. 39
51. Marzari, *Saggio medico-politico*, p. 38.
52. Fanzago, 'Cause della pellagra', p. 23; Marzari, *Saggio medico-politico*, pp. 41–2.
53. Marzari, *Saggio medico-politico*, p. 59.
54. F. Fanzago, *Istruzione catechistica sulla pellagra, divisa in tre dialoghi* (Venice: Francesco Andreola, 1816). In it, Fanzago characterized as a 'hornets' nest' the 'many debates [that] have arisen amongst those authors who have written on pellagra' (p. 9). The irony is that in today's general historical surveys of pellagra, Marzari is credited with being the first to espouse the deficiency theory. See, for example, K. Carpenter, *Pellagra* (Stroudsburg, PA: Hutchinson Ross, 1981), p. 3.
55. Fanzago, 'Cause della pellagra', pp. 29–30, 32–3.
56. Ibid., p. 36. Fanzago approvingly cites a study by a doctor of Gottingen named Welt, and discussed by his mentor Frank, which suggested that most diseases, excepting contagious ones, originated in the lower gut. J. Welt, *De exanthematum fonte abdominali* (Gottingen, 1784), in J. P. Frank, *Delectus opuscularum medicorum antehac in Germaniae diversis academiis editorum*, 12 vols (Ticini [Pavia]: P. Galeatii, 1785–93), vol. 4, p. 30.
57. Fanzago, 'Cause della pellagra', pp. 36–7.
58. Marzari, *Saggio medico-politico*, pp. 111–12.
59. Ibid., pp. 112–13.
60. Ibid., p. 116.
61. V. Chiarugi, *Saggio di ricerche sulla pellagra* (Florence: Pietro Allegrini, 1814), pp. 82–99. Chiarugi cites Fanzago's *Paralleli* of 1792 (pp. 62–3) but not his 1810 work, and does not cite Marzari.
62. V. Chiarugi, *Saggio teorico-pratico sulle malattie cutanee sordide, osservate nel Regio Ospedale di Bonifazio in Firenze* (Florence: Pietro Allegrini, 1799).
63. L. Marri Malacrida, E. Panconesi and K. Holubar, 'Vincenzo Chiarugi (1759–1820): The Academic Career of the First Professor of Skin Diseases', *Italian General Review of Dermatology*, 28:3 (1991), pp. 129–40; G. Mora, 'Vincenzo Chiarugi (1759–1820) and his Psychiatric Reform in Florence in the Late 18th Century', *Journal of the History of Medicine and Allied Sciences*, 14 (1959), pp. 424–33; U. Baldini, 'Vincenzo Chiarugi', *Dizionario biografico degli Italiani*, at http://www.treccani.it/biografie/ [accessed 12 May 2011].
64. Chiarugi, *Saggio di ricerche*, pp. 6–7.
65. V. Chiarugi, *Della pazzia in genere, e in specie. Trattato medico-analitico con una centuria di osservazioni*, 3 vols (Florence: Luigi Carlieri, 1793–4); Chiarugi, *Malattie cutanee sordide*. He refers to pellagra in the latter work, but only to list it as one of the diseases that he would not discuss, 'since during the last ten years I have never seen it in this hospital, where a large number of individuals suffering from chronic skin diseases are admitted for treatment every day' (Chiarugi, *Malattie cutanee sordide*, p. vii).

66. Chiarugi, *Saggio di ricerche*, pp. 14–16.
67. Ibid., p. 47. Chiarugi took nosology very seriously, having previously argued in his study of mental diseases for a set of terms with which everyone would associate the same meanings, instead of the prevailing uncertainty and confusion. E. Fischer-Homberger, 'Eighteenth-Century Nosology and its Survivors', *Medical History*, 14 (1970), pp. 397–403, on p. 399.
68. Chiarugi, *Saggio di ricerche*, pp. 17–30.
69. Ibid., p. 22.
70. Ibid., pp. 75–80.
71. Ibid., pp. 101–6; his discussion of diet is on pp. 113–15.
72. Ibid., pp. 44–5. The 'impetigo order' includes scrofula, scurvy, syphilis, elephantiasis and leprosy, although Cullen does not mention pellagra. J. Thompson (ed.), *The Works of William Cullen ... Containing his Physiology, Nosology, and First Line of the Practice of Physic*, 2 vols (Edinburgh: William Blackwood, 1827), vol. 1, p. 244.
73. Chiarugi, *Saggio di ricerche*, pp. 121–3.

5 Siena, 'The Moral Biology of "the Itch" in Eighteenth-Century Britain'

1. Westminster City Archives (WCA), St Margaret's Westminster, Workhouse Committee Minutes, 1730–6, E2634, 383–6.
2. Middlesex Sessions Papers, Justices Working Documents, 1782, *London Lives, 1690–1800*, LMSMPS507620014–15, at www.londonlives.org [accessed 1 May 2011].
3. *An Abstract of the Orders of St. Thomas's Hospital* (London, 1707), p. 1; *An Account of the Proceedings of the Governors of St. George's Hospital* (London, 1736), p. 4; *The Laws of the London Infirmary* (London, 1743), p. 8.
4. Early histories of dermatology excepted: W. A. Pusey, *The History of Dermatology* (Springfield, IL: Charles C. Thomas, 1933; repr. Baltimore, MD: AMS, 1979), pp. 44–6; and R. Friedman, *The Story of Scabies* (New York: Froben Press, 1947).
5. J. Quincy, *Lexicon Physico-Medicum* (London, 1787), p. 729.
6. D. Harley, 'Rhetoric and the Social Construction of Illness and Healing', *Social History of Medicine*, 12:3 (1999), pp. 407–35; and J. Arrizabalaga, 'Problematizing Retrospective Diagnosis in the History of Disease', *Asclepio*, 54:1 (2002), pp. 51–70.
7. J. Arrizabalaga, J. Henderson and R. French, *The Great Pox: The French Disease in Renaissance Europe* (New Haven, CT: Yale University Press, 1997), pp. 1–19; C. Stein, *Negotiating the French Pox in Early Modern Germany* (Burlington, VT: Ashgate, 2009), pp. 23–66.
8. M. J. Ratcliff, *The Quest for the Invisible: Microscopy in the Enlightenment* (Burlington, VT: Ashgate, 2009), p. 25.
9. K. Codell Carter, *Rise of the Causal Concept of Disease* (Burlington, VT: Ashgate, 2003), pp. 26–37. See also K. Ott, 'Contagion, Public Health and the Visual Culture of Nineteenth-Century Skin', in D. Serlin (ed.) *Imagining Illness: Public Health and Visual Culture* (Minneapolis, MN: University of Minnesota Press, 2011), pp. 85–107.
10. D. Ghesquier, 'A Gallic Affair: The Case of the Missing Itch-Mite in French Medicine in the Early Nineteenth Century', *Medical History*, 43:1 (1999), pp. 26–54, on p. 30.
11. R. Mead, 'An Abstract of Part of a Letter from Dr Bonomo to Sigmor Redi', *Philosophical Transactions*, 23:283 (1702), pp. 1296–9; G. Adams, *Micrographia Illustrata* (London, 1746), p. 101; H. Baker, *The Microscope Made Easy* (London, 1742), pp. 169–72.

12. C. Bissett, *Medical Essays and Observations* (Newcastle-upon-Tyne, 1766), pp. 262–3.

13. T. Lobb, *The Practice of Physic in General* (London, 1771), pp. 228–9.

14. P. L., *A Letter from an Apothecary in London* (London, 1752), pp. 16–25.

15. Ibid.

16. R. Wiseman, *Severall Chirurgicall Treatises* (London, 1676), p. 134; T. Willis, *Practice of Physick* (London, 1684), p. 156.

17. Wiseman, *Severall Chirurgicall Treatises*, p. 134.

18. P. L., *A Letter from an Apothecary*, p. 25.

19. H. Boerhaave, *Modern Practice of Physic*, 2 vols (London, 1746), vol. 2, pp. 188–212.

20. D. Turner, *De Morbis Cutaneis* (London, 1714). All references refer to the fuller 1736 fifth edition. On Turner, see P. K. Wilson, *Surgery, Skin and Syphilis: Daniel Turner's London (1667–1741)* (Amsterdam: Rodopi, 1999).

21. T. Spooner, *Short Account of the Itch* (London, 1714). All references refer to the fuller 1728 sixth edition.

22. Ibid., pp. 18–19.

23. D. Turner, *The Ancient Physician's Legacy Impartially Survey'd* (London, 1733), pp. 57–9.

24. Spooner, *Short Account*, pp. 26–27; Turner, *De Morbis Cutaneis*, pp. 50–8.

25. Spooner, *Short Account*, pp. 2–3.

26. Ibid., pp. 7, 9–10.

27. Ibid., p. 10.

28. Ibid., pp. 14–15.

29. Boerhaave, *Modern Practice of Physic*, p. 189.

30. Turner, *De Morbis Cutaneis*, p. 9.

31. Ibid., p. 49.

32. Wiseman, *Severall Chirurgicall Treatises*, p. 138. Francis Spilsbury quoted this passage much later in his *A Treatise on the Method of Curing the Gout, Scurvy, Leprosy, Elephantiasis, Evil, and other Cutaneous Eruptions* (London, 1775), p. 31.

33. B. Dominiceti, *Medical Anecdotes of the Last Thirty Years* (London, 1781), pp. 419–22.

34. J. Archer, *Secrets Disclosed of Consumptions Showing how to Distinguish between Scurvy and Venereal Disease* (London, 1684).

35. T. Trotter, *Observations on the Scurvy* (London, 1786), pp. 22–3; also also L. Mansey, *The Practical Physician* (London, 1800) p. 243.

36. R. Dickinson, *An Essay on Cutaneous Diseases* (London, 1800), p. 41; J. Lind, *A Treatise on the Scurvy* (London, 1772), pp. 37–9; L. Mardon, *The English Malady Removed* (London, 1769), p. 41.

37. J. Ball, *The Modern Practice of Physic* (London, 1762), pp. 253–4; N. D. Falck, *The Seaman's Medical Instructor* (London, 1774), p. 144.

38. Bissett, *Medical Essays and Observations*, pp. 226, 239, 260–8.

39. J. Astruc, *Treatise of the Venereal Disease*, 2 vols (London, 1737), vol. 1, p. 160, also pp. 59, 145. H. Boerhaave, *A Treatise on the Venereal Disease and its Cure* (London, 1729), pp. 13–16; J. Hunter, *A Treatise on the Venereal Disease* (London, 1786), p. 22.

40. Boerhaave, *A Treatise on the Venereal Disease*, p. 16.

41. J. Becket, *A New Essay on the Venereal Disease* (London, 1765), p. 8; P. Desault, *A Treatise on the Venereal Distemper* (London, 1738), pp. 10–30; J. Profily, *An Easy and Exact Method of Curing the Venereal Disease* (London, 1748), p. 101. Astruc refuted the theory in *Treatise of the Venereal Disease*, vol. 1, p. 150.

42. J. Hill, *Cases in Surgery* (Edinburgh, 1772), p. 228. Here, Hill summarized a dissertation that he himself critiqued.

43. C. Peter, *New Observations on the Venereal Disease* (London, 1704), p. 58; J. Cam, *A Dissertation on the Pox* (London, 1731), p. 111; R. Brookes, *The General Practice of Physic*, 2 vols (London, 1754), vol. 2, pp. 244–5.

44. Dominiceti, *Medical Anecdotes*, p. 419.

45. A. Foa, 'The New and the Old: The Spread of Syphilis, 1494–1530', in E. Muir and G. Ruggiero (eds), *Sex and Gender in Historical Perspective* (Baltimore, MD: Johns Hopkins University Press, 1990), p. 39.

46. G. Harvey, *Little Venus Unmask'd* (London, 1702), pp. 12–15, 129–30.

47. A. Duncan, *Medical Cases, Selected from the Records of the Public Dispensary at Edinburgh* (Edinburgh, 1778), p. 215.

48. Anon., *The Edinburgh Practice of Physic and Surgery* (London, 1800), p. 560.

49. H. Boerhaave, *Academical Lectures on the Lues Venerea* (London, 1763), pp. 5–6.

50. Spooner, *Short Account*, p. 54.

51. Spilsbury, *Treatise on the Method of Curing the Gout*, p. 44; see also Spooner, *Short Account*, pp. 45–7.

52. J. Leake, *Dissertation on the Properties and Efficacy of Lisbon Diet-Drink* (London, 1783), pp. 118–19.

53. J. G. Zimmermann, *A Treatise on Experience in Physic*, 2 vols (London, 1778), vol. 1, p. 29.

54. K. Siena, 'Pliable Bodies: the Moral Biology of Health and Disease', in C. Reeves (ed.), *A Cultural History of the Human Body in the Age of Enlightenment* (Oxford: Berg, 2010), pp. 33–52.

55. Spooner, *Short Account*, p. 3.

56. For the nineteenth century, see C. Hamlin, 'Predisposing Causes and Public Health in Early Nineteenth-Century Medical Thought', in *Social History of Medicine*, 5:1 (1992), pp. 43–70.

57. Siena, 'Pliable Bodies', pp. 39–42.

58. Willis, *Practice of Physick*, p. 156; and Spooner, *Short Account*, pp. 18–21.

59. P. L., *Letter from an Apothecary*, pp. 26, 34.

60. J. Quincy, *Medicina Statica* (London, 1720), p. 106.

61. Siena, 'Pliable Bodies', pp. 46–9.

62. Bissett, *Medical Essays and Observations*, pp. 259–60, 262–3, 268.

63. W. Salmon, *Praxis Medica. The Practice of Physick: or, Dr. Sydenham's Processus Integri, Translated out of Latin into English, with Large Annotations, Animadversions and Practical Observations on the Same* (London, 1716), p. 74; Packe, *Medela Chymica*, p. 80.

64. W. Buchan, *Domestic Medicine* (Dublin, 1796), p. 324.

65. Mansey, *The Practical Physician*, p. 405.

66. Spooner, *Short Account*, p. 4.

67. W. Ellis, *The Country Housewife's Family Companion* (London, 1750), pp. 262–5.

68. Middlesex Sessions Papers, Justices Working Documents, 25 February 1712, *London Lives, 1690–1800*, LMSMPS501280029, at www.londonlives.org [accessed 1 May 2011].

69. Middlesex Sessions Papers, Justices Working Documents, 14 October 1751 and 30 June 1753, *London Lives, 1690–1800*, LMSMPS504140053 and LMSMPS504290096–98, at www.londonlives.org [accessed 1 May 2011].

70. S. Connor, *The Book of Skin* (London: Reaktion, 2004), esp. pp. 73–94; and C. Benthein, *Skin: On the Cultural Border between the Self and the World* (New York: Columbia University Press, 2002), esp. pp. 37–62.

71. On beauty in the Enlightenment, see D. M. Turner, 'The Body Beautiful', in C. Reeves (ed.), *A Cultural History of the Human Body in the Age of Enlightenment* (Oxford: Berg, 2010), pp. 113–31.

72. Dickinson, *Essay on Cutaneous Diseases*, p. 51.

73. Ibid., p. 7.

74. Spilsbury, *Treatise on the Method of Curing the Gout*, pp. 27–8.

75. Ovid, *De arte amandi, and The Remedy of Love Englished* (London, 1701), p. 76.

76. K. Siena, 'The Foul Disease and Privacy: The Effects of Venereal Disease and Patient Demand on the Medical Marketplace in Early Modern London', *Bulletin of the History of Medicine*, 75:2 (2001), pp. 199–224.

77. P. L., *Letter from an Apothecary*, pp. 31–2; see also Spooner, *Short Account*, pp. 7, 43, 47.

78. Anon., *An Essay on the Ancient and Modern Use of Physical Necklaces for Children's Teeth* (London, 1726), p. 16. On this practitioner's business, see F. Doherty, *A Study in Eighteenth-Century Advertising Methods: The Anodyne Necklace* (Lewiston: Edwin Mellen Press, 1992).

79. Turner, *De Morbis Cutaneous*, p. 53; Bissett, *Medical Essays and Observations*, pp. 268–9; Buchan, *Domestic Medicine*, pp. 322–3.

80. Spooner, *Short Account*, p. 47, also pp. 40, 43, 55–6.

81. Packe, *Medela Chymica*, p. 81.

82. G. Wilson, *Reports of Cases Argued and Adjudged in the King's Courts at Westminster*, 2 vols (London, 1770), vol. 2, p. 403.

83. Ibid., pp. 403–4.

84. M. Nedham, *Christianissimus Christianandus* (London, 1678), p. 37; J. Shebbeare, *The Marriage Act*, 2 vols (London, 1754), vol. 1, pp. 233, 235.

85. L. Demaitre, *Leprosy in Premodern Medicine* (Baltimore, MD: Johns Hopkins University Press, 2007), pp. 5–8; A. Foa, *The Jews of Europe After the Black Death* (Berkeley, CA: University of California Press, 2000), p. 21.

86. B. Marten, *A New Theory of Consumptions* (London, 1720), pp. 65–6.

87. Turner, *De Morbis Cutaneous*, pp. 6–7.

88. B. Ramazzini, *A Treatise of the Diseases of Tradesmen* (London, 1705), pp. 187–8.

89. H. de Longeville, *Long Livers* (London, 1722), p. xxvi.

90. L. Colley, *Britons: Forging the Nation 1707–1837* (New Haven, CT: Yale University Press, 2005), pp. 101–45.

91. J. Makittrick Adair, *Unanswerable Arguments Against the Abolition of the Slave Trade* (London, 1790), p. 46.

92. 'The Union-Proverb', in O. Dykes, *English Proverbs, with Moral Reflexions* (London, 1709), pp. 6–7.

93. A. Scriblerus, *Gorgoneicon: Being a Supplement to Whistoneutes* (London, 1731), pp. xii–xiii.

94. Ibid., p. 21.

95. Ibid., p. 119.

96. Anon., *A Seventh Letter to the People of England* (London, 1758), p. 15.

97. Connor, *The Book of Skin*, pp. 235–6.

98. T. Bridges, *A Burlesque Translation of Homer* (London, 1772), p. 508.

99. J. Thistlethwaite, *The Consultation. A Poem. In Four Cantos. Canto I* (London, 1771), p. 64.

100. 'YUCK. f. [*jocken*, Dutch.] Itch', in S. Johnson, *A Dictionary of the English Language*, 2 vols (London, 1756), vol. 2, [n.p.]. The *New Oxford English Dictionary*'s entry for 'yuck' only dates the term to the mid-twentieth century.

101. N. Robinson, *A New Treatise of the Venereal Disease* (London, 1736), pp. 48–9.

102. Bissett, *Medical Essays and Observations*, p. 272; W. Rowley, *The Rational Practice of Physic*, 4 vols (London, 1793), vol. 4, pp. 511–12.

103. Anon., *Medical Essays and Observations, Published by a Society in Edinburgh*, 4 vols (Edinburgh, 1747), vol. 1, p. 67.

104. Hill, *Cases in Surgery*, pp. 229–30.

105. Ibid., pp. 256, 260.

106. B. Bell, *A Treatise on Gonorrhoea Virulenta, and Lues Venerea*, 2 vols (Edinburgh, 1797), vol. 2, pp. 442–57; this quotation on p. 446.

107. Buchan, *Domestic Medicine*, pp. 179, 182–3.

108. Benthien, *Skin*, esp. pp. 48–62.

109. Ibid., p. 102; see also D. Wahrman's comments on masquerade, *The Making of the Modern Self: Identity and Culture in Eighteenth-Century England* (New Haven, CT: Yale University Press, 2004), pp. 159–68, 255–61, 265–7.

6 Minard, 'Syphilis, Backwardness and Indigenous Skin Lesions through French Physicians' Eyes in the Colonial Maghreb, 1830–1930'

1. Y. Turin, *Affrontements culturels dans l'Algérie coloniale: écoles, médecines, religion, 1830–1880* (Algiers: ENAL, 1983).

2. C. Fredj, 'L'Algérie comme matrice des médecins de l'Armée (1830–1860)', in A. Messaoudi, D. Nordman, N. Oulebsir (eds), *Savoirs, institutions et disciplines en Méditerranée (1830–1930)*, forthcoming.

3. J. Arnould, 'Dermatologie africaine: la lèpre kabyle', *Recueil de mémoires de médecine, chirurgie et pharmacie militaires*, 3rd series, 7 (1862), pp. 338–56, on p. 354.

4. Ibid., p. 340.

5. P. M. E. Lorcin, 'Imperialism, Colonial Identity, and Race in Algeria, 1830–1870: The Role of the French Medical Corps', *Isis*, 90:4 (1999), pp. 653–79.

6. H. Gauthier, *Histoire de la syphilis en Afrique du Nord, plus particulièrement en Algérie* (Algiers: Imprimerie Jules Carbonel, 1931), pp. 107–11.

7. J. Foucqueron, 'Essai topographique et médical sur la régence d'Alger', *Recueil de mémoires de médecine, de chirurgie et de pharmacie militaires*, 34 (1833), pp. 1–104, on pp. 74–5.

8. Deleau and Ferrus, 'Constantine', *Mémoires de médecine, de chirurgie et de pharmacie militaires*, 52 (1842), pp. 230–92, on p. 262.

9. Cited by Turin, *Affrontements culturels dans l'Algérie coloniale*, p. 97.

10. M.-A. Vincent, *Exposé clinique des maladies des Kabyles traitées à l'hôpital militaire de Dellys* (Paris: J.-B. Baillère et Fils, 1862), p. 55.

11. J. Brault, 'Les lépreux en Algérie', *Archiv für Schiffs- und Tropen-Hygiene*, 12 (1908), pp. 205–28, on p. 207.

12. B. L. Grigsby, *Pestilence in Medieval and Early Modern English Literature* (New York: Routledge, 2004), pp. 68–77.

13. R. Edmond, *Leprosy and Empire: A Medical and Cultural History* (Cambridge: Cambridge University Press, 2006), pp. 110–19.

14. G. Lacapère, *La syphilis arabe (Maroc, Algérie, Tunisie)* (Paris: Doin, 1923), p. 2. 'Arabs' was often used as a generic term to refer to both Arabs and Kabyles.

15. D. Zanrè, 'French Diseases and Italian Reponses: Representations of the *mal francese* in the Literature of Cinquecento Tuscany', in K. Siena (ed.), *Sins of the Flesh: Responding to Sexual Disease in Early Modern Europe* (Toronto: Centre for Reformation and Renaissance Studies, 2005), pp. 187–208.

16. A. Hanoteau and A. Letourneux, *La Kabylie et les coutumes kabyles* (Paris: Bouchène, 2003 [1893]), p. 363.
17. N. L. Stepan, *Picturing Tropical Nature* (London: Reaktion Books, 2001), p. 171.
18. A. Marie, 'Paralysie générale et syphilis chez les Arabes', *La Syphilis, revue mensuelle de médecine spéciale*, 4 (1906), pp. 1–13, on p. 7.
19. Lacapère, *La syphilis arabe*, p. 49.
20. R. Gonssolin, *De la syphilis mutilante chez les indigènes musulmans de l'Afrique du Nord* (Lyon: Bosc Frères & Riou, 1926), p. 14.
21. J. L. Alibert, 'De la syphilis ulcérante', in *Monographie des dermatoses ou Précis théorique et pratique des maladies de la peau*, 2 vols (Paris: Daynac, 1832), vol. 2, pp. 380–6.
22. M. Worboys, 'Germs, Malaria and the Invention of Mansonian Tropical Medicine: From "Diseases in the Tropics" to "Tropical Diseases"', in D. Arnold (ed.), *Warm Climates and Western Medicine: the Emergence of Tropical Medicine, 1500–1900* (Amsterdam: Rodopi, 1996), pp. 181–207.
23. See D. C. Danielssen and W. Boeck, *Traité de la Spédalskhed ou éléphantiasis des Grecs* (Paris: J. B. Baillière, 1847); W. Boeck, *Traité de la Radesyge (syphilis tertiaire)* (Christiana: Johan Dahl, 1860). The skin symptoms of the 'radesyge', as described by Boeck, were very similar to those observed among 'syphilitics' of North Africa. See A. K. Lie, 'Origin Stories and the Norwegian Radesyge', *Social History of Medicine*, 20:3 (December 2007), pp. 563–79.
24. Catrin, 'Modifications apportées à la syphilis par les pays chauds', in F. J. van Leent, A. A. A. Guye, de Perrot and J. Zeeman (eds), *Congrès international de médecins des colonies, Amsterdam, septembre 1883* (Amsterdam: F. Van Rossen, 1884), pp. 280–9.
25. On patients suffering from general paralysis of insanity due to syphilis, see G. Davis, *'The Cruel Madness of Love': Sex, Syphilis and Psychiatry in Scotland, 1880–1930* (Amsterdam: Rodopi, 2008).
26. C. Taraud, *La prostitution coloniale: Algérie, Tunisie, Maroc, 1830–1962* (Paris: Payot, 2003); see also J. Clancy-Smith, 'Islam, Gender, and Identities in the Making of French Algeria, 1830–1962', in J. Clancy-Smith and F. Gouda (eds), *Domesticating the Empire: Race, Gender and Family Life in French and Dutch Colonialism* (Charlottesville, VA: University Press of Virginia, 1998), pp. 154–74.
27. Lacapère, *La syphilis arabe*, p. 11.
28. L. Duncan Bulkley, *Syphilis in the Innocent* (New York: Bailey & Fairchild, 1894), pp. 142–57.
29. J. L. Alibert, *Précis théorique et pratique sur les maladies de la peau*, 2 vols (Paris: Caille et Ravier, 1818), vol. 2, pp. 112–54.
30. J. Rollet, *Recherches sur plusieurs maladies de la peau réputées rares ou exotiques, qu'il convient de rattacher à la syphilis* (Paris: P. Asselin, 1861).
31. G. A. Paire, *Contribution à l'étude de la syphilis maligne précoce en Algérie* (Montpellier: Imprimerie Firmin, Montane et Sicardi, 1908), p. 45.
32. L. Raynaud, 'Revue des maladies cutanées et vénériennes signalées chez les indigènes algériens', *Journal des maladies cutanées et syphilitiques*, 9 (1897), pp. 65–80, on pp. 66–7.
33. C. J. Daga, 'Documents pour servir à l'histoire de la syphilis chez les Arabes', *Archives générales de Médecine* (September 1864), pp. 287–310, on p. 299.
34. At the same time, such traditions and habits of country folk were considered a means of contamination in Europe; see P. Baldwin, *Contagion and the State in Europe, 1830–1930* (Cambridge: Cambridge University Press, 1999), pp. 408–13.

35. J. Raux, 'Impressions de clinique arabe', Archives du Service de Santé des Armées, Val-de-Grâce (hereafter ASSA VDG), 68 (23).

36. 'The disease appeared to Europeans as an exact index of cultural deprivation', remarks L. Engelstein, in her article dedicated to non-venereal syphilis in Russia, 'Morality and the Wooden Spoon: Russian Doctors View Syphilis, Social Class, and Sexual Behavior, 1890–1905', in C. Gallagher and T. W. Laqueur (eds), *The Making of the Modern Body: Sexuality and Society in the Nineteenth Century* (Berkeley, CA: University of California Press, 1987), pp. 169–208, on p. 170.

37. Lacapère, *La syphilis arabe*, p. 2.

38. Edmond, *Leprosy and Empire*, p. 112.

39. Ibid., pp. 127–8.

40. See D. Pick, *Faces of Degeneration: A European Disorder, c.1848–c.1918* (Cambridge: Cambridge University Press, 1989); and A. Maxwell, *Picture Imperfect: Photography and Eugenics, 1870–1940* (Brighton: Sussex Academic Press, 2008).

41. C. C. Bernard, *La syphilis chez les Arabes au point de vue de l'hygiène publique et de la nécessité d'une hospitalisation entièrement indigène* (Algiers: Association ouvrière V. Aillaud et Cie, 1875), p. 9.

42. J. P. V. Licke, *Étude sur les accidents tertiaires de la syphilis, d'après des faits recueillis en Afrique sur des Indigènes* (Montpellier: Boehm, 1853), p. 8.

43. Ibid., p. 9.

44. See B. J. M. Peyronie, *Le traitement de la syphilis chez les indigènes en Tunisie* (Bordeaux: Imprimerie commerciale et industrielle, 1905); and P. Susini, *Quelques considérations sur la syphilis des indigènes d'Algérie* (Paris: Jouve & Cie, 1920).

45. L. Raynaud, 'Les maladies cutanées et syphilitiques au Maroc', *Journal des maladies cutanées et syphilitiques*, 13 (1902), pp. 1–9, on p. 1.

46. Hanoteau and Letourneux, *La Kabylie et les coutumes kabyles*, p. 368.

47. 'Rapport sur un nouveau mode de traitement de la syphilis chez les Arabes', Dellys (15 June 1862), ASSA VDG, 68 (32).

48. Arnould, 'Dermatologie africaine: la lèpre kabyle', p. 499.

49. Peyronie, *Le traitement de la syphilis chez les indigènes en Tunisie*, p. 40.

50. G. Marcou, *Leucomélanodermie syphilitique (Lèpre kabyle)* (Paris: Jouve et Boyer, 1898), p. 94. The *communes mixtes* were rural administrative districts where few Europeans lived.

51. B. Gaumer, *L'organisation sanitaire en Tunisie sous le Protectorat français (1881–1956): un bilan ambigu et contrasté* (Laval: Presses de l'Université de Laval, 2006), p. 157.

52. The same process of retreat of non-venereal 'syphilis' has also been observed in almost all other regions of the African continent, as was shown by M. Vaughan, 'Syphilis in Colonial East and Central Africa: The Social Construction of an Epidemic', in T. Ranger and P. Slack (eds), *Epidemics and Ideas: Essays on the Historical Perception of Pestilence* (New York: Cambridge University Press, 1992), pp. 269–302.

53. Lacapère, *La syphilis arabe*, p. 479.

54. L. M. Pautrier, 'Inspection des travailleurs indigènes'; Circular 399 Ci/7, 'Examen dermato-vénéréologique des travailleurs coloniaux et étrangers à leur arrivée et pendant leur séjour dans les usines', Archives of the Service Historique de l'Armée de Terre (SHAT), 9 NN 7/1053.

55. In fact, most of the North African immigrants treated for syphilis in Parisian clinics had contracted the disease in France; see C. D. Rosenberg, *Policing Paris: The Origins of Modern Immigration Control Between the Wars* (Ithaca, NY: Cornell University Press, 2006), p. 176.

56. On the manner by which tropical diseases were constructed as simultaneously specific to the colonies and potentially dangerous for the metropoles, see R. Edmond, 'Returning Fears: Tropical Disease and the Metropolis', in F. Driver and L. Martins (eds), *Tropical Visions in an Age of Empire* (Chicago, IL: University of Chicago Press, 2005), pp. 175–96.

57. E. H. Hudson, 'Treponematosis among the Bedouin Arabs of the Syrian Desert', *US Naval Medical Bulletin*, 26:4 (1928), pp. 817–25.

58. His studies culminated in a book: E. H. Hudson, *Non-Venereal Syphilis: A Sociological and Medical Study of Bejel* (Edinburgh: E. S. Livingstone, 1958).

59. E. H. Hudson, 'Treponematosis and African Slavery', *British Journal of Venereal Diseases*, 40 (1964), pp. 43–52. For a re-examination of this old controversy, see O. Dutour (ed.), *L'origine de la syphilis en Europe, avant ou après 1493? Actes du colloque international de Toulon, 25–28 novembre 1993* (Paris: Errance, 1994).

7 Vongsathorn, 'Discovering the "Leper": Shifting Attitudes towards Leprosy in Twentieth-Century Uganda'

1. C. Benthien, *Skin: On the Cultural Border between Self and the World* (New York: Columbia University Press, 2002), pp. 98–100; S. Connor, *The Book of Skin* (London: Reaktion Books, 2004), p. 147; E. Goffman, *Stigma* (London: Penguin Books, 1963), pp. 64–8.

2. S. Browne, *Leprosy in the Bible* (London: Christian Methodist Fellowship, 1970), p. 3; S. N. Brody, *The Disease of the Soul* (Ithaca, NY: Cornell University Press, 1974), p. 11; R. I. Moore, *The Formation of a Persecuting Society* (Oxford: Blackwell, 2007), p. 10; R. Edmond, *Leprosy and Empire* (New York: Cambridge University Press, 2006), pp. 1–3.

3. Z. Gussow and G. Tracy, 'Stigma and the Leprosy Phenomenon', *Bulletin of the History of Medicine*, 44:5 (1970), pp. 425–49.

4. Although a decision was made in 1948 at the Fifth International Leprosy Congress to substitute the term 'leprosy patient' for 'leper', for the sake of clarity and consistency, I will use the term 'leper' when it is important to an understanding of the historical context in which it was used.

5. T. Ranger, 'Godly Medicine', *Social Science and Medicine*, 15B (1981), pp. 261–2; M. Vaughan, *Curing Their Ills* (Stanford, CA: Stanford University Press, 1991), p. 56; D. Hardiman, 'Introduction', in D. Hardiman (ed.), *Healing Bodies, Saving Souls: Medical Missions in Asia and Africa* (Amsterdam: Rodopi, 2006), p. 5; C. Good, Jr, *The Steamer Parish* (London: University of Chicago Press, 2004), p. 2.

6. Vaughan, *Curing Their Ills*, pp. 69–70, 75.

7. 'Obituary: C. A. Wiggins', *British Medical Journal*, 1:5483 (5 February 1966), pp. 363–4, on p. 363; 'C. M. S. Leper Work', *Mission Hospital*, 31:348 (1927), p. 16.

8. K. Makower, *Not a Gap Year* (Eastbourne: Apologia Publications, 2008), pp. 22–4.

9. University of Birmingham Special Collections, Birmingham, Church Missionary Society Papers (hereafter CMS), Annual Letter, 1933, G3/AL Langley.

10. M. Louis, *Love is the Answer: The Story of Mother Kevin* (Dublin: Fallons, 1964), p. 49.

11. Bishop's House Archive, Jinja, Nyenga Leper Camp, Mother Kevin to Father Minderop, 31 May 1933.

12. Gussow and Tracy, 'Stigma and the Leprosy Phenomenon', p. 436.

13. 'The Spread of Leprosy', *The Times*, 13 June 1889, p. 10; H. B. Chapman, 'The Late Father Damien', *The Times*, 14 May 1889, p. 4.

14. 'The Alleged Case of Leprosy at the Meat Markets', *The Times*, 19 June 1889, p. 13.

15. Anon., 'London: Saturday, June 29, 1889', *The Lancet*, 133:3435 (29 June 1889), pp. 1309–12, on p. 1309.

16. J. Freeland, 'Notes on Leprosy', *British Medical Journal*, 2:1501 (5 October 1889), pp. 760–1; Anon., 'London: Saturday, June 29, 1889', *The Lancet*, 133:3435 (29 June 1889), pp. 1309–12, on p. 1309.

17. L. de la Marche, *La Lepre et les Leproseries* (Paris, 1892), in L. W. Mulhane, *Leprosy and the Charity of the Church* (Chicago, II., 1896), p. 75.

18. Z. Gussow and G. Tracy, 'The Use of Archival Materials in the Analysis and Interpretation of Field Data', *American Anthropologist*, 73:3 (1971), pp. 695–709, on p. 702.

19. E. L. McEwen, 'The Leprosy of the Bible in Its Medical Aspect', *Biblical World*, 38.3 (September 1911), pp. 194–202, on p. 194.

20. Anon., 'High Court of Justice', *The Times*, 17 May 1916, p. 3.

21. Browne, *Leprosy in the Bible*, p. 17.

22. Benthien, *Skin*, p. 126.

23. B. Russell (ed.), *St. John's Hospital for Diseases of the Skin* (Edinburgh: E. & S. Livingstone, 1963), p. 10.

24. R. M. Langley, 'Cleanse the Lepers', *Mission Hospital*, 33:431 (1933), pp. 312–16, on p. 312; R. M. Langley, 'The Hospital from a New Worker's Point of View', *Ruanda Notes*, 34 (1930), pp. 24–5, on p. 24.

25. L. Rogers and E. Muir, *Leprosy* (London: Simpkin, Marshall, Hamilton, Kent & Co., 1925), pp. 126–7.

26. Ibid., p. 51.

27. Langley, 'Cleanse the Lepers', p. 313.

28. A. C. S. Smith, 'Leprosy in Kigezi, Uganda Protectorate', *Mission Hospital*, 35:407 (1931), pp. 312–15, on p. 312.

29. Uganda National Archives, Entebbe, Uganda (hereafter UGA), J. R. Innes, 'Report No. 5', J6/25I.

30. UGA, Innes, 'Report No. 1', J6/25I; Innes, 'Report No. 3', J6/25I.

31. Smith, 'Leprosy in Kigezi', p. 312.

32. Ibid.

33. Innes, 'Leprosy in Uganda', *East African Medical Journal*, 27:7 (1950), pp. 278–83, on p. 281.

34. Smith, 'Leprosy in Kigezi', pp. 312–13.

35. CMS, Annual Letter, 1935, G3/AL Langley; 'The Healing Fellowship', *Mission Hospital*, 43:500 (1939), pp. 219–53, on p. 239.

36. M. M. Edel, *The Chiga of Western Uganda* (New York: Oxford University Press, 1957), pp. 129–72.

37. Edel, *The Chiga*, p. 124; P. Ngologoza, *Kigezi and its People* (Kampala: Fountain Publishers, 1998), pp. 19–20.

38. Edel, *The Chiga*, p. 130.

39. Langley, 'Cleanse the Lepers', p. 312; Langley, 'The Hospital', p. 24.

40. Smith, 'Leprosy in Kigezi', pp. 312–13.

41. L. E. S. Sharp, 'Kigezi', *Mission Hospital*, 32:364 (1928), pp. 103–6, on p. 103.

42. Langley, 'Cleanse the Lepers', p. 313.

43. Edel, *The Chiga*, pp. 33, 130, 144.

44. 'A Leper Settlement', *Uganda Herald*, 28 July 1933.

45. L. E. S. Sharp, 'Dr. Sharp's Account of the R.G.M.M. and Leprosy', *Ruanda Notes*, 26 (1928), pp. 5–6, on p. 5.
46. KDA, Kigezi DC to Western PC, 24 March 1927, Medical General, p. 103; United Kingdom National Archives, Annual Report of the Medical Department, Uganda Protectorate, 1931, CO 685/30, on pp. 99, 103; K. Vongsathorn, '"First and Foremost the Evangelist"? Mission and Government Priorities for Leprosy Treatment in Uganda, 1927–1948', *Journal of Eastern African Studies*, 40:5 (2012), pp. 863–78.
47. Sharp, 'Kigezi', p. 103.
48. CMS, Annual Letter, 1931, G3/AL Langley.
49. CMS, Annual Letter, 1934, G3/AL Martin.
50. R. R. Webster, 'At the Home Base', *Ruanda Notes*, 46 (1933), pp. 5–7, on pp. 5–6.
51. Interview with Mary Sharp, 3 November 2009.
52. Interviews with John and Vicent, 5 August 2011.
53. L. E. S. Sharp, 'Letter', *Ruanda Notes*, 41 (1932), pp. 9–11, on p. 10; Webster, 'At the Home Base', p. 6.
54. Webster, 'At the Home Base', p. 6.
55. L. E. S. Sharp, 'Plans for the Leper Work', *Ruanda Notes*, 30 (1929), pp. 5–9, on p. 9.
56. Interviews with John, Vicent and Jacqueline, 5 August 2011; KDA, Secretary General to Rwamuchucha, 6 September 1947, Resettlement of Bakiga; G. Carswell, *Cultivating Success in Uganda* (Oxford: James Currey, 2007), p. 61.
57. Interview with Pat Gilmer, 4 November 2009.
58. Sharp, 'Letter', p. 11.
59. CMS, Annual Letter, 1932, G3/AL Langley.
60. Interview with Vicent, 5 August 2011.
61. R. M. Langley, 'Report of the Leper Work, Bunyonyi', *Mission Hospital*, 41:479 (1937), pp. 316–19, on p. 318.
62. Interview with Pat Gilmer, 4 November 2009.
63. Ngologoza, *Kigezi and its People*, p. 70.
64. Interview with Pat Gilmer, 4 November 2009.
65. Gussow and Tracy, 'The Use of Archival Materials', p. 703.
66. M. Mallinga, 'Attitudes Towards Leprosy in Kumi District' (BA dissertation, Makerere University, 1980), pp. 38
67. Ibid., p. 41.
68. CMS, Wiggins to Hooper, 17 April 1930, G3/A10/m1A 1934–49.
69. Mallinga, 'Attitudes Towards Leprosy in Kumi District', pp. 47, 53, 59.
70. Interviews with Lawrence, Michael, Zerri, Sipola and Samson, 5 July 2010.
71. UGA, Innes, 'Report No. 3', J6/25I; Group interview, Buluba, 9 August 2011.
72. Jinja District Archives, Jinja, Uganda, Elliot to Chief Secretary, Entebbe, 1927, Medical: Leprosy.
73. Interview with Vincent, 28 April 2010.
74. Interview with Yoana, 26 April 2010.
75. UGA, Innes, 'Report No. 1', J6/25I.
76. J. Iliffe, *The African Poor* (Cambridge: Cambridge University Press, 1987), p. 216.
77. UGA, Innes, 'Report No. 12', J6/25I.
78. Iliffe, *The African Poor*, p. 153.
79. J. Orley, *Culture and Mental Illness* (Nairobi: East African Publishing House, 1970), pp. 38–9.
80. F. Walser, *Luganda Proverbs* (Berlin: Reimer, 1982).
81. Interview with Doreen, 30 April 2010.

8 McKay, 'Sex and Skin Cancer: Kaposi's Sarcoma Becomes the "Stigmata of AIDS", 1979–83'

1. R. Shilts, *And the Band Played On: Politics, People, and the AIDS Epidemic* (hereafter *ATBPO*) (New York: St Martin's Press, 1987), p. 198.

2. R. A. Shiels, 'A History of Kaposi's Sarcoma', *Journal of the Royal Society of Medicine*, 79 (September 1986), pp. 532–4, on p. 532.

3. M. Kaposi, 'Idiopathisches multiples Pigmentsarkomen der Haut', *Archiv Dermatol Syphilis*, 4 (1872), pp. 265–73; cited in G. Sternbach and J. Varon, 'Moritz Kaposi: Idiopathic Pigmented Sarcoma of the Skin', *Journal of Emergency Medicine*, 13:5 (1995), pp. 671–4, on p. 671.

4. *Philadelphia* (Tri-Star, 1993), J. Demme (dir.).

5. C. Patton, 'Visualizing Safe Sex: When Pedagogy and Pornography Collide', in D. Fuss (ed.), *Inside/Out: Lesbian Theories, Gay Theories* (London: Routledge, 1991), pp. 373–86, on p. 383.

6. See also D. Crimp, 'How To Have Promiscuity in an Epidemic', in D. Crimp (ed.), *AIDS: Cultural Analysis, Cultural Activism* (Cambridge, MA: MIT Press, 1988), pp. 237–71.

7. I explored this topic extensively in my doctoral research: R. A. McKay, 'Imagining "Patient Zero": Sexuality, Blame, and the Origins of the North American AIDS Epidemic' (PhD thesis, University of Oxford, 2010). For an excellent general discussion, see P. Wald, *Contagious: Cultures, Carriers, and the Outbreak Narrative* (London: Duke University Press, 2008), pp. 213–63.

8. 'Patient Zero', *60 Minutes*, CBS, 15 November 1987; 'Patient Zero', *People*, 28:26 (28 December 1987), p. 47.

9. 'Quotes of the Week', *U.S. News & World Report*, 103:16 (19 October 1987), p. 7.

10. For the development of the biomedical 'facts' of HIV/AIDS, see G. Oppenheimer, 'In the Eye of the Storm: The Epidemiological Construction of AIDS', in E. Fee and D. M. Fox (eds), *AIDS: The Burdens of History* (Berkeley, CA: University of California Press, 1988), pp. 267–300; S. Epstein, *Impure Science: AIDS, Activism, and the Politics of Knowledge* (Berkeley, CA: University of California Press, 1996), pp. 45–78.

11. The oral history interviews undertaken for my doctoral research were deposited at the British Library's Sound Archive.

12. D. Conn, interview, Halifax, Canada, 25 July 2008.

13. C. M. Mathieson and H. J. Stam, 'Renegotiating Identity: Cancer Narratives', *Sociology of Health & Illness*, 17:3 (1995), pp. 283–306, on p. 302.

14. '*Pneumocystis* Pneumonia – Los Angeles', *Morbidity and Mortality Weekly Report*, 30 (1981), pp. 250–2.

15. D. Juranek, Kaposi's Sarcoma in Male Homosexuals, memo, 11 June 1981, William Darrow's Personal Papers, Miami, Florida, AIDS Task Force: 1981, pp. 2–3.

16. R. Redford, 'Notes for Richard McKay', in McKay, 'Imagining "Patient Zero"', p. 348.

17. Redford, 'Memories of Gaetan' [email to R. A. McKay] (7 January 2008), rich.mckay@history.ox.ac.uk [accessed 7 January 2008].

18. D. M. Auerbach, et al., 'Cluster of Cases of the Acquired Immune Deficiency Syndrome: Patients Linked By Sexual Contact', *American Journal of Medicine*, 76:3 (March 1984), pp. 487–92.

19. A. R. Moss, 'AIDS without End', *New York Review of Books*, 35:19 (1988), p. 60.

20. P. A. Lanzaratta, 'Why Me?', *Christopher Street*, 63 (April 1982), p. 16.

21. S. Sontag, *Illness as Metaphor and AIDS and Its Metaphors* (New York: Picador USA, 1990), p. 40.

22. N. Fain, 'Is Our Lifestyle Hazardous To Our Health? Part II', *The Advocate*, 1 April 1982, p. 17.

23. Cartoons and articles in New York City's *Christopher Street* throughout 1982 illustrate this range of responses.

24. A. Silversides, *AIDS Activist: Michael Lynch and the Politics of Community* (Toronto: Between the Lines, 2003), pp. 29–41; Epstein, *Impure Science*, pp. 55–66.

25. The figure of 600 cases comes from W. P. McCarthy and G. T. Pack, 'Malignant Blood Vessel Tumors', *Surgery, Gynecology & Obstetrics*, 91 (1950), pp. 465–82; cited in Sternbach and Varon, 'Moritz Kaposi', p. 672.

26. For example, 'Kaposi's Sarcoma: How to Recognize It … How to Fight It' (San Francisco, CA: Kaposi's Sarcoma Foundation, *c.* 1982); Steven P. Borkovic, 'Kaposi's Sarcoma in Gay Men' (San Francisco, CA: Ad Hoc Committee on Kaposi's Sarcoma, Bay Area Physicians for Human Rights, *c.* 1982); for both pamphlets, see San Francisco GLBT Historical Society, AIDS Ephemera Collection, Box C, Educ/Prevent Other Ephemera.

27. N. Fain, 'Is Our Lifestyle Hazardous To Our Health?', *The Advocate*, 18 March 1982, p. 17.

28. M. Conant, interview, San Francisco, CA, USA, 27 July 2007.

29. S. Nichols, 'For Patients, for Ourselves', *New York Native*, 11–24 October 1982, p. 15.

30. Lanzaratta, 'Why Me?', p. 15.

31. 'A Warning to Gay Men with AIDS', *New York Native*, 22 November–5 December 1982, p. 16. See also Epstein, *Impure Science*, pp. 58–66.

32. R. Berkowitz and M. Callen, *How to Have Sex in an Epidemic: One Approach* (New York: News from the Front Publications, 1983), pp. 8, 10.

33. M. Fuerst, '"Shell-Shocked" Gays Told "Wear Condoms": Homosexual Practices Linked to Kaposi's Risk', *Medical Post*, 19:8 (1983), p. 8.

34. See also R. Berkowitz, *Stayin' Alive: The Invention of Safe Sex: A Personal History* (Oxford: Westview Press, 2003), pp. 137–8.

35. Shilts, *ATBPO*, p. 413.

36. Friedman-Kien, quoted in R. Bayer and G. Oppenheimer, *AIDS Doctors: Voices from the Epidemic: An Oral History* (Oxford: Oxford University Press, 2000), p. 61.

37. L. Mass, 'KS: Latest Developments', *New York Native*, 24 August–6 September 1981, p. 12.

38. Shilts, *ATBPO*, p. 247.

39. R. Shilts, Bob Tivey interview notes, *c.* 1986, Randy Shilts Papers (GLC 43), San Francisco Public Library, James C. Hormel Gay and Lesbian Center, Books, *ATBPO*, Box 2, folder 23: Patient Zero.

40. Conant, interview.

41. M. S. Vos, *Denial and Quality of Life in Lung Cancer Patients* (Amsterdam: Pallas Publications – Amsterdam University Press, 2009).

42. Shilts, *ATBPO*, p. 200.

43. S. E. Dritz and M. F. Silverstein, *The AIDS Epidemic in San Francisco: The Medical Response, 1981–1984, Vol. I* [online transcript], 35–6 (updated 1995), at http://content.cdlib.org/ark:/13030/kt2m3n98v1/ [accessed 10 August 2006].

44. In particular, see M. Lynch, 'Living with Kaposi's', *Body Politic*, 88 (November 1982), pp. 31–7; B. Lewis, 'The Real Gay Epidemic: Panic and Paranoia', *Body Politic*, 88 (November 1982), pp. 38–40.

45. Lynch, 'Living with Kaposi's', p. 37.

46. S. Macdonell, interview, Vancouver, Canada, 11 June 2008.

47. Shilts, *ATBPO*, p. 208.

48. R. Crane to Board of Directors, memo, 15 November 1982, UCSF Library and Center for Knowledge Management, Archives and Special Collections, University of California, San Francisco, San Francisco AIDS Foundation Records (MSS 94-60), Carton 2, folder 2/10: Monthly Reports to Board 1982: Sept.–Dec., Foundation Program Activities, p. 1.

49. Conant to Crane, letter, 11 November 1982, SFAF records, Carton 2, folder 2/32: Letters and Announcements.

50. Crane to Board, p. 2.

51. Conant to Crane, letter, 11 November 1982.

52. Conant, interview.

53. N. Siraisi, *Medieval and Early Renaissance Medicine: An Introduction to Knowledge and Practice* (London: University of Chicago Press, 1990), pp. 101–4.

54. S. Connor, *The Book of Skin* (Ithaca, NY: Cornell University Press, 2004), pp. 20–1.

55. For a discussion of the highly sexualized environment of the airline industry in the 1960s and 1970s, see, for example, K. M. Barry, *Femininity in Flight: A History of Flight Attendants* (London: Durham University Press, 2007), pp. 174–5.

56. A. C. Morton, *Airline Guide to Stewardess and Steward Careers*, ed. M. R. Tingley (10th edn; Miami Springs, FL: Passenger and Inflight Service Magazine, 1977), p. 92.

57. Morton, *Airline Guide*, p. 19; J. Miller, interview, Vancouver, Canada, 10 June 2008.

58. Morton, *Airline Guide*, p. 9.

59. J. Smith, *How To Be a Flight Stewardess or Steward: A Handbook and Training Manual for Airline Cabin Attendants* (3rd revised edn; Van Nuys, CA: Pan American Navigation Service, Inc., 1978), p. 23; italics in original.

60. Redford, 'Notes', in McKay, 'Imagining "Patient Zero"', p. 353.

61. Miller, interview.

62. S. Rose, 'Historic AIDS Memento will be Auctioned for ASG', *Provincetown Banner*, 21 October 2004, at http://www.provincetownbanner.com/article/features_article/_/30070/Features/10/21/2004 [accessed 27 April 2010].

63. L. J. Laubenstein, et al., 'Treatment of Epidemic Kaposi's Sarcoma with Etoposide or Combination of Doxorubicin, Bleomycin, and Vinblastine', *Journal of Clinical Oncology*, 2:10 (October 1984), pp. 1115–20; see also Berkowitz, *Stayin' Alive*, p. 94.

64. R. Bisson, interview, Vancouver, Canada, 21 August 2008.

65. J. W. Bean, 'Coverups', *New York Native*, 5 December 1983, p. 18. Simon Garfield describes the importance of camouflaging KS lesions to later patients in the UK in *The End of Innocence: Britain in the Time of AIDS* (London: Faber & Faber, 1995), pp. 158–9.

66. Stewart, interview.

67. Gay Men's Health Crisis, 'AIDS? What You Should Know about our Health Emergency ...', *c.* October 1982, leaflet, San Francisco GLBT Historical Society, AIDS Ephemera Collection, Box C, Educ/Prevent Other Ephemera.

9 Newsom Kerr, '"An Alteration in the Human Countenance": Inoculation, Vaccination and the Face of Smallpox in the Age of Jenner'

1. R. J. Thornton, 'Second Letter to Mr. Tilloch on the Cow-Pock', *Philosophical Magazine*, 20 (1805), pp. 143–52, on pp. 143–6.

2. Quoted in C. Creighton, *A History of Epidemics in Britain, Vol. II* (Cambridge: Cambridge University Press, 1894), pp. 452–3.

3. Ibid., p. 530.
4. J. R. Smith, *The Speckled Monster: Smallpox in England, 1670–1970, with Particular Reference to Essex* (Chelmsford: Essex Record Office, 1987), p. 20.
5. J. Moore, *The History of the Small-Pox* (London, 1815), pp. 237–8.
6. D. Hartley, *Some Reasons Why the Practice of Inoculation Ought to be Introduced into the Town of Bury at Present* (1733), quoted in P. Razzell, *The Conquest of Smallpox: The Impact of Inoculation on Smallpox Mortality in Eighteenth Century Britain* (2nd edn; London: Caliban Books, 2003), p. 62.
7. Moore, *The History of the Small-Pox*, p. 251. See also M. May, 'Inoculating the Urban Poor in the Late Eighteenth Century', *British Journal for the History of Science*, 30 (1997), pp. 291–305.
8. Razzell, *The Conquest of Smallpox*, pp. 32–3; Smith, *The Speckled Monster*, pp. 68–91.
9. 'Uninterested Spectator', *A Letter to J. V. Lettsom M.D. Occasioned by Baron Dimsdale's Remarks* (London, 1779), quoted in D. Shuttleton, *Smallpox and the Literary Imagination, 1660–1820* (Cambridge: Cambridge University Press, 2007), pp. 37–8.
10. J. Mackenzie, *History of Health* (1760), quoted in W. Buchan, *Domestic Medicine* (16th edn; London, 1798), p. 232.
11. Quoted in Smith, *The Speckled Monster*, p. 72.
12. W. Lipscombe, 'Beneficial Effects of Inoculation', in *Poems and Translations* (London, 1830), pp. 18–24.
13. I. Grundy, 'Medical Advance and Female Frame: Inoculation and its After-Effects', *Lumen*, 13 (1994), pp. 13–42, on p. 15. See also Shuttleton, *Smallpox and the Literary Imagination*; F. Nussbaum, 'Scarred Women: Frances Burney and Smallpox', in *The Limits of the Human: Fictions of Anomaly, Race, and Gender in the Long Eighteenth Century* (Cambridge: Cambridge University Press, 2003), pp. 109–32.
14. Buchan, *Domestic Medicine*, p. 233.
15. T. Dimsdale, *Thoughts on General and Partial Inoculations* (London, 1776), pp. 35–41. Houses for inoculation were not conceived of as 'isolation' facilities in a modern sense, but rather as centres of sociability for upper-class patients, who could expect pleasant diversions during the potentially stressful procedure. Shuttleton, *Smallpox and the Literary Imagination*, p. 38; Smith, *The Speckled Monster*.
16. Buchan, *Domestic Medicine*, p. 220.
17. S. R. Duncan, et al., 'The Dynamics of Smallpox Epidemics in Britain, 1550–1800', *Demography*, 30:3 (1993), pp. 405–23; D. Brunton, 'Smallpox Inoculation and Demographic Trends in Eighteenth-Century Scotland', *Medical History*, 36:4 (1992), pp. 403–29; Razzell, *The Conquest of Smallpox*.
18. J. Baron, *The Life of Edward Jenner*, 2 vols (London, 1838), vol. 2, p. 263.
19. Quoted in Razzell, *The Conquest of Smallpox*, pp. 72–3, 101.
20. Dr Bradley, 'An Account of the Publications and Experiments on the Cow-Pox', *Medical and Physical Journal*, 1:1 (1799), p. 1.
21. Smith, *The Speckled Monster*, p. 20.
22. Buchan, *Domestic Medicine*, p. 232.
23. 'Willan and Others on Vaccination', *The Edinburgh Review*, 9:12 (1806–7), pp. 32–66, on p. 50.
24. F. Zampieri, A. Zanatta and M. Rippa Bonati, 'Iconography and Wax Models in Italian Early Smallpox Vaccination', *Medicine Studies*, 2:4 (2011), pp. 213–27.
25. Woodville's letter to Jenner, 25 January 1799, in Baron, *Life of Jenner*, vol. 1, pp. 307–8.
26. J. McVail, 'Cow-Pox and Small-Pox: Jenner, Woodville, and Pearson', *British Medical Journal*, 1847 (23 May 1896), pp. 1271–4.

27. E. Jenner, *Further Observations on the Variolae Vaccinae, or Cow Pox* (London, 1799), p. 5.
28. B. Waterhouse, *A Prospect for Exterminating the Small Pox, Part II* (Cambridge, MA: Harvard University Press, 1802), p. 78. Waterhouse indicates that he relayed Jenner's representations to President Thomas Jefferson, Dr Benjamin Rush and Dr John Redman Coxe.
29. Baron, *Life of Jenner*, vol. 1, pp. 565–83. Infighting caused the breakup of this group and the formation of the quasi-governmental National Vaccine Establishment in 1809. D. Brunton, *The Politics of Vaccination: Practice and Policy in England, Wales, Ireland, and Scotland, 1800–1874* (Woodbridge: Boydell & Brewer, 2008), p. 15.
30. Quoted in R. J. Thornton, *Vaccinae Vindicia; or, Defence of Vaccination* (London: H. D. Symonds, 1806), pp. 4–5.
31. W. Blair, *The Vaccine Contest* (London: J. Murray, 1806), p. 69.
32. 'Pamphlets on Vaccination', *Edinburgh Review*, 15:30 (1810), pp. 322–51, on p. 338. See also S. Nunn, '"Wonderful Effects!!!": Graphic Satires of Vaccination in the First Decade of the Nineteenth Century', in D. M. Turner and K. Stagg (eds), *Social Histories of Disability and Deformity* (New York: Routledge, 2006), pp. 79–94; Smith, *Speckled Monster*, pp. 95–107.
33. J. Adams, *A Popular View of Vaccine Inoculation* (London: R. Phillips, 1807), p. 143.
34. Blair, *The Vaccine Contest*, p. vii.
35. The print is widely available to view online: J. Gillray, *The Cow-Pock, or, The Wonderful Effects of the New Inoculation! Vide the Publications of the Anti-Vaccine Society* (London, 1802).
36. J. Coakley Lettsom, *Expositions of the Inoculation of the Small-Pox, and of the Cow-Pox* (2nd edn; London, 1806), pp. 6, 9.
37. W. Aitkin, *The Science and Practice of Medicine, Vol. I* (London: Charles Griffin, 1863), p. 270.
38. W. Rowley, *Cow-Pox Inoculation no Security Against Small-Pox Infection* (London: J. Barfield, 1805), pp. 2–3, 8.
39. A French medical text described at least seventy different varieties of scars attendant upon vaccination. *Royal Commission to Inquire into Vaccination, Fourth Report*, c.6527 (London: HMSO, 1893), p. 97.
40. C. R. Aikin's short book of 1801 reportedly sold in the thousands. A second edition with updated plates was published the next year. Aikin, *A Concise View of All the Most Important Facts which have Hitherto Appeared Concerning the Cow-Pox, Second Edition, Corrected and Enlarged* (London: R. Phillips, 1801).
41. J. D. Fisher, *Description of the Distinct, Confluent, and Inoculated Smallpox, Varioloid Disease, Cow Pox, and Chicken Pox, Illustrated by Thirteen Plates* (Boston, MA: Wells and Lilly, 1829), pp. 58–9. See also Aikin, *A Concise View*, pp. 97–8.
42. Fisher, *Description*, pp. 59–60.
43. J. Bushby, quoted in 'Letter from Dr. Thornton to Mr. Tilloch on the Cow-Pox', *Philosophical Magazine*, 20 (1805), pp. 36–60, on p. 51.
44. This perhaps deliberately echoes John Dyer's 1726 poem 'Grongar Hill' and its corporeal metaphor for urban-rural contrast: 'The town and village, dome and farm, / Each give each a double charm, / As pearls upon an Ethiop's arm.'
45. Shuttleton, *Smallpox and the Literary Imagination*.
46. R. Bloomfield, *Good Tidings; or, News from the Farm, A Poem* (London, 1804), p. 19. See T. Fulford and D. Lee, 'The Jenneration of Disease: Vaccination, Romanticism, and Revolution', *Studies in Romanticism*, 39:11 (2000), pp. 139–63; D. Lee and T. Fulford,

'The Beast Within: The Imperial Legacy of Vaccination in History and Literature', *Literature and History*, 9:1 (2000), pp. 1–23; S. White, 'Rural Medicine: Robert Bloomfield's "Good Tidings"', *Romanticism*, 9:2 (2003), pp. 141–56.

47. Bloomfield, *Good Tidings*, p. 29.
48. R. T. Thornton, *Facts Decisive in Favour of the Cow-Pock: Including an Account of the Inoculation of the Village of Lowther* (London, 1802), p. 130.
49. [T. Paytherus?], *Vaccinia: Or, the Triumph of Beauty* (London, 1806), pp. 11–13.
50. J. Ring, 'Comments on the Cow-Pox', *Medical and Physical Journal*, 2:6 (1799), pp. 25–9, on p. 27.
51. J. Ring, *A Treatise on the Cow-Pox; Containing the History of Vaccine Inoculation* (London: J. Johnson, 1803), p. 1036.
52. Iconoclastes, *Pethox Parvus. Dedicated, without Permission, to the Remnant of Blind Priests of that Idolatry* (London, 1807), reviewed in *The British Critic*, 30 (1808), pp. 564–5.
53. Bloomfield, *Good Tidings*, p. 27.
54. For example, see Report of Royal Jennerian Society (4 December 1805) in Blair, *The Vaccine Contest*, p. 80.
55. Blair, *The Vaccine Contest*, pp. 85–6. In 1807, according to the hospital's records, 4,594 persons were inoculated, of which 4,246 were released and requested to return twice a week to be inspected. 'Mr. Blair's Hints for the Consideration of Parliament', *Medical and Physical Journal*, 19:112 (June 1808), pp. 556–62. Under pressure, the hospital discontinued out-patient inoculation in 1807, with inmates permitted to be given the smallpox until about 1821. Creighton, *A History of Epidemics in Britain, Vol. II*, p. 586.
56. Brunton, *The Politics of Vaccination*, pp. 16–18; *Hansard's Parliamentary Debates, Vol. 26* (London, 1814), cols 987–9.
57. *Rex v. Vantandillo*. G. Maule and W. Selwyn, *Reports of Cases Argued and Determined in the Court of King's Bench, Vol. 4* (London, 1817), pp. 74–7. For the treatment of medieval leprosy and the problematic legal nature of sequestration, see C. Rawcliffe, *Leprosy in Medieval England* (Rochester, NY: Boydell Press, 2006).
58. *Rex v. Burnett*. The defendant received six months' imprisonment. Maule and Selwyn, *Reports of Cases*, pp. 273–4.
59. R. J. Thornton, 'Letter from Dr. Thornton on the Cow-Pox', *Philosophical Magazine*, 20 (1805), p. 37.
60. *Select Poems &c. by the late John Dawes Worgan* (London, 1810), pp. 205–6, 208, 210.
61. 'Third Festival of the Royal Jennerian Society', *Gentleman's Magazine*, 75 (June 1805), pp. 521–6, on p. 525.
62. 'Report from the National Vaccine Establishment', *Annual Register, 1822* (London, 1823), p. 513.
63. 'Vaccine Institution', *London Medical Gazette* (19 May 1838), p. 349.
64. Rev. Mr Marks, quoted in J. Cribb, *Small-Pox and Cow-Pox: Comprehending a Concise History of those Diseases* (Cambridge, 1825), pp. 20–1.
65. S. Percy and R. Percy, *London, or Interesting Memorials of its Rise, Progress and Present State*, 3 vols (London: T. Box, 1824), vol. 3, pp. 155–6.
66. *The Art of Beauty; or, The Best Methods of Improving and Perceiving the Shape, Carriage, and Complexion. Together with, The Theory of Beauty* (London: Knight and Lacey, 1825), p. 169.

10 Fend, 'Portraying Skin Disease: Robert Carswell's Dermatological Watercolours'

1. E. Ackerknecht, *Medicine at the Paris Hospital, 1794–1848* (Baltimore, MD: John Hopkins Press, 1967), p. xi; M. Foucault, *The Birth of the Clinic: An Archeology of Medical Perception*, trans. A. M. Sheridan Smith (London: Tavistock, 1973), p. 59. See also C. Hannaway and A. La Berge, 'Paris Medicine: Perspectives Past and Present', in C. Hannaway and A. La Berge (eds), *Constructing Paris Medicine* (Amsterdam: Rodopi, 1998), p. 5.

2. M. Foucault, *La naissance de la clinique: une archéologie du regard médical* (Paris: Presses universitaires de France, 1963), p. 59, uses the expression 'des maladies dont le porteur est indifférent', which is not literally translated in Smith's version (as above).

3. See S. Jacyna, 'Robert Carswell and William Thomson at the Hôtel-Dieu of Lyons: Scottish Views of French Medicine', in R. French and A. Wear (eds), *British Medicine in the Age of Reform* (London: Routledge, 1991), pp. 110–35.

4. For some general information on this fund and for a complete list of the drawings, see the website of UCL Special Collections, at http://www.ucl.ac.uk/Library/special-coll/carswellrest.shtml and http://www.ucl.ac.uk/Library/special-coll/carswell.shtml [both accessed 3 December 2012]. For an early scholarly account of the collection, see H. Reckert, *Das unbekannte Werk des Pathologen Robert Carswell (1793–1857)* (Köln: Kölner Medizinhistorische Beiträge; vol. 22, 1983).

5. Letter by Robert Carswell to the University of London Council, 21 December 1827, UCL College Correspondence 304, here quoted from the documentary material on the collection pulled together by Susan Stead: *Carswell Collection Catalogue*. Copyright UCL Collections.

6. Numbers F.d. 44 to F.d. 1031 in UCL Special Collections. A small number of the drawings under the rubric 'Skin' were made between 1832 and 1837 in London.

7. See Hannaway and La Berge, 'Paris Medicine', pp. 1–70, on the myth of early nineteenth-century medicine in Paris created by some of the protagonists of the medical reforms themselves and still perpetuated by seminal studies such as Erwin Ackerknecht's, and which has been critiqued by historians of medicine over the past two decades. Also, see their article for an assessment of the historiography.

8. D. E. Manuel (ed.), *Walking the Paris Hospitals: Diary of an Edinburgh Medical Student 1834–1835* (London: Wellcome Trust Centre for the History of Medicine at UCL, 2004).

9. Ibid., p. 45.

10. J. L. Alibert, *Description des maladies de la peau observées à l'hôpital Saint-Louis.* (Paris: Barrois, 1806), p. i. If not indicated otherwise, translations from the French are mine.

11. J. L. Alibert, *Monographie des dermatoses où précis théorique et pratique des maladies de la peau* (Paris: Chez le Docteur Daynac, éditeur, 1832), p. xiv.

12. For the passage quoted above and Alibert's use of the metaphor of the theatre, see L. S. Jacyna, 'Pious Pathology: J. L. Alibert's Iconography of Disease', in C. Hannaway and A. La Berge (eds), *Constructing Paris Medicine* (Amsterdam: Rodopi, 1998), p. 190.

13. G. Deleuze in the chapter 'Strata or Historical Formations: The Visible and the Articulable', in *Foucault*, trans. Seán Hand and foreword by Paul Bové (Minneapolis, MN: University of Minnesota Press, 1986), p. 49.

14. See the chapter 'Surface of Recognition' in M. Te Hennepe, *Depicting Skin: Visual Culture in Nineteenth-Century Medicine* (Wageningen: Ponsen & Looijen, 2007), pp. 21–53; and, more generally, C. Benthien, *Skin: On the Cultural Border between Self and the World* (New York: Columbia University Press, 2002 [first German edn 1999]), pp. 53–62.

15. See Te Hennepe, *Depicting Skin*, pp. 23–48.

16. Alibert, *Description*, p. xx.
17. So the title of one of Alibert's books: *Nosographie naturelle: ou maladies du corps distribuées par famille* (Paris: Caille & Ravier, 1817).
18. L. Daston and P. Galison, *Objectivity* (New York: Zone Books, 2007), p. 82.
19. Alibert, *Description*, p. vi.
20. Te Hennepe, *Depicting Skin*, pp. 44–8.
21. R. Willan, *On Cutaneous Diseases* (London: Printed for J. Johnson, 1808), pp. viii [originally published in four volumes as *Description and Treatment of Cutaneous Diseases*, 1798–1808].
22. Ibid., p. x–xiv and Plate I. All images from dermatological atlases discussed here are accessible via the Wellcome Images database, at http://images.wellcome.ac.uk [accessed 3 December 2012].
23. Willan, *Cuteaneous Diseases*, p. 26 and Plate IV, fig. 2.
24. Ibid., p. 23.
25. For example, thirty-three out of the fifty-five illustrations from Alibert's 1806 *Description* focus on the head and bust.
26. Te Hennepe, *Depicting Skin*, pp. 44–5.
27. L. T. Biett, *Abrégé pratique des maladies de la peau ... d'après les documents puisés dans les leçons cliniques de M. le Biett*, ed. A. Cazenave and H. E. Schedel (Paris: Béchet Jeune, 1828), pp. xi–xii and xv–xvi.
28. P. F. Rayer, *Traité théorique et pratique des maladies de la peau, fondé sur des nouvelles recherches d'anatomie et de physiologie pathologiques* (Paris: J. B. Baillière; Londres: Même Maison; Bruxelles: Depot de Librairie Médicale Française, 1826–7). See also Te Hennepe, *Depicting Skin*, pp. 38–41.
29. As is the case of the copy owned by the Wellcome Library (shelfmark: B 43118/B/1 Atlas).
30. R. Carswell, *Notebook*, pp. 103–5. UCL Special Collections. '[?]' has been inserted to indicate illegible words.
31. Alibert, *Description*, pp. ix–xiii.
32. Foucault, *Birth of the Clinic*, chapter 7 'Seeing and Knowing', p. 112. See also Foucault, *Naissance*, p. 113. Smith translates Foucault's 'tableau' as 'picture', and the word can indeed designate both table and picture; in this case, however, as Foucault talks about a structure that is both visual and verbal, 'table' seems to be the more appropriate translation.
33. Ibid., p. 113.
34. Foucault, *La naissance de la clinique*.
35. Alibert, *Description*, p. xxi. See also Jacyna, *Pious Pathology*, pp. 191–2.
36. J. L. Alibert, *Clinique de l'hôpital Saint-Louis, ou traité complet des maladies de la peau* (Paris: B. Corman et Blanc, 1833), Plate VIII.
37. Ibid., p. 73.
38. Alibert, *Description*, plate 41.

11 Angel, 'Atavistic Marks and Risky Practices: The Tattoo in Medico-Legal Debate, 1850–1950'

1. E. Berchon, *Histoire Medicale du Tatouage* (Paris, 1869), p. 96.
2. For a detailed analysis of the criminological interest in tattooing during the nineteenth century, see J. Caplan, '"National Tattooing": Traditions of Tattooing in Nineteenth-Century Europe', in J. Caplan (ed.), *Written on the Body: The Tattoo in European and American History* (Princeton, NJ: Princeton University Press, 2000), pp. 156–73.
3. Ibid., p. 158.

4. D. Horn, *The Criminal Body: Lombroso and the Anatomy of Deviance* (New York: Routledge, 2003), p. 9.
5. Ibid., p. 10
6. Ibid., p. 8.
7. Ibid.
8. See J. Canales and A. Herscher, 'Criminal Skins: Tattoos and Modern Architecture in the Work of Adolf Loos', *Architectural History*, 48 (2005), pp. 235–56.
9. See S. Ottermann, 'On Display: Tattooed Entertainers in America and Germany', in Caplan (ed.), *Written on the Body*, pp. 193–211. See also D. MacDougall, 'The Visual in Anthropology', in M. Banks and H. Morphy (eds), *Rethinking Visual Anthropology* (New Haven, CT: Yale University Press, 1997), pp. 276–95.
10. See D. Horn, *The Criminal Body: Lombroso and the Anatomy of Deviance* (New York: Routledge, 2003), pp. 48–54; D. Pick, *Faces of Degeneration: A European Disorder, c.1848–c.1918* (Cambridge: Cambridge University Press, 1989), pp. 109–52; and Caplan, 'National Tattooing', pp. 156–73.
11. C. Lombroso, 'The Savage Origin of Tattooing', *Popular Science Monthly*, 48 (1896), pp. 793–803, on p. 802.
12. '[L]e milieu social est le bouillon de culture de la criminalité; le microbe, c'est le criminel, un élément qui n'a d'importance que le jour où il trouve le bouillon qui le fait fermenter' (my translation). A. Lacassagne, 'Les transformations du droit pénal et les progrès de la médecine légale, de 1810 à 1912', *Archives d'anthropologie criminelle* (1913), pp. 321–64, on p. 364.
13. J. Fleming, 'The Renaissance Tattoo', in Caplan (ed.), *Written on the Body*, pp. 61–82, on p. 64.
14. Lombroso, 'The Savage Origin', p. 802.
15. M. Foucault, *Discipline and Punish* (1975; London: Penguin 1991), pp. 23, 29–30, 135–56.
16. C. Lombroso, *L'uomo delinquente* (Milan, 1876).
17. M. F. Hutin, 'Recherches sur les Tatouages', *Annali di Medicina Navale* (September–October 1866), pp. 10–11.
18. See G. Long and L. Rickman, 'Infectious Complications of Tattoos', *Clinical Infectious Diseases*, 18:4 (1994), pp. 610–19, on pp. 612–13, for summary tables of medical literature dealing with tattooing and infection with syphilis and tuberculosis.
19. F. R. Barker, 'Notes of Cases on an Outbreak of Syphilis Following on Tattooing', *British Medical Journal*, 1:1479 (1889), pp. 985–9, on p. 985.
20. Ibid., p. 986.
21. See A. Lacassagne, *Les Tatouages Étude Anthropologique et Médico-Légale* (Paris, 1881).
22. J. Bradley, 'Body Commodification?', in Caplan (ed.), *Written on the Body*, pp. 136–55, on p. 143.
23. A. Gell, *Wrapping in Images: Tattooing in Polynesia* (Oxford: Oxford University Press, 1993), p. 20.
24. Pulmonary tuberculosis.
25. D. W. Collings and W. Murray, 'Three Cases of Inoculation of Tuberculosis from Tattooing', *British Medical Journal*, 1:1796 (1895), pp. 1200–1, on p. 1200.
26. F. F. Maury and C. W. Dulles, 'Syphilis Communicated by Tattooing', *American Journal of the Medical Sciences*, 75 (1878), pp. 44–62, on p. 62.
27. G. Rosen, *A History of Public Health* (New York: Johns Hopkins University Press, 1993), p. 308.

28. It is perhaps fair to say that an attitude of ambivalence towards the regulation of tattoo-ing predominated in the USA during this period. For example, following an apparent outbreak of hepatitis caused by tattooing in New York City, on 1 November 1961 the Board of Health closed down all tattoo studios as a danger to health. However, following a legal appeal by the tattoo artists whose livelihoods were affected, the decision was later reversed in 1962. See R. W. B. Scutt and C. Gotch, *Art, Sex and Symbol: The Mystery of Tattooing* (New York: Cornwall Books, 1986), p.136.

29. See R. L Stauter, 'Tattooing: The Protection of Public Health', *Health Matrix*, 6:2 (1988), pp. 51–9.

30. Professor of English, novelist and tattooist Samuel Steward discusses the oral culture of tattooing folklore within the context of the Chicago and Oakland tattoo communities during the mid-twentieth century. He writes somewhat disparagingly that 'the rumours, half-facts, and downright untruths arrive from two sources: the clientele and the tat-toodlers [*sic*] themselves ... Not understanding the *why* of many things ... the tattoo artist – gifted with the wondrous imagination of con-men – are very quick to create logical-sounding stories about the art itself'. S. Steward, *Bad Boys and Tough Tattoos: A Social History of the Tattoo, with Gangs, Sailors and Street Corner Punks, 1950–1965* (New York: Harrington Park Press, 1990), p. 82.

31. Writing in 1912, the tattooist Louis Morgan details his method of maintaining sanitary working practices: 'Keep the needles thoroughly clean by washing in strong antisep-tic, such as bichloride of mercury or carbolic acid. Wash the acid off well in clear water and dry with a clean cloth. Then dip in vaseline. When a tattoo is finished wash it with witch-hazel and alcohol in equal parts, and apply some kind of antiseptic healing salve.' L. Morgan, *The Modern Tattooist* (Berkeley, CA: Courier Publishing Company, 1912), pp. 59–60. The business cards of early twentieth-century tattooists often made a point of advertising the cleanliness of their studios and practices. Morgan's own card from 1912 (which is reproduced on the cover *The Modern Tattooist*) advertises his 'Thoroughly Antiseptic Method'. Similar examples are found on Herb Antes's card (1940s): 'Lat-est Equipment and Sanitary Methods Used'; and later on Rex Bennett's card (1960s): 'World's Most Sterile Tattoo Studio'. Reproductions of both these cards appear in *Lyle Tuttles's Business Card Collection*, pamphlet available at www.tattooarchive.com [accessed 23 August 2011].

32. See A. Parry, *Tattoo: Secrets of A Strange Art* (New York: Dover, 2006), pp. 122–41; and W. D. Hambly, *The History of Tattooing* (1925; New York: Dover, 2009), pp. 109–60.

33. C. S. Myers, 'Contributions to Egyptian Anthropology: Tatuing', *Journal of the Anthro-pological Institute of Great Britain and Ireland*, 33 (1903), pp. 82–9, on p. 82.

34. Ibid., p. 85.

35. Ibid., p. 86.

36. Ibid., p. 87.

37. W. Blackman, *The Fellāhīn of Upper Egypt* (Cairo: American University in Cairo Press, 1927), p. 53.

38. Parry, *Tattoo: Secrets of a Strange Art*, p. 136.

39. Ibid., p.137; L. Morgan, *Modern Tattooist*, p. 34.

40. Steward, *Bad Boys and Tough Tattoos*, p. 82.

41. Cinnabar, or cinnabarite (red mercury(II) sulfide (HgS), native vermilion), is the com-mon ore of mercury.

42. For adverse skin reactions to mercury-based tattoo pigments, see F. G. Novy, 'A General-ized Mercurial (Cinnabar) Reaction Following Tattooing', *Archives of Dermatology and*

Syphilology, 49 (1944), pp. 172–3; and F. E. S. Keiller and R. P. Warin, 'Mercury Dermatitis in a Tattoo', *British Medical Journal*, 1:5020 (1957), p. 678.

43. G. H. Belote, 'Tattoo and Syphilis', *Archives of Dermatology and Syphilology*, 18:2 (1928),
    pp. 200–9, on p. 203.

44. Novy, 'Generalized Mercurial (Cinnabar) Reaction', pp. 172–3.

45. For an account of his technique, see C. Butler Savory, 'Hypodermic Medication in Skin
    Disease', *British Medical Journal*, 1:1998 (1899), pp. 904–5, on p. 904.

46. Ibid., pp. 904–5.

47. See R. Turell and A. W. Martin Marino, 'Technic of Tattooing with Mercury Sulphide
    for Pruritus Ani', *Annals of Surgery*, 115:1 (1942), pp. 126–30.

48. See also N. Lake, 'Tattooing in Service of Surgery', *British Medical Journal*, 1:5079
    (1958), pp. 1084–7.

49. S. J. Reiser, *Technological Medicine: The Changing World of Doctors and Patients* (New
    York: Cambridge University, 2009), p. 186.

50. Ibid., p. 187.

51. See A. C. S. Hobson et al., 'Tattooing as Possible Means of Transmitting Viral Hepatitis',
    British Medical Journal, 1:4768 (1952), pp. 1111–12; and B. F. Smith, 'Occurrence of
    Hepatitis in Recently Tattooed Service Personnel', *JAMA*, 144:13 (1950), pp. 1074–6.

52. See Long and Rickman, 'Infectious Complications of Tattoos', p. 616. See also R. L.
    Braithwaite et al., 'Risks Associated with Tattooing and Body Piercing', *Journal of Public
    Health Policy*, 20:4 (1999), pp. 459–70; and T. C. Abiona et al., 'Body Art Practices
    Among Inmates: Implications for Transmission of Bloodborne Infections', *American
    Journal of Infection Control*, 38:2 (2010), pp. 121–9. It is interesting to note that poten-
    tial cases of HIV infection inoculated by tattooing are frequently associated with
    criminals, despite the lack of empirically proven links; this is perhaps a lingering contem-
    porary manifestation of the 'doubly pathological' signification of tattooing which links
    criminality with disease.

53. Steward, *Bad Boys and Tough Tattoos*, p. 164.

54. R. L. Stauter, 'Laws Regulating Tattooing' (letter), *American Journal of Public Health*,
    79:9 (1989), pp. 1308–9.

12 Woloshyn, '"Kissed by the Sun": Tanning the Skin of the Sick with Light Therapeutics, *c.* 1890–1930'

1. J. H. Kellogg, *Light Therapeutics: A Practical Manual of Phototherapy for the Student
   and the Practitioner*, 2nd edn (Battle Creek: Modern Medicine Publishing Company,
   1927), p. 43.

2. For a popular history of tanning, see the following: P. Ory, *L'invention du bronzage* (Paris:
   Éditions Complexe, 2008); B. Andrieu, *Bronzage: une petite histoire du soleil et de la peau*
   (Paris: CNRS Éditions, 2008); B. Cormack, *A History of Holidays, 1812–1990* (Lon-
   don: Routledge and Thomas Cook Archives, 1998); M. Blume, *Côte d'Azur: Inventing the
   French Riviera* (London: Thames and Hudson, 1992); R. Mighall, *Sunshine: One Man's
   Search for Happiness* (London: John Murray, 2008); R. Dyer, *White* (London and New
   York: Routledge, 1999); K. Dutton, *The Perfectible Body: The Western Ideal of Physical
   Development* (London: Cassell, 1995); I. Littlewood, *Sultry Climates: Travel and Sex since
   the Grand Tour* (London: John Murray, 2001). In these works, sun-tanning is historically
   positioned as novel and fashionable, with little discussion of primary medical material.

3. For a British context, see: Mighall, *Sunshine*; I. Zweiniger-Bargielowska, *Managing the Body: Beauty, Health, and Fitness in Britain, 1880–1939* (New York: Oxford University Press, 2010); S. Carter, *Rise and Shine: Sunlight, Technology and Health* (Oxford: Berg, 2007); R. Hobday, *The Healing Sun* (Forres: Findhorn Press, 1999); and R. Hobday, *The Light Revolution* (Forres: Findhorn Press, 2006). For a French context, see: Ory, *L'invention du bronzage*; Andrieu, *Bronzage*; A. Ouédraogo, 'Food and the Purification of Society: Dr Paul Carton and Vegetarianism in Interwar France', *Social History of Medicine*, 14:2 (2001), pp. 223–45; and A. Baubérot, *Histoire du Naturisme: Le mythe du retour à la nature* (Rennes: Presses Universitaires de Rennes, 2004). For a German context, see: M. Hau, *The Cult of Health and Beauty in Germany: A Social History, 1890–1930* (Chicago, IL: University of Chicago Press, 2003); and M. Möhring, 'Working Out the Body's Boundaries: Physiological, Aesthetic, and Psychic Dimensions of the Skin in German Nudism, 1890–1930', in C. Forth and I. Crozier (eds), *Body Parts: Critical Explorations in Corporeality* (Lanham, MD: Lexington Books, 2005), pp. 229–46.

4. French physicians' beliefs in the national, social potential of heliotherapy – to improve racial health by means of positive eugenics, following Neo-Lamarkism – is the subject of my forthcoming publication, 'Regenerative Tanning: Pigmentation, Racial Health and the *cure de soleil* on the Côte d'Azur, c. 1890–1936', in F. Brauer and S. Keshavjee (eds), *Picturing Evolution and Extinction: Regeneration and Degeneration in Modern Visual Culture* (Newcastle upon Tyne: Cambridge Scholars Publishing, 2013).

5. Finsen (Denmark) and Rollier (Switzerland) are the historical linchpins of light therapeutics, but heliotherapy was also contemporaneously developing along the Côte d'Azur: see my forthcoming article, '*Le pays du soleil*: The Art of Heliotherapy on the Côte d'Azur', *Social History of Medicine* (2013).

6. M. K. Kassabian, *Röntgen Rays and Electro-Therapeutics, with Chapters on Radium and Phototherapy* (Philadelphia, PA: J. B. Lippincott Company, 1907), p. 517.

7. C. W. Allen, *Radiotherapy and Phototherapy* (New York: Lea Brothers & Co., 1904), pp. 450–1.

8. N. R. Finsen, 'The Red Light Treatment of Small-Pox', *British Medical Journal*, 2:1823 (7 December 1895), pp. 1412–14, on p. 1414.

9. Allen, *Radiotherapy and Phototherapy*, p. 427.

10. M. Morris and S. E. Dore, 'Further Remarks on Finsen's Light and X-Ray Treatment in Lupus and Rodent Ulcer', *British Medical Journal*, 1:2161 (31 May 1902), pp. 1324–8, on p. 1325. See also the descriptions in Anon., 'The "Light Treatment" at the London Hospital', *British Medical Journal*, 1:2061 (30 June 1900), pp. 1595–7.

11. For a description of Finsen's experiments, see E. Millioz, *De l'héliothérapie locale comme traitement des tuberculoses articulaires* (Lyon: Bourgeon, 1899), p. 49.

12. H. Bach, *Irradiation with the Alpine Sun Quartz Lamp*, trans. R. King Brown (Slough: Sollux Publishing Co., 1931), p. 36.

13. Kellogg, *Light Therapeutics*, p. 36.

14. C. W. Saleeby, *Sunlight and Health* (London: Nisbet & Co. Ltd, 1923), pp. 20–1.

15. 'Si la pigmentation ne s'accentue pas, le pronostic est des plus graves'; Dr F. Chiaïs, 'La cure solaire directe', in *Troisième Congrès Français de Climatothérapie et d'Hygiène Urbaine* (Cannes: n.p., 1907), p. 30.

16. 'la pigmentation est le baromètre de la cure solaire'; L. Landouzy, cited in J. A. C. Lamaison, *De l'Héliothérapie dans la Tuberculose* (Bordeaux: Barthélemy & Clédes, 1913), p. 25.

17. Kellogg, *Light Therapeutics*, p. 43.

18. Ibid., p. 41.

19. A. Rollier, *Heliotherapy* (London: Oxford Medical Publications, 1923), pp. 17, 31, 43, and Saleeby's foreword, p. xvii, respectively.

20. 'L'accentuation de la coloration pigmentaire est un signe d'augmentation de l'activité nutritive et par conséquent de la vigueur'; A. Monteuuis, *L'Usage Chez Soi des Bains d'Air, de Lumière et de Soleil* (Nice: Librairie Visconti, 1911), p. 125.

21. Möhring, 'Working Out the Body's Boundaries', p. 243, n. 51.

22. In a French publication, Kellogg asserted that 'Le plus puissant de tous les désinfectants naturels; il n'est pas de germe morbide qui résiste aux rayons directs du soleil, choléra, consomption, diphtérie, fièvres scarlatine et typhoïde, et autres maladies'. J. H. Kellogg, *Hygiène populaire et Moniteur de la santé* (Bâle: Librairie Polyglotte, 1897), p. 108. On light as bactericidal: 'Le sang absorbe, il est vrai, une grande partie des rayons violets, mais le chimisme de la lumière n'est pas entièrement épuisé à son contact, et ses propriétés stimulantes et bactéricides ont une zone de pénétration plus étendue'. Dr Gilli, 'La Cure solaire pratique en phtisiothérapie', in *Premier Congrès Français de Climatothérapie et d'Hygiène Urbaine* (Monaco: Imprimerie de Monaco, 1904), pp. 455–62, on p. 456.

23. A. Downes and T. P. Blunt, 'Researches on the Effect of Light upon Bacteria and Other Organisms', *Proceedings of the Royal Society of Medicine*, 26 (1877), pp. 488–500.

24. See Zweiniger-Bargielowska's *Managing the Body*; Hau's *The Cult of Health and Beauty*; and Baubérot's *Histoire du Naturisme*.

25. Sir J. H. Gauvain, 'Foreword', in Rollier, *Heliotherapy*, p. xi.

26. Monteuuis, *L'Usage Chez Soi*, p. 42.

27. See the original pair, plate XL, and plates XLI, CIV, CV and CVI in A. Rollier, *La cure de soleil* (Paris: Baillière & Fils; Lausanne: Constant Tarin, 1914). Case notes in Rollier's *Heliotherapy* date the 'before' photo to 1908 and the 'after' photo to 1910 (pp. 130–2).

28. Rollier, *Heliotherapy*, p. 145.

29. Saleeby, 'Foreword', in ibid, p. xv.

30. See Möhring, 'Working Out the Body's Boundaries', especially p. 238.

31. Ibid., pp. 271–2.

32. Kellogg, *Light Therapeutics*, p. 41.

33. T. M. Madden, *On Change of Climate. A Guide for Travellers in Pursuit of Health* (London: T. Cautley Newby, 1864), p. 30.

34. For more on the 'imprinting', transformative power of the Riviera's climate, see my 'Aesthetic and Therapeutic Imprints: Artists and Invalids on the Côte d'Azur, c. 1890–1910', *Nineteenth-Century Art Worldwide*, 11:1 (2012), at http://www.19thc-artworldwide.org/index.php/spring12/aesthetic-and-therapeutic-imprints-artists-and-invalids-on-the-cote-dazur-c-18901910 [accessed 20 February 2012], and 'La Côte d'Azur: the *terre privilégié* of Invalids and Artists, c. 1860–1900', *French Cultural Studies*, 20:4 (2009), pp. 383–402.

35. Alexander A. Knox wrote, 'Invalids come to such a place as this [Algiers] for various reasons; but I suppose that consumption, that terrible scourge of Northern Europe, is the chief amongst these'. A. Knox, *The New Playground or Wanderings in Algeria* (London: Kegan Paul, Trench & Co., 1883), p. 98.

36. See C. Bronne, *Rilke, Gide et Verhaeren: Correspondance inédite* (Paris: Messein, 1955), p. 48.

37. A. Gide, *L'Immoraliste (The Immoralist)* (1902), trans. D. Bussy (Harmondsworth: Penguin Books Ltd, 1981), p. 55. This passage has been identified as the first evidence of sun-tanning in French literature, twenty years before its supposed beginnings with Coco Chanel, by J. Weightman, 'The Solar Revolution: Reflections on a Theme in French literature', *Encounter*, 35 (1970), pp. 9–18.

38. Pemble notes that contemporaneous British tourists in the Mediterranean also viewed the tanned skins of peasants and labourers of southern Europe as healthy and sexually attractive, adding that 'This tawny flesh suggested life and health. It was the antithesis of the waxen whiteness of sickness and death'. J. Pemble, *The Mediterranean Passion: Victorians and Edwardians in the South* (Oxford: Clarendon Press, 1987), p. 125. Significantly, tanned skin in this context denoted the working classes, marking out peasants from the middle or upper-class tourists. Mary Blume similarly compared Chanel's tan to that of a cabin boy (*Côte d'Azur*, p. 74), another obvious reference to class differences (an act of imitation à la Gide, perhaps). The patients of Rollier, Bernhard, Monteuuis, Kellogg and others, however, were fee-paying clients who spent many months at their sanatoria, and thus were from the affluent classes. However Rollier was known to have facilities for the poor as well. The question of class itself is complex when it comes to analyzing the images; somehow I doubt these clients would have consented to being photographed nude (as in Figure 12.4). The therapeutics of tanning during this period complicates the popular belief that bronzed skin was a visual marker *only* of the lower (implicitly healthy) classes.

39. See Monteuuis's description of the 'direct bath', in A. Monteuuis, *Air, Light and Sun Baths in the Treatment of Chronic Complaints*, trans. F. Rothwell (London: John Bale, Sons & Danielsson, Ltd, 1907), pp. 54–5.

40. Champel is not far from Geneva, near Lake Léman. Leysin is located at the other end of Lake Léman, between Champel and Lecco. I am not suggesting that Gide was a visitor to Rollier's facilities in Leysin, or even that he was aware of this particular physician or resort. I am, however, arguing that Gide was among a contemporaneous network of Europeans that perceived Alpine sunshine in the Swiss mountains as beneficial to the tubercular patient, and that at the forefront of this network were heliotherapists.

41. A. Gide, *Si le grain ne meurt... (If it die...)* (1920), trans. D. Bussy (Harmondsworth: Penguin Books Ltd, 1982), p. 264.

42. C. Benthien, *Skin: On the Cultural Border between Self and the World*, trans. T. Dunlap (New York: Columbia University Press, 2002), p. 220.

43. Saleeby, *Sunlight and Health*, p. 68.

44. Kellogg, *Light Therapeutics*, p. 42.

45. O. Bernhard, *Light Treatment in Surgery*, trans. R. King Brown (London: Edward Arnold & Co., 1926), p. 67.

46. Möhring, 'Working Out the Body's Boundaries', p. 238.

47. One of the founders of the American eugenics organization, the Race Betterment Foundation (1906), Kellogg was a keen advocate of natural therapeutics, of which sunlight was a major component, and his medical practices must be contextualized within his larger social aims. See J. Hodges, 'Dealing with Degeneracy: Michigan Eugenics in Context' (PhD dissertation, Michigan State University, 2001), as well as Zweiniger-Bargielowska's *Managing the Body* for the eugenic beliefs of life reform practitioners in Britain, and Hau's *The Cult of Health and Beauty* for those in Germany.

48. See Hau, *The Cult of Health and Beauty*, p. 178.

49. Kellogg, *Light Therapeutics: A Practical Manual of Phototherapy for the Student and the Practitioner* (Battle Creek, MI: Good Health Publishing Company, 1910), pp. 23–4.

13 Stark, '"Classic, Characteristic or Typical": The Skin and the Visual Properties of External Anthrax Lesions

1. W. Budd, 'Additional Note on the Occurrence of Malignant Pustule in England', *British Medical Journal* (30 May 1863), pp. 557–8, on p. 557.

2. S. Shadorny and N. Rosenstein, 'Anthrax', in R. B. Wallace (ed.), *Public Health and Preventive Medicine* (New York: McGraw-Hill Medical, 2008), pp. 427–30, on p. 428.

3. Turnbull refers to the 'characteristic eschar' of external anthrax. See P. C. B. Turnbull, 'Introduction: Anthrax History, Disease and Ecology', in T. M. Koehler (ed.), *Anthrax* (Berlin; London: Springer, 2002), pp. 1–20, on p. 1.

4. S. D. Jones, *Death in a Small Package: A Short History of Anthrax* (Baltimore, MD: Johns Hopkins University Press, 2010).

5. A. Bartholomaeus, *De Proprietatibus Rerum: John Trevisa's Translation of Bartholomaeus Anglicus 'De proprietatibus rerum', a Critical Text*, 2 vols (Oxford: Clarendon Press, 1975), vol. 1, p. 418.

6. S. D. Jones and P. M. Teigen, 'Anthrax in Transit: Practical Experience and Intellectual Exchange', *Isis*, 99:3 (2008), pp. 455–85.

7. Anthrax has been the subject of a number of disease biography treatments in recent years. See Jones, *Death in a Small Package*; and R. M. Swiderski, *Anthrax: A History* (Jefferson, NC: McFarland, 2004).

8. See, for example, W. A. Pusey, *The History of Dermatology* (New York: AMS Press, 1979). The disease can also be contracted through inhalation or ingestion of material contaminated with the spores of *Bacillus anthracis*. The cutaneous form of the disease is the least fatal, but still causes death in around 20 per cent of cases if left untreated. J. A. Witkowski and L. C. Parish, 'The Story of Anthrax from Antiquity to the Present: A Biological Weapon of Nature and Humans', *Clinics in Dermatology*, 20 (2002), pp. 336–42.

9. C. Benthien, *Skin: On the Cultural Border between Self and the World*, trans. T. Dunlap (New York: Columbia University Press, 2002), p. 1.

10. For a consideration of the distinction between 'normal' and 'pathological', see G. Canguilhem, *The Normal and the Pathological*, trans. C. R. Fawcett and R. S. Cohen (New York: Zone Books, 1991).

11. A. Besson, *Technique Microbiologique et Serotherapique* (Paris: J. B. Baillière, 1898), p. 227.

12. F. W. Eurich, 'Some Notes on Industrial Anthrax: Its Diagnosis and Treatment', *British Medical Journal* (8 July 1933), pp. 50–3, on p. 51.

13. S. Connor, *The Book of Skin* (Ithaca, NY: Cornell University Press, 2004), p. 154. Skin colour has also been linked with generalized ideas of ill health, otherness and monstrosity. See J. Halberstam, *Skin Shows: Gothic Horror and the Technology of Monsters* (Durham, NC: Duke University Press, 1995), p. 7

14. Connor, *The Book of Skin*, p. 154.

15. Exodus 11:9–10.

16. J. H. Dirckx, 'Virgil on Anthrax', *American Journal of Dermatopathology*, 3 (1981), pp. 191–5.

17. Jones, *Death in a Small Package*, pp. 19–24.

18. K. Codell Carter, *The Rise of Causal Concepts of Disease: Case Histories* (Aldershot: Ashgate, 2003).

19. J. B. Morrell, 'Wissenschaft in Worstedopolis: Public Science in Bradford, 1800–1850', *British Journal for the History of Science*, 18:1 (1985), pp. 1–23; T. Southey, *The Rise, Pro-*

gress and Present State of Colonial Sheep & Wools (London: Effingham Wilson, 1951), p. 16.

20. J. A. Jowitt, 'Textiles and Society in Bradford and Lawrence, USA, 1880–1920', *Bradford Antiquary*, 5 (1991), pp. 3–24, at http://www.bradfordhistorical.org.uk/antiquary/third/vol05/textiles.html#bref23 [accessed 4 July 2011].

21. J. A. Jowitt and R. K. S. Taylor (eds), *Bradford, 1880–1914: The Cradle of the Independent Labour Party* (Leeds: University of Leeds, 1980); D. M. Jones, 'The Liberal Press and the Rise of Labour: A Study with Particular Reference to Leeds and Bradford, 1850–1895' (PhD thesis, University of Leeds, 1973).

22. D. James, 'William Byles and the *Bradford Observer*', in D. G. Wright and J. A. Jowitt (eds), *Victorian Bradford: Essays in Honour of Jack Reynolds* (Bradford: City of Bradford Metropolitan Council, Libraries Division, 1982), pp. 115–36; D. Jones, 'The Liberal Press and the Rise of Labour: A Study with Particular Reference to Leeds and Bradford, 1850–1895' (PhD dissertation, University of Leeds, 1973).

23. Dr J. H. Bell, notebook concerning anthrax epidemic in Bradford, West Yorkshire Archive Service (hereafter WYAS), Bradford, DB15/C5.

24. Bradford Medico-Chirurgical Society, *Report of the Commission on Woolsorters' Diseases* (Bradford: Toothill, 1882).

25. J. N. C. Davies-Colley, 'Notes of Two Cases of Malignant Pustule, Together with a Table of Seventeen Cases which have been Treated at Guy's Hospital', *Medico-Chirurgical Transactions*, 65 (1882), pp. 237–56, on pp. 239 and 242.

26. Davies-Colley, 'Notes of Two Cases of Malignant Pustule', p. 245.

27. J. H. Hemming, 'Two Cases of "Charbon" or "Malignant Pustule" Directly Inoculated from a Cow Suffering with "Splenic Fever:" Recovery', *British Medical Journal* (20 September 1884), p. 560.

28. A. E. Barker, 'On Some Points Regarding the Distribution of Bacillus Anthracis in the Human Skin in Malignant Pustule', *Medico-Chirurgical Transactions*, 69 (1886), pp. 127–34, on pp. 129–30.

29. J. H. Bell, 'On Oedematous and Erysipelatous Anthrax', *British Medical Journal* (20 July 1901), pp. 133–5, on p. 135.

30. J. Connal Wilson, 'Case of Anthrax in which the Infection Arose from a Hitherto Undescribed Source', *British Medical Journal* (21 December 1901), pp. 1804–5, on p. 1804.

31. R. Lawford Knaggs, 'A Case of Multiple Malignant Pustules (Anthrax)', *British Medical Journal* (20 July 1901), p. 135; J. C. Sturdy, 'A Case of Anthrax with Extensive Meningeal Haemorrhage', *British Medical Journal* (20 July 1901), pp. 135–6; W. Morrant Baker, 'A Case of Anthrax or Charbon, with External Symptoms (Malignant Pustule): Excision: Recovery', *British Medical Journal* (14 June 1884), pp. 1134–5.

32. H. L. Burrell, 'Report of a Case of Anthrax', *Annals of Surgery*, 18:6 (1893), pp. 605–22, on p. 612.

33. I. Mortimer and J. Melling, '"The Contest between Commerce and Trade, on the One Side, and Human Life on the Other": British Government Policies for the Regulation of Anthrax Infection and the Wool Textile Industries, 1880–1939', *Textile History*, 31:2 (2000), pp. 222–36.

34. Anthrax Investigation Board Minutes (hereafter AIB Minutes), WYAS, 17 July 1905, WYB111/1/2/15.

35. AIB Minutes, WYAS, 20 July; 30 October 1905, WYB111/1/2/15.

36. Anthrax Investigation Board, 'First Annual Report' (1906), CHSTM Anthrax Papers (hereafter CHSTM), uncatalogued, University of Manchester.

37. Ibid. Eurich analyzed over 14,000 samples of wool, dust and hair sent to him by man-ufacturers, and built up a complex classification system of fleeces according to their perceived risk.

38. Anthrax Investigation Board, 'Second Annual Report' (1907), CHSTM.

39. Anthrax Investigation Board, 'Tenth Annual Report' (1915), CHSTM, pp. 13–14.

40. Ibid., p. 14.

41. A therapeutic anti-anthrax serum from Italy – Sclavo's serum – was employed very widely in British cases of the disease from 1905. Eurich was a particularly strong advocate of the serum, as was Thomas Morison Legge. See T. Carter., 'Anthrax: A Global Problem with an Italian Cure', in A. Grieco, S. Iavicoli and G. Berlinguer (eds), *Contributions to the History of Occupational and Environmental Prevention* (Amsterdam: Elsevier, 1999), pp. 247–51.

42. *Annual Report of the Chief Inspector of Factories and Workshops for the Year 1906* (Lon-don: HMSO, 1907) [Cd. 3586], p. 289. Thanks to Tim Carter for drawing my attention to this reference.

43. 'Anthrax Research: The Work of the Investigation Board: Criticism by Mr Jowett M.P.', *Bradford Daily Telegraph*, 19 December 1910, p. 6; 'The Anthrax Board's Work: Attack by Mr. Jowett: Trades Council Members Withdraw', *Yorkshire Daily Observer*, 30 Janu-ary 1911, p. 5.

44. *Report of the Departmental Committee Appointed to Inquire as to Precautions for Prevent-ing Danger of Infection by Anthrax in the Manipulation of Wool, Goat Hair, and Camel Hair*, 3 vols (London: HMSO, 1918), vol. 2, pp. 3–4.

45. F. W. Eurich, 'Anthrax in the Woollen Industry, with Special Reference to Bradford', *Pro-ceedings of the Royal Society of Medicine*, 6 (1913), pp. 219–40, on p. 227.

46. M. Bligh, *Dr. Eurich of Bradford* (London: Clarke, 1960).

47. Anthrax Investigation Board, 'Eleventh Annual Report' (1916), CHSTM, p. 4.

48. Ibid.

49. Eurich, 'Some Notes on Industrial Anthrax', p. 51.

50. Anthrax Investigation Board, 'First Annual Report', p. 12.

51. 'Anthrax Poster' (London: HMSO, 1927), Papers of Dr Donald Hunter (1898–1977) (hereafter Hunter Papers), Wellcome Library, CMAC PP/HUN/B/17.

52. J. F. Stark, 'A Poster of Pustules: Representations of Early Twentieth Century Industrial Anthrax in Britain', *Endeavour*, 35:1 (2011), pp. 22–9.

53. 'Dermatitis: Cautionary Notice' (London: HMSO, 1928), Hunter Papers, CMAC PP/HUN/B/17; 'Effects of Chrome on the Skin' (London: HMSO, 1917), Hunter Papers, CMAC PP/HUN/B/17; Stark, 'A Poster of Pustules', pp. 27–8.

54. F. W. Eurich, 'Industrial Health and Disease. VI – Anthrax', *Welfare Work*, 7:82 (1926), pp. 182–4, on p. 183.

55. Ibid., on pp. 182–3.

56. Mortimer and Melling, 'The Contest between Commerce and Trade'.

57. Peter Bartrip has argued that 'it is probable that the disease would have all but disap-peared even if the entire paraphernalia of inquiry, legislation and inspection [had] never been'. See P. W. J. Bartrip, *The Home Office and Dangerous Trades in Victorian and Edwardian Britain* (Amsterdam: Rodopi, 2002), on p. 257.

58. 'The Government Wool Disinfecting Station (Home Office) Bacteriological Records Book', National Archives, Kew, LAB 46/48.

59. Royal Mail Films, *Men in Danger* (1939), at http://edina.ac.uk/purl/isan/0013-0000-2893-0000-0-0000-0000-0 [accessed 12 March 2011]; D. Hunter, 'Devices for the

Protection of the Worker against Injury and Disease', *British Medical Journal* (25 February 1950), pp. 449–54, on p. 453.

60. Hunter, 'Devices for the Protection of the Worker', p. 453.

61. T. M. Loudon to R. W. Pearman, 14 October 1952, National Archives, Kew, AY 4/1025.

62. Pearman to Loudon, 25 October 1952, National Archives, Kew, AY 4/1025.

63. Loudon to Pearman, 7 November 1952, National Archives, Kew, AY 4/1025.

64. G. W. Millington and N. J. Levell, 'Vitiligo: The Historical Curse of Depigmentation', *International Journal of Dermatology*, 46 (2007), pp. 990–5.

65. Connor, *The Book of Skin*, p. 154.

66. N. G. Jablonski, *Skin: A Natural History* (Berkeley, CA: University of California Press, 2006) p. 95; Benthien, *Skin*.

67. O. Braun-Falco, G. Plewig, H. H. Wolff and W. H. C. Burgdorf, *Dermatology*, 2nd edn (Berlin: Springer, 2000), p. 6.

68. Eurich, 'Industrial Health and Disease', p. 183.

69. Canguilhem, *The Normal and the Pathological*.

Wilson, 'Afterword: Reading the Skin, Discerning the Landscape: A Geo-historical Perspective of our Human Surface'

1. The framework for this chapter was originally presented as the opening keynote address of the October 2010 'Scratching the Surface' Conference, the gathering that served as the nidus towards generating the chapters in this volume. Upon reflection, Kevin Siena and Jonathan Reinarz's 'Introduction' to this volume proffered such an expansive and all-encompassing skin-like covering of the subject that my remarks have been recast in the form of an Afterword. Specific suggestions that the editors provided regarding the transformation of this chapter are much appreciated.

2. A slight modification of Richard Hartshorne's helpful definition of geography in *Perspective on the Nature of Geography* (Chicago, IL: Rand McNally and Company, Monograph No. 1, 1959), p. 21.

3. For a popular account of 'Our Skin as an Eco-System', see M. Andrews, *The Life that Lives on Man* (London: Faber and Faber, 1976), pp. 26–44. See also M. J. Marples, 'Life on the Human Skin', *Scientific American*, 220 (1969), pp. 108–15.

4. Among the expanding scholarship in this field, see D. Livingston, *Putting Science in Its Place: Geographies of Scientific Knowledge* (Chicago, IL: University of Chicago Press, 2003); H. Michie and R. R. Thomas (eds), *Nineteenth-Century Geographies: The Transformation of Space from the Victorian Age to the American Century* (New Brunswick, NJ: Rutgers University Press, 2003); N. A. Rupke (ed.), *Medical Geography in Historical Perspective*, *Medical History*, supplement no. 20 (London: Wellcome Trust Centre for the History of Medicine at UCL, 2000); E. Dyck and C. Fletcher (eds), *Locating Health: Historical and Anthropological Investigations of Place and Health* (London: Pickering & Chatto, 2010); and the many provocative and inspirational works of University of Wisconsin-Madison Geography Professor Emeritus, Yi-Fu Tuan.

5. M. Flanagan and A. Booth, *Re: Skin* (Cambridge, MA: MIT Press, 2006), p. 11.

6. Jay Prosser introduces this term in his 'Skin Memories', in S. Ahmed and J. Stacey (eds), *Thinking Through the Skin* (London: Routledge, 2001), pp. 52–68, on pp. 65–7. There, he talks of Dennis Potter's use of this term as the name of a bar frequented by the psoriasis-suffering detective, Philip Marlowe, in his 1986 television remake of *The Singing Detective*.

7. Flanagan and Booth, *Re: Skin*, p. 12.

8. The Swiss-American geo-historian, Arnold Henri Guyot, introduced the correlative methods of Carl Ritter to the United States. For an extract of Guyot's influential geo-historical writing *The Earth and Man*, see 'Guyot: Geography as a Correlative Science', in W. Warntz and P. Wolff (eds), *Breakthroughs in Geography* (New York: Plume, 1971), pp. 133–50.

9. C. Benthien, *Skin: On the Cultural Border between Self and World* (New York: Columbia University Press, 2002), p. 53.

10. S. Connor, *The Book of Skin* (Ithaca, NY: Cornell University Press, 2004), p. 139.

11. T. Unwin, *The Place of Geography* (Harlow: Longman, 1992), as cited by D. T. Herbert and J. A. Matthews, 'Geography: Roots and Continuities', in J. A. Matthews and D. T. Herbert (eds), *Unifying Geography: Common Heritage, Shared Future* (London: Routledge, 2004), pp. 3–18, on p. 3.

12. A. R. H. Baker, *Geography and History: Bridging the Divide* (Cambridge: Cambridge University Press, 2003), pp. 162–63.

13. Twentieth-century geo-history is frequently depicted under the regional, yet panoramic, concept of areal differentiation.

14. N. G. Jablonski, *Skin: A Natural History* (Berkeley, CA: University of California Press, 2006), p. 121.

15. Ibid., p. 2.

16. See G. Keynes's edited 'Notes for a Lecture on the Skin by Sir Thomas Brown, Kt., MD', *St Bartholomew's Hospital Reports*, 57 (1924), pp. 108–13, on p. 111.

17. A. Ravogli, 'History of Dermatology', *Medical Life*, 33 (1926), pp. 492–538, on p. 492.

18. D. Wilson, 'New Technologies Revitalize the Ancient Field of Geography', *Chronicle of Higher Education*, 29 November 1996, p. A23.

19. M. Lappé, *The Body's Edge: Our Cultural Obsession with the Skin* (New York: Henry Holt, 1996), p. 6.

20. Mercurialis was a colleague of renowned anatomist Andreas Vesalius, whose *De Humani Corporis Fabrica* (1543) revolutionized the approach to anatomical dissection and remapped understandings of human structure-function relationships. For a review of Mercurialis, see R. L. Sutton, 'Diseases of the Skin: Mercurialis, 1572', *Archives of Dermatology*, 94 (1966), pp. 763–72.

21. J. Moscoso, 'Hidden in Plain View: The Skin in Science and Culture', in *'Skin' Exhibition Guide* (London: Wellcome Collection, 2010), pp. 3–4, on p. 3.

22. Moscoso, 'Hidden in Plain View', p. 5.

23. Jablonski, *Skin*, pp. 4–5. It was likely much later that human-centred thinkers would openly question, 'Who am I without my skin?'

24. For an overview of the sixteenth-century beginnings of this geo-historical representation of syphilis, see N. D. Cook, *Born To Die: Disease and New World Conquest, 1492–1650* (Cambridge: Cambridge University Press, 1998), p. 27.

25. T. S. Turner addressed the concept of skin as a 'frontier of the social self' in his anthropological work on the Amazonian Kayapó tribe, 'The Social Skin', in C. B. Burroughs and J. D. Ehrenreich (eds), *Reading the Social Body* (Iowa City, IA: University of Iowa Press, 1993), pp. 15–39. Among the voluminous research on syphilis in history, two works of special note relative to this chapter are C. Quétel's *History of Syphilis* (Oxford: Polity Press, 1990); and K. P. Siena's *Venereal Disease: Hospitals and the Urban Poor: London's 'Foul Wards', 1600–1800* (Rochester, NY: University of Rochester Press, 2004).

26. Turner's venereal disease writings are central to P. K. Wilson's 'Exposing the "Secret Disease": Recognizing and Treating Syphilis in Daniel Turner's London', in L. Merians (ed.), *Venereal Disease in Eighteenth-Century France and Great Britain* (Lexington, KY: University Press of Kentucky, 1996), pp. 68–84.

27. See P. K. Wilson's '"Out of Sight, Out of Mind?": The Daniel Turner–James Blondel Dispute over the Power of the Mother's Imagination', *Annals of Science*, 49 (1992), pp. 63–85; and 'Eighteenth-Century "Monsters" and Nineteenth-Century "Freaks": Reading the Maternally-Marked Child', *Literature and Medicine*, 21 (2002), pp. 1–25.

28. For more on Cowper's depiction of the skin, see P. K. Wilson's 'William Cowper's Anatomy of the Skin', *International Journal of Dermatology*, 31 (1992), pp. 361–3.

29. For further explanation of Turner's role of the skin, see P. K. Wilson, 'Imaging the Human Body: A Surgical Perspective of the Skin in the Enlightenment', in Y. Otsuka, S. Sakai and S. Kuriyama (eds), *Medicine and the History of the Body* (Tokyo: Ishiyaku EuroAmerica, 1999), pp. 339–55; and P. K. Wilson, *Surgery, Skin and Syphilis: Daniel Turner's London (1667–1741)* (Amsterdam and Atlanta, GA: Rodopi Press, Wellcome Institute of the History of Medicine Series, 1999).

30. S. M. Squier discusses the important concept of liminality in *Liminal Lives: Imagining the Human at the Frontiers of Biomedicine* (Durham, NC: Duke University Press, 2004).

31. Flanagan and Booth, *Re: Skin*, p. 12.

32. H. S. Purdon, 'Brief Historical Sketch of Dermatology, Classification of Skin Diseases, General Remarks on the Anatomy of the Skin', *Journal of Cutaneous Medicine*, 4 (1871), pp. 203–7, on p. 206.

33. F. H. Garrison, 'The Skin as a Functional Organ of the Body', *Bulletin of the New York Academy of Medicine*, 9 (1933), pp. 417–32, on pp. 428–9.

34. J. Thomson, *An Account of the Life, Lectures, and Writings of William Cullen*, 2 vols (Edinburgh: W. Blackwood & Sons, 1859), vol. 2, p. 37.

35. For excellent reviews of dermatologic classification systems from Plenck through the nineteenth century, see E. B. Bronson, 'The Classification of Skin Disease', *Journal of Cutaneous and Genito-Urinary Diseases*, 5 (1887), pp. 371–81, 427–33, on pp. 371–2. See also J. T. Crissey and L. C. Parish, *The Dermatology and Syphilology of the Nineteenth Century* (New York: Praeger, 1981); and B. S. Potter, 'Bibliographic Landmarks in the History of Dermatology', *Journal of the American Academy of Dermatology*, 48 (2003), pp. 919–32.

36. R. Willan, *Description and Treatment of Cutaneous Diseases* (London: J. Johnson, 1798). For an overview of Willan, see J. Lane, 'Robert Willan', *Archives of Dermatology and Syphilology*, 13 (1926), pp. 737–59.

37. Bronson, 'The Classification of Skin Disease', p. 372.

38. Though helpful as pictorial identifiers in many instances, atlases did not always clearly delineate patterns of disease on all colours of skin. Of somewhat more limited use than atlases, wax models also became popular visual mappings of skin disease. See L. C. Parish, G. Worden, J. A. Witowski, A. Scholz and D. H. Parish, 'Wax Models in Dermatology', *Transactions and Studies of the College of Physicians of Philadelphia*, 13 (1991), pp. 29–74. Alicia Imperiala describes recent aims of digital skin mapping in 'Seminal Space: Getting Under the Digital Skin', in M. Flanagan and A. Booth (eds), *Re: Skin*, pp. 265–91.

39. Alexander John Balmanno Squire deserves considerable recognition for his milestone, *Photographs (Coloured from Life) of the Diseases of the Skin* (London: J. Churchill and Sons, 1864–6). Among the considerable work on the importance of images to scientific and medical imaging of this era, see, in particular, L. Jordanova, *Sexual Visions: Images of Gender in Science and Medicine between the Eighteenth and Twentieth Centuries*

(Madison, WI: University of Wisconsin Press, 1989); and J. Tucker, 'The Historian, the Picture, and the Archive', *Isis*, 97 (2006), pp. 111–20.

40. Bronson, 'The Classification of Skin Disease', p. 373.

41. Ibid.; J.-L.-M. Alibert, *Monographie des Dermatoses* (Paris: Germer Ballière, 1832).

42. C.-A. Lorry, *Tractatus de Morbis Cutaneis* (Paris: Cavelier, 1777). Sir Thomas Brown had previously referred to the skin, particularly the cutis, as an organ in a 1676 lecture delivered at Chirurgeons' Hall, London. See Keynes, 'Notes for a Lecture on the Skin', p. 111. Lorry expanded upon the skin as an organ which interacted with other bodily organs in contrast to the long-held view of the skin as mere enclosure.

43. For a general overview, see C. I. Armstrong's *Romantic Organicism: From Idealist Origins to Ambivalent Afterlife* (New York: Palgrave Macmillan, 2003); as well as D. R. Stoddart's chapter, 'Organicism and Ecosystem as Geographical Models', in his *On Geography and Its History* (Oxford: Basil Blackwell, 1986), pp. 230–70.

44. For recent work on Humboldt's *Cosmos* lectures and writing, see G. Helferich, *Humboldt's Cosmos* (New York: Gotham Books, 2005); and P. Werner, *Himmel und Erde. Alexander von Humboldt und sein Kosmos* (Berlin: Akademie Verlag, 2004).

45. For an enriching review of contemporary skin microscopy, see M. te Hennepe's 'Depicting Skin: Microscopy and the Visual Articulation of Skin Interior 1820–1850', in R. van de Vall and R. Zwijnenberg (eds), *The Body Within: Art, Medicine and Visualization* (Leiden: Brill, 2009), pp. 51–65.

46. Skin and touch have played an important role in physical diagnosis, as S. L. Gilman notes in 'Touch, Sexuality and Disease', in W. F. Bynum and Roy Porter (eds), *Medicine and the Five Senses* (Cambridge: Cambridge University Press, 1993), pp. 198–224. See also M. M. Smith's chapter, 'Touching', in his *Sensing the Past: Seeing, Hearing, Smelling, Tasting, and Touching in History* (Berkeley, CA: University of California Press, 2007), pp. 93–116.

47. For further interest, see E. M. Liebow, *Dr. Joe Bell: Model for Sherlock Holmes* (Madison, WI: Popular Press, 2007).

48. For further summary, see A. E. Rodin and J. D. Key, *Medical Casebook of Doctor Arthur Conan Doyle: From Practitioner to Sherlock Holmes and Beyond* (Malabar, FL: Robert E. Krieger, 1984), pp. 223–25.

49. Connor opens his *The Book of Skin* (p. 9) with this reminder of the skin's increasing popularity and visibility. Connor (p. 26) explicitly draws 'cosmeceutical' from M. Serres, *Les Cinq Sens* (Paris: Hachette, 1998). For relevant work on cosmetics and skin, see G. Kay, *Dying to Be Beautiful: The Fight for Safe Cosmetics* (Columbus, OH: Ohio State University Press, 2005). Modifying the portrayal of one's self through the appearance of the skin is inherent within elective plastic surgeries. For recent foundational historical work on this subject, see E. Haiken, *Venus Envy: A History of Cosmetic Surgery* (Baltimore, MD: Johns Hopkins University Press, 1997); S. L. Gilman, *Making the Body Beautiful: The Cultural History of the Aesthetic Surgery* (Princeton, NJ: Princeton University Press, 2000); and V. Blum, *Flesh Wounds: The Culture of Cosmetic Surgery* (Berkeley, CA: University of California Press, 2003). For a psychoanalytic approach to elective skin alteration, see A. Lemma, *Under the Skin: A Psychoanalytic Study of Body Modification* (London: Routledge, 2010).

50. See, for example, A. DuCille, *Skin Trade* (Cambridge, MA: Harvard University Press, 1996); M. P. Guterl, *The Color of Race in America 1900–1940* (Cambridge, MA: Harvard University Press, 2001); and K. C. Cheng, 'Demystifying Skin Color and "Race"', in R. E. Hall (ed.), *Racism in the 21st Century: An Empirical Analysis of Skin Color* (New York: Springer, 2008), pp. 3–23.

51. W. Penfield and T. Rasmussen, *The Cerebral Cortex of Man* (New York: Macmillan, 1950).
52. J. J. Keegan and F. D. Garrett, 'The Segmental Distribution of the Cutaneous Nerves in the Limbs of Man', *Anatomical Record*, 102 (1948), pp. 409–37.
53. Flanagan and Booth, *Re: Skin*, p. 3. For more on the cultural codification of skin, see Benthien, *Skin*.
54. Lappé, *The Body's Edge*, p. x.
55. C. Classen (ed.), *The Book of Touch* (Oxford: Berg, 2005).

INDEX

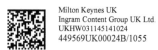

Milton Keynes UK
Ingram Content Group UK Ltd.
UKHW031145141024
449569UK00024B/1055